Breast Cancer Survivorship

Alistair Ring • Marina Parton
Editors

# Breast Cancer Survivorship

## Consequences of early breast cancer and its treatment

Springer

*Editors*
Alistair Ring
The Royal Marsden NHS Foundation Trust
Sutton
UK

Marina Parton
The Royal Marsden NHS Foundation Trust
London
UK

ISBN 978-3-319-41856-8 ISBN 978-3-319-41858-2 (eBook)
DOI 10.1007/978-3-319-41858-2

Library of Congress Control Number: 2016959600



Printed on acid-free paper

This Springer imprint is published by Springer Nature
The registered company is Springer International Publishing AG Switzerland
The registered company is Gewerbestrasse 11, 6330 Cham, Switzerland

# Foreword

Over the past few decades, the great strides in early detection and treatment of breast cancer have led to a growing population of survivors of the disease. Breast cancer survivors comprise a diverse group of individuals with unique concerns and needs. Internationally, there is wide variation both culturally and with regard to access to optimal screening and treatment, as well as supportive care resources that lead to substantial heterogeneity in care and outcomes. Nevertheless, identifying and addressing the universal concerns and common issues facing patients after the diagnosis of breast cancer are of utmost importance to the common goal of breast cancer care mitigating not only the mortality but the morbidity, both medical and psychosocial, of the disease and associated treatment. Further, with increased globalization, especially in the fields of medicine and communications, patients living with, through, and beyond breast cancer seem to have much more in common than not, particularly women living in developed nations.

In this well-crafted book edited by Drs. Ring and Parton, salient issues are identified and reviewed, with an eye toward educating clinicians about optimal strategies from which their breast cancer survivor patients may benefit. Equally important is the attention paid to practices where evidence for benefit is lacking and debunking preconceived notions that can lead to suboptimal care, such as the practice of screening for systemic recurrence in an early stage breast cancer survivor. Chapters cover the main domains of cancer survivorship care including detection of recurrence and new disease, as well as extensive attention to the detection, management, and prevention of important long-term late effects. The authors also address the increasingly important area of modification of health behaviors such as diet and physical activity to improve symptoms, emotional well-being, and potentially disease outcomes. Finally, this text, which is devoted to practical ways to set up clinics to deliver survivorship care, provides valuable models that clinicians can adopt and adapt to improve the day-to-day care provided in their health systems for the growing number breast cancer survivors living in and receiving care in diverse settings.

2016, Boston, MA, USA

Ann H. Partridge, MD, MPH
Director, Adult Survivorship Program
Dana-Farber Cancer Institute
Associate Professor of Medicine
Harvard Medical School

# Preface

Breast cancer is the most commonly diagnosed cancer in women, with 1.67 million women estimated to be diagnosed with breast cancer globally every year [1]. Many of these women are diagnosed with localized (early) breast cancer and are treated with curative intent. Fortunately, over the last few decades, there have been significant improvements in long-term survival rates. As a result, there are many more women living with a history of invasive breast cancer, with an estimated 570,000 breast cancer survivors thought to be living in the UK and 3.1 million women in the USA [2, 3].

However women with a prior diagnosis of early breast cancer remain at risk of relapse, may be continuing on treatment and surveillance, and may also be experiencing long-term sequelae of breast cancer or its treatment. Despite this, the majority of these women have been discharged from routine follow-up in breast surgical and cancer units. As a result, breast cancer survivors come into contact with a variety of healthcare professionals who may be less familiar with the issues and needs of this patient population.

We recognize this challenge in our clinical practices and from our discussions with our patients, and as a result set out to write a comprehensive overview regarding the care of women with a diagnosis of early breast cancer following completion of their initial hospital-based treatment. In doing this, we have drawn on a multidisciplinary authorship reflecting the necessary relevant expertise but also the different perspectives such that a holistic picture of management is provided.

We hope that this book provides a useful reference document and source of practical advice for the health care professional involved in the care of breast cancer survivors.

Surrey UK
May 2016

Alistair Ring
Marina Parton

## References

1. Ferlay J, Soerjomataram I, Ervik M, Dikshit R, Eser S, Mathers C, Rebelo M, Parkin DM, Forman D, Bray F. GLOBOCAN 2012 v1.0, Cancer Incidence and Mortality Worldwide: IARC CancerBase No. 11 [Online]. GLOBOCAN: Breast Cancer Estimated Incidence, Mortality and Prevalence Worldwide in 2012. 2012. http://globocan.iarc.fr/Pages/fact_sheets_cancer.aspx. Accessed 24 Sept 2015.
2. Maddams J, Brewster D, Gavin A, Stewart J, Elliott J, Utley M, Moller H. Cancer prevalence in the United Kingdom: estimates for 2008. Br J Cancer. 2009;101:541–47.
3. The American Cancer Society. Cancer treatment and survivorship facts & figures 2014–2015. 2014. http://www.cancer.org/acs/groups/content/@research/documents/document/acspc-042801.pdf. Acessed 21 Jan 2016

# Acknowledgments

The editors and authors are grateful to their patients and colleagues who have inspired them to write this book in order to improve the care of women diagnosed with early breast cancer. Dr. Ring and Dr. Parton would also like to acknowledge the support of the Royal Marsden National Institute for Health Research Biomedical Research Centre for Cancer and the Cridlan Fund which has supported the education and research endeavors of the editors and many of the authors of this text.

# Contents

# Contributors

**Steven Allen, MBBS, MRCS, FRCR** Imaging Department, The Royal Marsden NHS Foundation Trust, London, UK

**Nawa Mustafa Amin, BSc (Hons), MSc, MBBS, MRCP** The Royal Marsden NHS Foundation Trust, Surrey, UK

**Anne C. Armstrong, MB, ChB, PhD** The Christie NHS Foundation Trust, Wilmslow, Manchester, UK

**Marta Capelan, MD** Breast Unit, The Royal Marsden NHS Foundation Trust, Surrey, UK

**Narda Chaabouni** The Breast Unit, The Royal Marsden NHS Foundation Trust, Surrey, UK

**Georgios Christopoulos, MD, MRCOG** Department of Reproductive Medicine Hammersmith and Queen Charlotte's Hospitals, Imperial College Healthcare NHS Trust, London, UK

**Nicola Cunningham, BSc (Hons) Physiotherapy, PGCert** Senior Project Manager (Patient Experience Programme and MSCC) & AHP Lead, London Cancer Alliance, London, UK

**Omar S. Din, MBChB, MSc, MC, MRCP, FRCR** Consultant in Clinical Oncology, Weston Park Hospital Sheffield, Sheffield, UK

**Kate Downey, BSc, MBBS, MD, FRCR** Imaging Department, The Royal Marsden NHS Foundation Trust, Surrey, UK

**Natalie Doyle, DNurs, MSc, BSc** The Royal Marsden NHS Foundation Trust, London, UK

**Lone Gothard, HND** Division of Radiotherapy and Imaging, The Institute of Cancer Research, London, UK

**Helena Harder, PhD, MSc, BSc** Brighton & Sussex Medical School, Sussex Health Outcomes Research & Education in Cancer (SHORE-C), University of Sussex, Brighton, East Sussex, UK

**Mark Harries, MA, FRCP, PhD** Department of Medical Oncology, Guy's and St Thomas' Hospital, London, UK

**Richard Henry, MSc, BSc, BA** Queens University Belfast, School of Nursing and Midwifery, Medical Biology Centre, Belfast, UK

**Valerie A. Jenkins, DPhil BSc** Brighton & Sussex Medical School, Sussex Health Outcomes Research & Education in Cancer (SHORE-C), University of Sussex, Brighton, East Sussex, UK

**Zoe Kemp, BSc, MBBS, PhD** The Royal Marsden NHS Foundation Trust, London, UK

**Belinda Kingston, MBChB, BSc** The Royal Marsden NHS Foundation Trust, London, UK

**Anna M Kirby, BA, MB, BChir, MA, MRCP, FRCR, MD** Royal Marsden NHS Foundation Trust & Institute of Cancer Research, Surrey, UK

**Amy Kwan, MBBS, BSc** Department of Medical Oncology, Weston Park Hospital, Sheffield, South Yorkshire, UK

**Stuart Lavery, MBBCh, MSc, MRCOG** Department of Reproductive Medicine Hammersmith and Queen Charlotte's Hospitals, Imperial College Healthcare NHS Trust, London, UK

**Alexander Lyon, MA, BM, BCh, PhD, FRCP** Royal Brompton Hospital, London, UK

**Anne Mc Loughlin, BSc (Hons), MSc** The Royal Marsden NHS Foundation Trust, London, UK

**Helen Mitchell, BSc (Hons), MA, MSc, DMedEth** Department of Clinical Oncology, The Christie NHS Foundation Trust, Withington, Manchester, UK

**Christos Nikolaou** Department of Oncology Guy's Hospital, London, UK

**Rachel L. O'Connell, MBBS, BSc, MRCS** The Royal Marsden NHS Foundation Trust, Surrey, UK

**David Okonji, MBBCh, MRCP, FRACP** The Royal Marsden NHS Foundation Trust, Surrey, UK

**Nilesh Pareek, MA (Hons) Cantab, MBBS, MRCP** Department of Cardiology, Royal Brompton and Harefield Foundation NHS Trust, London, UK

**Felicity Paterson, MBBS, BSc** Department of Clinical Oncology, The Royal Marsden NHS Foundation Trust, Surrey, UK

**Stefania Redana, MD, PhD** The Royal Marsden NHS Foundation Trust, Surrey, UK

**Alistair Ring, MA, FRCP, MD** The Royal Marsden NHS Foundation Trust, Surrey, UK

**Nicola Roche, MB, BCh, BAO, MCh, FRCS** The Royal Marsden NHS Foundation Trust, London, UK

**Jennifer E. Rusby, BM, BCh, DM, FRCS** The Royal Marsden NHS Foundation Trust, Surrey, UK

**Clare Shaw, BSc (Hons) Nutrition, PhD, RD** Department of Nutrition and Dietetics, The Royal Marsden NHS Foundation Trust, London, UK

**Navita Somaiah, DPhil, FRCR, MD, MBBS** Division of Radiotherapy and Imaging, The Institute of Cancer Research and The Royal Marsden NHS Foundation Trust, London, UK

**Susannah Stanway, MBChB, MD, MRCP, MSc** The Breast Unit, The Royal Marsden NHS Foundation Trust, Surrey, UK

**Richard Towers, DNurs, MSc, BSc (Hons), RN** Royal Marsden NHS Foundation Trust, London, UK

**Matthew C. Winter, MB, ChB, MSc, MD, FRCP** Hospitals NHS Foundation Trust, Sheffield, South Yorkshire, UK

**Belinda Yeo, FRACP, MBBS, BA** Olivia Newton-John Cancer Research Institute, Melbourne, Australia

# Chapter 1
# Introduction

**David Okonji and Alistair Ring**

**Abstract** Breast cancer is the second most common cancer in the world and the most common cancer to be diagnosed in women. In the UK, there has not only been a 6 % increase in the incidence of breast cancer over the last 10 years, but also a doubling of survival rates in the last 40 years. This improvement in outcomes has been contributed to by the evolving management of the disease. The majority of women diagnosed with early breast cancer (Stages I-III) undergo surgery as their primary treatment modality. After surgery adjuvant therapy may then be used to treat occult micrometastatic disease and reduce the risks of local and distant recurrence. Reductions in mortality rates with the addition of chemotherapy (20–40 %), trastuzumab (up to 40 %), endocrine therapy (approximately 30 %) and radiotherapy (approximately 5 %) are observed. Hence, in 2010 in the UK, there were more than half a million "breast cancer survivors": women living with a past history of breast cancer. This number is projected to reach nearly 2 million by 2040. In current breast surgical and oncological practice many of these women will be discharged from routine follow-up. However, these patients will not only continue to require monitoring for recurrence but also for the potential long term sequelae of their prior breast cancer treatment.

**Keywords** Breast Cancer • Epidemiology • Adjuvant • Surgery • Chemotherapy • Trastuzumab • Endocrine therapy • Radiotherapy

## Breast Cancer Incidence and Mortality

Breast cancer is the second most common cancer in the world and the most common cancer to be diagnosed in women with an estimated 1.67 million new breast cancer cases diagnosed in 2012 [1]. Incidence rates vary considerably across the

D. Okonji, MBBCh, MRCP, FRACP (✉) • A. Ring, MA, FRCP, MD
Breast Unit, The Royal Marsden NHS Foundation Trust, Surrey, UK
e-mail: david.okonji@rmh.nhs.uk; Alistair.ring@rmh.nhs.uk



A. Ring, M. Parton (eds.), *Breast Cancer Survivorship*,
DOI 10.1007/978-3-319-41858-2_1

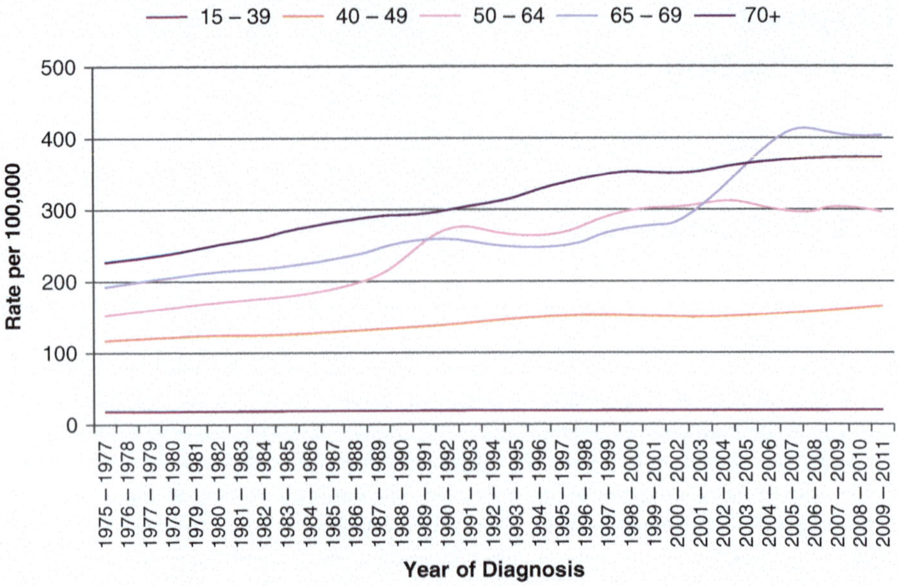


**Fig. 1.1** European Age standardized incidence rates per 100,000 population for UK women from 1975 to 2011 (Adapted from Cancer Research UK [2]. Available at: http://www.cancerresearchuk.org/health-professional/cancer-statistics/statistics-by-cancer-type/breast-cancer/incidence-invasive#heading-Two. Accessed 15 Oct 2015)

world regions, ranging from 27 per 100,000 in Africa and Eastern Asia to 96 per 100,000 in Western Europe. In the UK, in 2011, the age-standardized incidence of breast cancer was approximately 125 per 100,000 meaning that the lifetime risk for women in the UK of being diagnosed with breast cancer was 1 in 8 [2]. Over the last 10 years the incidence of breast cancer has increased by 6 % in the UK (Fig. 1.1).

Despite these increases in incidence, the number of women dying from breast cancer has been decreasing since the 1970s (Fig. 1.2). Overall there has been doubling of survival rates from breast cancer in the last 40 years from 40 to 80 % [2]. Approximately 80 % of women diagnosed with early stage breast cancer in the UK are expected to survive their disease by more than 10 years, with 65 % expected to have an overall survival of 20 years or more [2].

These improvements in survival are likely to be due to a number of reasons, including earlier diagnosis (through screening programs) better surgical techniques and the increasing use of adjuvant therapies to reduce the risks of disease recurrence.

## Prevalence of Breast Cancer Survivors

An inevitable consequence of the increased breast cancer incidence combined with improved survival rates is that there will be more "breast cancer survivors": women living with a past history of breast cancer. In 2010, there were estimated to be

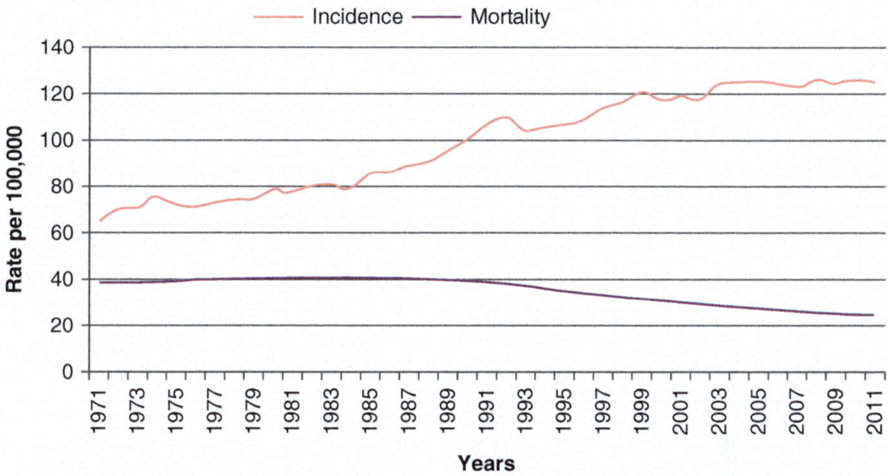


**Fig. 1.2** Breast cancer incidence and mortality rates for woman in England from 1971 to 2011 (Adapted from Office for National Statistics, 2015: Part of Cancer Statistics Registrations, England (Series MB1), No. 42, 2011 Release. Released: 27 Sept 2013 [Online]. Available at: http://www.ons.gov.uk/ons/rel/vsob1/cancer-statistics-registrations--england--series-mb1-/no--42--2011/sty-breast-cancer-survival.html)

570,000 female breast cancer survivors in the UK, and this is projected to reach nearly 1.7 million by 2040 [3]. In the US, it was estimated that there were more than 3.1 million women living with a history of invasive breast cancer in 2014, with this number projected to increase to 3.9 million by 2024 [4].

This large and increasing population of breast cancer survivors represent a heterogeneous group in terms of their personal characteristics (age, co-morbidities, race and social situation), as well as tumor characteristics (stage and biological type) and the treatments received. These factors influence the survivor's prognosis, her experience of treatment and ultimately the impact on her life.

## Population Characteristics of Breast Cancer Survivors

Age is a significant risk factor for breast cancer (Fig. 1.3). The largest increase in incidence rates in the last 3 years has been seen in those over 50 years of age (Fig. 1.1), with 80% of new diagnoses made in this group. This in part may be a reflection of the advent of the mammographic screening program [2]. Over one third of women diagnosed with breast cancer in the UK are aged 70 or older at the time of diagnosis, and given the aging of the population, the number of older women diagnosed with breast cancer is increasing rapidly [5].

As a result many breast cancer survivors are likely to be older, meaning an increased likelihood of pre-existing co-morbidities and reductions in functional status which will have implications for the survivorship population's ongoing needs [6].

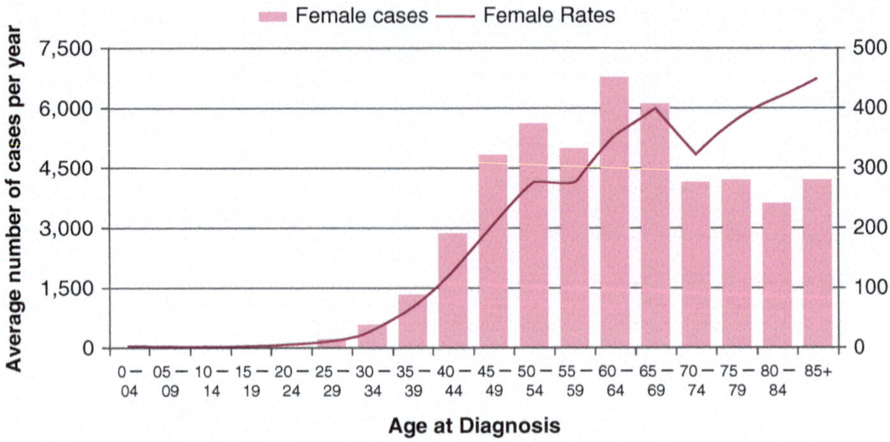


**Fig. 1.3** UK Average number of new female breast cancer cases per year & ages specific incidence rates per 100,000 Population from 2009 to 2011 (Adapted from Cancer Research UK, 2015 [Online] [2]. Available at: http://www.cancerresearchuk.org/health-professional/cancer-statistics/statistics-by-cancer-type/breast-cancer/incidence-invasive#heading-One. Accessed 15 Oct 2015)

Obesity is also a risk factor for breast cancer and rates of obesity in the UK (and much of the developed world) are increasing. In the UK in 2011 only 39 % of women had a healthy Body Mass Index (BMI: 18.5 to < 25) [7]. In one UK study nearly half of women aged 40 or under when diagnosed with breast cancer were overweight (BMI ≥ 25 or < 30) or obese (BMI > 30) at diagnosis [8]. Obesity is recognized to be associated with a worse outcome from breast cancer, and the management of obesity and advice around exercise and diet will become increasingly important amongst breast cancer survivors [9] (Chaps. 8 and 9).

In the UK, there is a racial disparity in breast cancer incidence with the highest incidence rate seen in Caucasians at 122–126 per 100,000, followed by that in those of Afro-Caribbean decent at 69–108 per 100,000 with the lowest in Asians at 60–92 per 100,000 [10]. Similar patterns are seen in the US [11]. From the socioeconomic perspective, there is an inverse relationship between breast cancer incidence and income, with 14 % lower incidence rates seen in socially deprived areas between 1996 and 2010 [12]. However, African-American race and low socioeconomic group are associated with late stage at presentation, which may in part account for the worse survival rates seen in these groups [13]. Recognition of the differing social and cultural needs of breast cancer survivors will be central to effective planning of the ongoing healthcare needs of this population.

## Tumor Characteristics

Breast cancer is described in terms of histo-pathological variables which influence treatment recommendations and outcome. These are divided into breast cancer stage and breast cancer biology.

**Table 1.1** Breast cancer staging by TNM

| Stage | Primary tumor size | Nodal involvement | Metastases |
|---|---|---|---|
| I | T1 | N0 | M0 |
| II | T1 | N1 | M0 |
| | T2 | N0-1 | M0 |
| | T3 | N0 | M0 |
| III | T0-2 | N2 | M0 |
| | T3 | N1-3 | M0 |
| | T4 | N0-3 | M0 |
| IV | Any T | Any N | M1 |

Key:

| Staging | | Pathological description |
|---|---|---|
| Tumor size | T1 | ≤20 mm |
| | T2 | >20 mm but ≤50 mm |
| | T3 | >50 mm |
| | T4 | Any size with direct extension to the chest wall or overlying skin |
| N-stage | N0 | No histologically detected node metastases |
| | N1 | Metastases in 1–3 axillary nodes |
| | N2 | Metastases in 4–9 axillary nodes |
| | N3 | Metastases in ≥10 axillary nodes or in infraclavicular nodes |
| M-stage | M1 | Detectable distant metastatic disease |

Adapted from https://cancerstaging.org/references-tools/quickreferences/Documents/BreastMedium.pdf. Accessed on 25 Jan 2016



## *Breast Cancer Stage*

Breast cancer staging takes into account: Tumor size (**T**), and involvement of axillary lymph Nodes (**N**) and presence of distant Metastases in any other part of the body (**M**) [14]. Clinical, radiological and pathological parameters can be utilized to determine overall TNM stage, and more often than not a combination of all three are used to provide prognostic information. Table 1.1 describes the Stages I-IV of breast cancer based on pathological TNM staging:

In England in 2013, 44 % of women were diagnosed with stage I disease, 40 % stage II and 10 % stage III. Six percent of women were diagnosed with Stage IV or distant metastatic disease at presentation [12]. The importance of stage is that it describes the risks of recurrence and prognosis. Hence for women who are diagnosed with stage I breast cancers nearly all women (99 %) will survive for 5 years or more after diagnosis. For stage II breast cancers 93 % will survive for 5 years or more after diagnosis, and for stage III breast cancer the rate is 72 % [15]. Nonetheless it is important to recognize that the risks of relapse extend beyond 5 years, such that patients may relapse many years following their initial diagnosis and treatment.

Women who present with stage IV (metastatic) breast cancer or develop stage IV disease having been diagnosed and treated for earlier stages of breast cancer in the past are not regarded as curable. The aims of treatment here are to prolong survival and to maintain quality of life. The median survival for women under these circumstances varies considerably according to breast cancer subtype, performance status and disease burden at presentation: but based on clinical trial data median survival may be estimated as between 1 and 5 years [16–18]. This patient population are not the topic of this book: these patients have specific treatment needs around prolongation of survival and maintenance quality of life, which are distinct to the needs of women with stage I-III breast cancer who are treated in a potentially curative setting.

## *Breast Cancer Biology*

In addition to stage, a breast cancer may also be described in terms of key biological features. These include tumor grade, estrogen receptor (ER) and progesterone receptor (PR) status and expression of HER2.

Hormone receptor (ER and PR) status plays both prognostic and predictive roles in breast cancer outcomes. Women with ER positive breast cancer have a better 5-year overall survival than women with ER negative breast cancer (85 % vs 68 % in one population studied) [19]. This may be partly explained by the association of ER negative status with high tumor grade and HER2 expression (see below) and contributed to by the fact that women with ER negative disease do not benefit from adjuvant endocrine therapy [20]. In the UK in 2007, hormone receptor status was available for 61 % of surgically treated invasive breast cancers [21]. Of these 84 % were ER positive, a similar incidence to the US SEER database for 2010, where the rate was 82.7 % [22].

In the UK and SEER databases, 15 % of patients presenting with early breast cancer over-expressed the HER-2 receptor (as defined by immunohistochemistry for the receptor or gene amplification). Women with so-called "HER2 positive" breast cancer have an increased risk of relapse [23, 24]. However, the advent of a monoclonal antibody directed to HER2 (trastuzumab, also known as Herceptin®) provides the opportunity to use a targeted therapy to reduce the risks of relapse in this population [25, 26]. As such HER2 status is a key prognostic and predictive variable in planning the management of early breast cancer.

Approximately, 10 % of patients present with breast cancer which does not express either hormone receptor (ER or PR) or HER2 [22, 27]. This is a disease subtype where endocrine therapy and trastuzumab are not indicated and where the risk of relapse is high [28].

A consideration of the stage and biology of breast cancer is therefore central to predicting the risks of recurrence (discussed in more details in Chap. 2). It is vital to be able to predict this as accurately as possible, as it influences treatment recommendations and may also affect life choices for that patient following completion of initial treatment.

## Treatment Overview for Early Breast Cancer

Breast cancer survivors may have experienced a range of treatments which, aside from the impact of the diagnosis and risks of recurrence have significant implications for experience of life beyond a diagnosis of early breast cancer. In 2008 in the UK alone, it was estimated that 44,000 women would benefit from rehabilitative support following completion of their treatment [29].

### *Surgery*

The majority of women diagnosed with early breast cancer undergo surgery as their primary treatment modality. This can either be in the form of breast conserving surgery (wide local excision) or a mastectomy. In the UK in 2007, 50,286 women were diagnosed with invasive or non-invasive breast cancer; of those women 82 % underwent surgery (57 % underwent breast conserving surgery and the remainder mastectomy). Breast conserving surgery was more common in women with screen-detected breast cancers, which tended to be smaller [21]. Breast reconstruction may be offered at the time of mastectomy or delayed until primary surgery and adjuvant therapies have been completed. (Delayed breast reconstruction and the need for surgery for other indications in breast cancer survivors are discussed in Chap. 12).

Surgery to the breast is performed in conjunction with some form of axillary procedure. This is necessary to confirm the stage of the breast cancer (see section "Introduction" in Chap. 4). This can be in the form of sentinel lymph node biopsy (SLNB) or axillary node dissection. SLNB is usually considered in women with clinically and radiologically negative nodes pre-operatively. It is a means to try to restrict more extensive axillary surgery to those patients who definitely need it. A blue dye usually in conjunction with a radioisotope is injected into the breast prior to surgery, enabling identification of the first draining node of the region of the breast. This node (the "sentinel" node) is therefore representative of the rest of the axillary lymph node basin. If on subsequent pathological examination or real-time examination (using molecular assays or frozen sections) this node is involved a completion axillary node dissection is considered. Although the necessity of completion dissection in all patients with positive sentinel nodes is debated [30], and a number of ongoing trials are addressing this issue. Those women who have pathologically confirmed axillary lymph node involvement prior to breast surgery, or are deemed to warrant further axillary surgery following a SLNB, are offered axillary lymph node dissection. This involves a more extensive procedure (defined anatomically into levels I, II and III), with a higher risk of late complications, including pain, hypersensitivity and lymphedema (Chap. 11).

## *Adjuvant Chemotherapy*

Women with early breast cancer who have had apparent removal of all macroscopic disease by surgery, may eventually relapse with stage IV breast cancer and die from metastatic disease. This is thought to occur as a result of occult micrometastatic disease, which may already be present at the time of surgery. For this reason, adjuvant systemic therapy may be considered to reduce the risks of disease recurrence. A meta-analysis of several trials has shown that 6 months of anthracycline-based chemotherapy following surgical resection of early breast cancer results in approximately 40 % reduction in mortality rates from breast cancer in women less than 50 years of age and a 20 % reduction in those between 56 and 69 years [31]. A further large meta-analysis subsequently demonstrated that the addition of taxane-based chemotherapy to anthracycline chemotherapy resulted in a further 15 % reduction in breast cancer mortality rates [32].

The absolute benefits of chemotherapy are determined by disease stage and biology. Therefore it is only women whose breast cancer is at a higher risk of recurrence who are offered chemotherapy as these women derive the greatest absolute benefits. As a result of the EBCTCG analyses most women who receive chemotherapy are offered poly-chemotherapy with anthracyclines (epirubicin or doxorubicin), taxanes (docetaxel or paclitaxel) or combinations of the two classes of agent. Treatment is administered intravenously on a day unit basis for 3–6 months. Aside from the immediate side-effects, breast cancer survivors may at risk of long-term side-effects from adjuvant chemotherapy exposure. These may include impact on fertility and induction of the menopause (Chaps. 13 and 15), cardiac toxicity (Chap. 16), risk of secondary malignancy (Chap. 17), and cognitive changes (Chap. 18).

## *Adjuvant Trastuzumab (Herceptin®)*

The previously poor prognosis associated with HER2 positive breast cancer has been improved by adjuvant trastuzumab. When trastuzumab (a monoclonal antibody targeted to HER2), has been added either concomitantly or sequentially to adjuvant chemotherapy, up to 39 % reduction in the mortality rates have been achieved [25, 26]. These original trials compared 1 year of trastuzumab with no additional therapy, and as such the standard treatment duration of trastuzumab was established as 1 year. Long term follow-up of the HERA trial [33] did not demonstrate benefit of longer (2 years) of therapy, and currently trials are examining if shorter durations may be effective [34, 35]. One year of trastuzumab involves intravenous or subcutaneous treatment given once every 3 weeks for 18 doses. In terms of day to day side-effects most patients tolerate trastuzumab very well, with a small risk of hypersensitivity reactions when the drug is first administered. However, there is a risk of cumulative cardiac toxicity which is of long-term relevance to breast cancer survivors (see Chap. 16).

## *Adjuvant Radiotherapy*

Adjuvant radiotherapy is the current standard of care for patients with early breast cancer following breast-conserving surgery, and in patients with a high risk of local recurrence following mastectomy. According to the Oxford overview analysis: 5-year local recurrence risks were 7 vs 26 % (2P < 0.00001) and 15-year breast cancer mortality risks 30.5 vs 35.9 % (2P = 0.0002) in those who underwent radiotherapy following breast conserving surgery compared with those under-going surgery alone [36]. Radiotherapy following breast-conserving surgery was associated with similar proportional reductions in local recurrence across all age groups. However, the absolute benefits of treatment were smaller in older patients as their overall risk of local recurrence was less, and there may be a population of older patients with low risk breast cancer where radiotherapy may be safely omitted [36, 37]. Adjuvant breast radiotherapy is usually administered as daily treatment (Monday to Friday) over 3 weeks in a cancer center. However, some patients are also given a boost to the tumor bed and may receive more prolonged courses, and a variety of different schedules are in routine clinical use or being examined in clinical trials. Some patients may receive radiotherapy to the loco-regional lymph node groups as well as to the breast or chest wall. Adjuvant radiotherapy may be associated with post-treatment changes in the breast or lymph node groups (Chap. 11) and potentially contribute to risks of cardiac toxicity (Chap. 16) and secondary malignancy (Chap. 17).

## *Adjuvant Endocrine Therapy*

The majority of breast cancers are estrogen receptor (ER) positive. In those women with ER positive breast cancer, adjuvant endocrine therapy is routinely offered. The addition of endocrine therapy following either adjuvant chemotherapy and/or radiotherapy confers a further 31 % reduction in mortality rates [31]. Historically the selective estrogen receptor modulator tamoxifen has been the mainstay of treatment in premenopausal women, although increasingly ovarian function suppression is being offered. In post-menopausal women aromatase inhibitors are the agents of choice (Chap. 6). Women may be advised to take adjuvant endocrine therapy for up to 10 years, and side-effects, which may manifest as menopausal symptoms (Chap. 13) or impact on bone health (Chap. 14) may be challenging for many patients and are key considerations for many breast cancer survivors.

## Summary

The focus of this book is patients with earlier stages of breast cancer (stage I-III) where the goal of treatment is cure. It is in this setting where the ongoing monitoring for recurrence and the longer term sequelae of the diagnosis and treatment are most relevant. In current breast surgical and oncological practice many of these women are discharged from routine follow-up. These patients may subsequently come into contact with a variety of healthcare professionals who may be less familiar with the issues and needs of this patient population. This book will therefore provide a framework to guide health care professionals in the care of early breast cancer survivors.

## References

1. Ferlay J, Soerjomataram I, Ervik M, Dikshit R, Eser S, Mathers C, Rebelo M, Parkin DM, Forman D, Bray F. GLOBOCAN 2012 v1.0, Cancer Incidence and Mortality Worldwide: IARC CancerBase No. 11 [Online]. GLOBOCAN: Breast Cancer Estimated Incidence, Mortality and Prevalence Worldwide in 2012. 2012. http://globocan.iarc.fr/Pages/fact_sheets_cancer.aspx. Accessed 24 Sept 2015.
2. Cancer Research UK. Breast Cancer Statistics-[Online]. 2015. http://www.cancerresearchuk.org/health-professional/cancer-statistics/statistics-by-cancer-type/breast-cancer. Accessed 21 Sept 2015.
3. Maddams J, Utley M, Møller H. Projections of cancer prevalence in the United Kingdom, 2010–2040. Br J Cancer. 2012;107(7):1195–202. doi:10.1038/bjc.2012.366. Epub 2012 Aug 14.
4. The American Cancer Society. Cancer treatment and survivorship facts & figures 2014–2015. 2014. http://www.cancer.org/acs/groups/content/@research/documents/document/acspc-042801.pdf. Acessed 21 Jan 2016.
5. Sinha R, Coyle C, Ring A. Breast cancer in older patients: national cancer registry data. Int J Clin Pract. 2013;67(7):698–700.
6. Parks RM, Lakshmanan R, Winterbottom L, Al Morgan D, Cox K, Cheung KL. Comprehensive geriatric assessment for older women with early breast cancer – a systematic review of literature. World J Surg Oncol. 2012;10(88):1–9.
7. Health and Social Care Information Centre, L. S. Statistics on obesity, physical activity and diet: England, 2013, National Health Service and The Information Centre for Health and Social Care [Online]. 2013. http://www.hscic.gov.uk/catalogue/PUB10364/obes-phys-acti-diet-eng-2013-rep.pdf. Accessed 21 Jan 2016.
8. Copson ER, Cutress RI, Maishman T, Eccles BK, Gerty S, Stanton L, et al. Obesity and the outcome of young breast cancer patients in the UK: the POSH study. Ann Oncol. 2015;26(1):101–12.
9. Chan DSM, Vieira AR, Aune D, Bandera EV, Greenwood DC, McTiernan A, et al. Body mass index and survival in women with breast cancer—systematic literature review and meta-analysis of 82 follow-up studies. Ann Oncol. 2014;25(10):1901–14.
10. Collaborative Group on Hormonal Factors in Breast Cancer. Breast cancer and breastfeeding: collaborative reanalysis of individual data from 47 epidemiological studies in 30 countries, including 50302 women with breast cancer and 96973 women without the disease. The Lancet. 2002;360(9328):187–95.

11. Smigal C, Jemal A, Ward E, Cokkinides V, Smith R, Howe HL, et al. Trends in breast cancer by race and ethnicity: update 2006. CA Cancer J Clin. 2006;56(3):168–83.
12. Cancer Research UK & the National Cancer Intelligence Network. Cancer by deprivation in England: incidence, 1996–2010, mortality 1997–2011. London: PHE Publications; 2014.
13. Lannin DR, Mathews HF, Mitchell J, Swanson MS, Swanson FH, Edwards MS. Influence of socioeconomic and cultural factors on racial differences in late-stage presentation of breast cancer. JAMA. 1998;279(22):1801–7.
14. Edge SB, David R, Compton, CC, Fritz AG. Greene FL. Trotti A. Cancer staging posters: breast cancer staging. [Online]. 2009. https://cancerstaging.org/references-tools/quickreferences/Documents/BreastMedium.pdf.
15. The American Cancer Society. Breast cancer: survival by stage. 2015. http://www.cancer.org/cancer/breastcancer/detailedguide/breast-cancer-survival-by-stage. Accessed 21 January 2016.
16. Tutt A, Ellis P, Kilburn L, Gilett C, Pinder S, Abraham J, et al. Abstract S3-01: the TNT trial: a randomized phase III trial of carboplatin (C) compared with docetaxel (D) for patients with metastatic or recurrent locally advanced triple negative or BRCA1/2 breast cancer (CRUK/07/012). Cancer Res. 2015;75(Suppl 9):S3-01-S3-.
17. Mehta RS, Barlow WE, Albain KS, Vandenberg TA, Dakhil SR, Tirumali NR, et al. Combination anastrozole and fulvestrant in metastatic breast cancer. New Eng J Med. 2012;367(5):435–44.
18. Swain S, Kim S, Cortes J, Ro J, Semiglazov V, Campone M, et al. Final overall survival (Os) analysis from The cleopatra study of first-line (1l) Pertuzumab (Ptz), Trastuzumab (T), and Docetaxel (D) In Patients (Pts) With Her2-Positive Metastatic Breast Cancer (Mbc). Ann Oncol. 2014;25(Suppl 4).
19. Bentzon N, Düring M, Rasmussen BB, Mouridsen H, Kroman N. Prognostic effect of estrogen receptor status across age in primary breast cancer. Int J Cancer. 2008;122(5):1089–94.
20. Early Breast Cancer Trialists' Collaborative Group (EBCTCG). Tamoxifen for early breast cancer: an overview of the randomised trials. The Lancet. 1998;351(9114):1451–67.
21. Lawrence GKO, Lagord C, Cheung S, Sidhu J, Sagar C. Second all breast cancer report: focussing on inequalities: variation in breast cancer outcomes with age and deprivation 2011 [Online]. http://www.ncin.org.uk/view?rid=612. Accessed 14 Oct 2015.
22. Howlader N, Altekruse SF, Li CI, Chen VW, Clarke CA, Ries LAG, et al. US incidence of breast cancer subtypes defined by joint hormone receptor and HER2 status. Journal of the National Cancer Institute. 2014;106(5).
23. Slamon DJ, Clark GM, Wong SG, Levin WJ, Ullrich A, McGuire WL. Human breast cancer: correlation of relapse and survival with amplification of the HER-2/neu oncogene. Science. 1987;235(4785):177–82.
24. Seshadri R, Firgaira FA, Horsfall DJ, McCaul K, Setlur V, Kitchen P. Clinical significance of HER-2/neu oncogene amplification in primary breast cancer. The South Australian Breast Cancer Study Group. J Clin Oncol. 1993;11(10):1936–42.
25. Perez EA, Romond EH, Suman VJ, Jeong J-H, Davidson NE, Geyer CE, et al. Four-year follow-up of Trastuzumab plus adjuvant chemotherapy for operable human epidermal growth factor receptor 2–positive breast cancer: joint analysis of data from NCCTG N9831 and NSABP B-31. J Clin Oncol. 2011;29(25):3366–73.
26. Goldhirsch A, Gelber RD, Piccart-Gebhart MJ, de Azambuja E, Procter M, Suter TM, et al. 2 years versus 1 year of adjuvant trastuzumab for HER2-positive breast cancer (HERA): an open-label, randomised controlled trial. The Lancet. 2013;382(9897):1021–8.
27. Jack RH, Davies EA, Renshaw C, Tutt A, Grocock MJ, Coupland VH, et al. Differences in breast cancer hormone receptor status in ethnic groups: A London population. Eur J Cancer. 2013;49(3):696–702.
28. Dent R, Trudeau M, Pritchard KI, Hanna WM, Kahn HK, Sawka CA, et al. Triple-negative breast cancer: Clinical features and patterns of recurrence. Clin Cancer Res. 2007;13(15):4429–34.
29. Maher J, McConnell H. New pathways of care for cancer survivors: adding the numbers. Br J Cancer. 2011;105 Suppl 1:S5–10.

30. Giuliano AE, Hunt KK, Ballman KV, et al. Axillary dissection vs no axillary dissection in women with invasive breast cancer and sentinel node metastasis: a randomized clinical trial. JAMA. 2011;305(6):569–75.
31. Early Breast Cancer Trialists' Collaborative Group (EBCTCG). Effects of chemotherapy and hormonal therapy for early breast cancer on recurrence and 15-year survival: an overview of the randomised trials. The Lancet. 2005;365(9472):1687–717.
32. Early Breast Cancer Trialists' Collaborative Group. Comparisons between different polychemotherapy regimens for early breast cancer: meta-analyses of long-term outcome among 100,000 women in 123 randomised trials. The Lancet. 2012;379(9814):432–44.
33. Smith I, Procter M, Gelber RD, Guillaume S, Feyereislova A, Dowsett M, et al. 2-year follow-up of trastuzumab after adjuvant chemotherapy in HER2-positive breast cancer: a randomised controlled trial. The Lancet. 2007;369(9555):29–36.
34. Guarneri V, Frassoldati A, Bruzzi P, D'Amico R, Belfiglio M, Molino A, et al. Multicentric, randomized phase III trial of two different adjuvant chemotherapy regimens plus three versus twelve months of Trastuzumab in patients with HER2-positive breast cancer (Short-HER Trial; NCT00629278). Clin Breast Cancer. 2008;8(5):453–6.
35. Pivot X, Romieu G, Debled M, Pierga J-Y, Kerbrat P, Bachelot T, et al. 6 months versus 12 months of adjuvant trastuzumab for patients with HER2-positive early breast cancer (PHARE): a randomised phase 3 trial. Lancet Oncol. 2013;14(8):741–8.
36. Clarke M, Collins R, Darby S, Davies C, Elphinstone P, Evans V, Godwin J, Gray R, Hicks C, James S, MacKinnon E, McGale P, McHugh T, Peto R, Taylor C, Wang Y. Effects of radiotherapy and of differences in the extent of surgery for early breast cancer on local recurrence and 15-year survival: an overview of the randomised trials. The Lancet. 2005;366(9503):2087–106.
37. Kunkler IH, Williams LJ, Jack WJL, Cameron DA, Dixon JM. Breast-conserving surgery with or without irradiation in women aged 65 years or older with early breast cancer (PRIME II): a randomised controlled trial. Lancet Oncol. 2015;16(3):266–73.

# Part I
# Disease Recurrence

# Chapter 2
# Predicting Risk of Disease Recurrence

**Belinda Yeo**

**Abstract** Most patients with early breast cancer do not recur after treatment with multimodality therapy. A minority of patients remain at significant risk of relapse and for some, this risk persists up to and beyond 10 years after diagnosis. Decision tools and genomic assays assist in stratifying patients into low and high risk so that adjuvant treatment intensity and its potential toxicities can be limited to those who have the most to gain from them. Definitive treatment for the intermediate risk patients remains uncertain. The four main breast cancer subtypes show distinct patterns and timing of recurrence although these may change over time as better adjuvant systemic and targeted agents begin to change the natural history of recurrent breast cancer.

**Keywords** Breast cancer recurrence • Risk stratification • Decision-aids • Late relapse

## Introduction; What Does Recurrence Mean?

In the setting of a patient being diagnosed and treated for early breast cancer, the term ‘recurrence’ usually describes a time-dependent event in which the cancer relapses. This may be identified when a patient presents with symptoms that warrant investigation, symptomatic recurrence, or it may be found asymptomatically, usually in the context of imaging being performed for another reason. Other than dedicated breast imaging usually with mammography, current guidelines do not recommend the routine radiological surveillance of patients in follow up to detect asymptomatic recurrence, as this does not impact on overall survival. It should be acknowledged however that if a survival advantage is identified through the detection and treatment of biochemical and/or oligometastatic relapse, future surveillance guidelines may need to be adjusted accordingly.

B. Yeo, FRACP, MBBS, BA
Olivia Newton-John Cancer Research Institute, Melbourne, Australia
e-mail: belinda.yeo@onjuri.org.au

 
A. Ring, M. Parton (eds.), *Breast Cancer Survivorship*,
DOI 10.1007/978-3-319-41858-2_2

**Table 2.1** Common terminology used to describe endpoints in breast cancer

| Acronym | Endpoint |
|---|---|
| BCSS | breast cancer specific survival |
| iDFS | invasive disease free survival |
| dDFS | distant disease-free survival |
| RFS | relapse free survival |
| LRFS | locoregional relapse-free survival |
| RFI | recurrence-free interval |
| BCFI | breast cancer-free interval |
| DRFI | distant recurrence-free interval |
| PFS | progression-free survival |
| TTP | time to progression |

Recurrence may occur locoregionally and/or with distant metastases. Local recurrence describes relapse in the ipsilateral breast, whereas regional recurrence includes nodal involvement of the ipsilateral axilla, supraclavicular, infraclavicular or internal mammary chain, as well as contralateral breast disease. Distant recurrence (DR) or metastatic disease denotes relapse in any organ outside the breast (e.g. lung, liver, brain, bones) as well as distant lymph nodes and skin involvement.

The distinction between these types of recurrence is significant for the reason that whilst locoregional relapse may be treated with curative intent, it is unusual to achieve a cure once distant metastatic disease is established. Table 2.1 shows some of the common terminology used to describe time to event endpoints in breast cancer studies [1].

## What Are the Risks of Recurrence?

As shown in Fig. 2.1, despite an increasing incidence of breast cancer, outcomes have improved for all breast cancer subtypes [2]. From a recent review of epidemiological data from the USA (SEER), overall survival rates have improved from 74 % in 1975 through 1977 to 90 % in 2003 through 2009 [3].

In 2016, the majority of woman treated with early breast cancer will be cured with multimodality therapy. This is likely in part due to breast cancer screening, although there remains some controversy about its impact on overall survival [4–6]. Improvements in systemic therapy, namely endocrine therapy, chemotherapy and targeted agents, have significantly improved long term survival and decreased recurrence rates for all subtypes of early breast cancer [2].

The Early Breast Cancer Trialists' Collaborative Group (EBCTG) have shown in their long-term follow up analysis that 5 years of adjuvant tamoxifen compared with no endocrine therapy nearly halves the risk of recurrence and reduces chance of dying from breast cancer by about a third [7]. More recently in their meta-analyses from over 30,000 women treated within a randomized trial comparing the aromatase inhibitors (AIs) with tamoxifen, they demonstrated a further 30 %

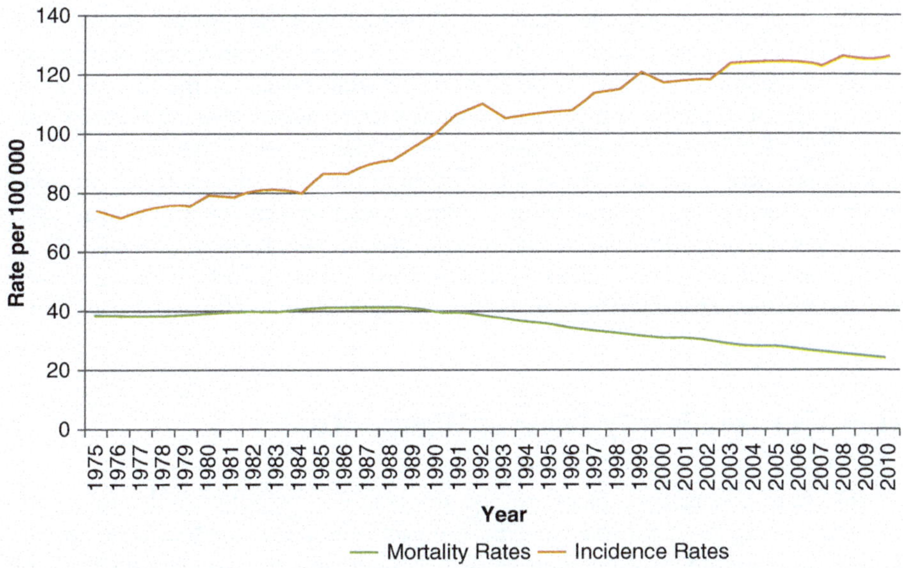


**Fig. 2.1** Breast cancer incidence and mortality rates in UK over the past 30 years (Adapted from Cancer Research UK statistics, Available from www.cancerresearchuk.org)

proportional reduction in recurrence achieved with the AIs compared with tamoxifen and a 15 % reduction in breast cancer mortality [8]. Combination adjuvant chemotherapy reduces the relative risk of death from breast cancer by about a third [9]. For woman with HER2 positive breast cancer, 1 year of adjuvant trastuzumab nearly halves the relative risk of recurrence as well as improving overall survival by 34 % [10, 11].

Adjuvant radiotherapy after breast conserving surgery significantly reduces the risk of locoregional or distant recurrence at 10 years (absolute reduction 15·7 %, 2p < 0·00001) as well as breast cancer mortality (absolute reduction 3·8 %, 2p = 0·00005) [12]. EBCTCG have also shown that post-mastectomy radiotherapy reduces recurrence and breast cancer mortality in a subset of women with positive lymph nodes [13].

## Why Do We Need to Better Identify the Risk of Recurrence?

Many of our adjuvant therapies have unpleasant and in some cases severe side effects. Polychemotherapy is well known to cause short-term toxicities including alopecia, fatigue, nausea and vomiting, and yet, many patients receive adjuvant chemotherapy for only small improvements in survival. Hence it is important to identify which patients have a significant risk of recurrence and may warrant chemotherapy, to justify the these side effects.

Whilst adjuvant endocrine therapy (ET) is offered to almost all women with hormone receptor (HR) positive early breast cancer, it too has potential side effects. Given the demonstrated benefit of 10 years of adjuvant endocrine therapy when compared with stopping at 5 years from trials such as MA17 [14], aTTom [15] and ATLAS [16], it is a current research priority to identify which patients may be at risk of long term relapse as those who will have the most to gain from extending treatment out to a decade. In addition, recent results from the SOFT [17] and TEXT [18] trials, designed to evaluate the role of ovarian suppression alongside ET in premenopausal, demand further research into risk stratifying which young women justify this more intensive therapy [19].

## How Can We Identify Those at Highest Risk?

In this era of personalized medicine, the aim is to use our adjuvant therapies judiciously, treating those who have the most to gain from them, and sparing those who have little or nothing to gain, their burden. Traditionally this risk stratification has relied upon estimating a woman's risk of recurrence based on clinicopathological factors such as tumor size, grade and nodal status. However it is well recognized that breast tumor biology also drives risk.

## Intrinsic Subtypes

Gene expression studies have identified at least four 'intrinsic' breast cancer subtypes: luminal A, luminal B, HER2-enriched and basal-like [20, 21]. Such studies have helped to differentiate between the two major groups of ER positive breast cancer. Luminal A tumors are characterized by high expression of ER and progesterone (PgR) receptor and low proliferation and have the best prognosis of all the intrinsic subtypes; whilst luminal B tumors exhibit lower ER and PgR expression and high expression of proliferation genes [20]. Luminal B tumors are considered a more aggressive phenotype compared with Luminal A, with higher rates of relapse [22] and are hence more likely to be treated with adjuvant chemotherapy.

Patients diagnosed with luminal A tumors have the highest rates of survival at 10 years, compared to luminal B, HER2 enriched and basal-like subtypes [23]. In a historical series of nearly 4000 women with breast cancers diagnosed between 1986 and 1992, 70 % of patients with luminal A tumors were alive at 10 years compared with between 46 and 62 % for the other subtypes [24]. It is worth noting that these outcomes describe a series of patients treated prior to the routine use of taxanes and HER2 directed therapy. From the HERA trial, recurrence rates in the trastuzumab-treated arm were significantly improved: the rate of local recurrence was 3.7 %, regional recurrence 1.4 % and distant recurrence 13.4 % at 8 years [25].

**Table 2.2** Comparison of information required in decision tools for adjuvant decision-making

| Characteristic | NPI | AoL | Predict | IHC4+C |
|---|---|---|---|---|
| Mode of detection | – | – | ✓ | – |
| Patient age | – | ✓ | ✓ | ✓ |
| Tumor size | ✓ | ✓ | ✓ | ✓ |
| Grade | ✓ | ✓ | ✓ | ✓ |
| Nodal status | ✓ | ✓ | ✓ | ✓ |
| ER | – | ✓ | ✓ | ✓ |
| PgR | – | – | – | ✓ |
| HER2 | – | – | ✓ | ✓ |
| ET for 5 years | | ✓ | ✓ | ✓ |
| Ki67 | – | – | ✓ | ✓ |
| Chemo/no chemo | – | ✓ | ✓ | – |
| Available online | ✓ | ✓ | ✓ | – |
| Prognostic info | ✓ | ✓ | ✓ | ✓ |
| Predictive info | – | ✓ | ✓ | – |

## Prognostic Versus Predictive Tests

Prognostic information gives an estimation of prognosis or in the case of breast cancer, the risk of recurrence, based on clinical or biological characteristics, usually in an untreated patient. It can be helpful risk stratifying patients for treatment decisions. Predictive information describes the likely benefit of treatment on the tumor. Whilst most molecular and non-molecular decision aids offer prognostic information only, some provide predictive information as to the relative benefit of treatment. The commonly used decision aids and molecular risk prognostic and predictive assays are described below.

## Non-molecular Decision Aids

There are several decision tools that use clinicopathological and immunohistochemical information provided in routine clinical practice for prognostication (Table 2.2). All three of these tools were developed in patients prior to the widespread use of aromatase inhibitors.

### *Nottingham Prognostic Index*

Nottingham Prognostic Index (NPI) is a prognostic tool originally developed in the 1980s using a retrospective analysis of nearly 400 woman with primary operable breast cancer [26]. It uses tumor size (in centimeters), grade and nodal status to risk stratify patients into good (≤3.4), moderate (3.4–5.4) and poor (>5.4) prognostic risk groups, corresponding to survival estimates of 80 %, 42 % and 13 % respectively [27].

## *Adjuvant! Online*

Adjuvant! Online (AoL) is a prognostic tool using tumor size, grade, nodal status as well as ER status (positive or negative) and clinical characteristics of patient age and underlying comorbidities, to estimate the 10 year risk of recurrence and overall survival [28]. It is based on SEER data and has been independently validated by Olivotto el al. in over 4000 stage 1 and 2 breast cancer patients [29]. It also serves as a predictive tool estimating the additional benefit of endocrine therapy and chemotherapy based on data from the EBCTCG [30]. It is still widely used by clinicians for adjuvant decision-making and is freely available online (www.adjuvantonline.com).

## *Predict*

Predict is an online prognostic model used to predict overall survival using tumor size, grade, nodal status, ER, and Ki67 ("positive or negative") as well as the patient age at diagnosis. It was developed in 5694 woman from a UK cancer registry diagnosed with EBC between 1999 and 2003 and was validated in an independent UK breast dataset of 5468 diagnosed in the same years [31]. It has also been validated in a Canadian dataset [32] and has been updated to include HER2 status [33]. An interesting feature of the model is that it adjusts for the mode of detection of breast cancer (screen vs. symptomatically detected), showing an inferior stage-for-stage survival for patients with a symptomatic presentation [34].

## *The IHC4+C Score*

The IHC4+C score is a prognostic tool that estimates the residual risk of distant recurrence at 10 years in postmenopausal women with HR positive breast cancer that have received 5 years of endocrine therapy. It incorporates both immunohistochemical parameters of estrogen receptor (ER), progesterone receptor (PgR), HER2 and the proliferation marker, Ki67, as well as the clinicopathological parameters of tumor size, grade, nodal status and type of endocrine therapy administered for 5 years (tamoxifen vs. aromatase inhibitor).

The IHC4+C score was developed from a retrospective analysis of 1125 patients with ER positive disease from the TransATAC cohort who did not receive

**Table 2.3** Molecular tools currently commercially available for the prediction of recurrence

| Test | Description | Test output |
|---|---|---|
| Oncotype DX RS | 21 gene-based expression profile; FFPE (RNA) | Low, intermediate and high risk scores |
| Prosigna ROR | 50 gene-based expression profile using Ncounter (RNA) | ROR scores, intrinsic subtypes |
| Endopredict | 12 gene-based expression profile using qRT-PCR; FFPE (RNA) | Low risk vs. high risk scores |
| Mammaprint | 70-gene-based expression profile, microarray; Fresh tissue (DNA) | Low vs. high risk scores |
| BCI | Multi-gene assay (HOXB13:IL17BR+MGI) using qRT-PCR; FFPE (RNA) | Low vs. high risk scores for each assay |

Modified from Sestak and Cuzick [38]

chemotherapy and validated in an independent Nottingham cohort of 786 patients. It has been shown in a retrospective study to perform similarly to the Oncotype DX Recurrence Score in predicting distant recurrence [35]. In a prospective decision impact study in a clinically relevant population, use of the IHC4+C score has been shown to significantly reduce adjuvant chemotherapy recommendations [36]. Further work is on going to produce standardized input for the IHC4 algorithm before it can be used routinely throughout the UK [37].

## Commercially Available Molecular Assays

Table 2.3 identifies five of the molecular and multigene scores now available to the clinician, most of which aim to provide better prognostication for the individual patient's risk of relapse [38]. Despite their availability these remain inaccessible to the majority of patients treated for early breast cancer largely due to cost.

### *Recurrence Score*

Oncotype DX Recurrence Score (RS) is a 21 gene assay is based on the gene expression using RNA extracted from FFPE tissue. It was originally developed using quantitative reverse transcription (qRT) PCR on 447 breast cancers, of which 223 were from NSABP-20, a phase III adjuvant clinical trial examining the benefit of chemotherapy in addition to tamoxifen in node negative, HR positive breast cancer [39]. From an original list of 250 candidate genes associated with survival, 16 genes (and 5 housekeeper genes) were selected weighted by proliferation, HER2 and ER signaling [40]. The RS numerically ranges from 0 to 100, with low (RS < 18), intermediate (RS 18–30) and high (RS > 30) risk categories. RS has been independently validated the NSABP-B14 and TransATAC [41] cohorts. There is no consensus as to the optimal treatment for those in the intermediate-risk range and clinical trials are currently underway to address this uncertainty (Table 2.4). RS is the most widely used genomic breast cancer assay in the United States and is endorsed by the American Society of Clinical Oncology (ASCO) [42], St Gallen [43] and most recently by NICE for the United Kingdom [44].

Two main studies have assessed the RS in its ability to predict chemotherapy benefit. Paik et al. reported that RS predicts magnitude of chemotherapy benefit in a study using 651 node negative patients from NSABP-B20. Patients with a high recurrence score had a large benefit from chemotherapy (relative risk, 0.26; 95% CI, 0.13–0.53) whilst patients with low-RS did not [45]. In a population of 367 woman with node positive breast cancer from the SWOG-8814, Albain et al. reported a benefit of chemotherapy in those tumors with a high RS (HR 0.59, CI 0.35–1.01, p=0.033) and no significant benefit in patients with a low RS (HR 1.02, CI 0.54–1.93, p=0.97) [46].

## *Prosigna® ROR*

The identification of four intrinsic subtypes (luminal A, B, HER2-like, basal) was identified through gene expression profiling examining nearly 2000 genes in 84 breast cancers [47] and shown to be predictive of relapse-free and overall survival [20]. From this original set 50 genes, involved in proliferation, estrogen regulation, HER2, and basal and myoepithelial characteristics were selected [21] that showed prognostic significance for relapse-free survival [40]. Neilsen et al. validated the PAM50 intrinsic subtyping using qRT-PCR in 786 ER positive patients treated with tamoxifen [48]. In a premenopausal population from the prospective phase III MA12 trial, comparing tamoxifen versus placebo, 398 breast tumors were subtyped using the PAM50 assay and shown to be prognostic for both DFS and OS (P=0.0003 and P=0.0002 respectively) [49].

Prosigna, licensed in 2012, is the commercially available prognostic assay based on the PAM50 gene signature using the nCounter Analysis System developed by NanoString Technologies. The risk of recurrence (ROR) score is derived from an algorithm based on the PAM50 gene signature, intrinsic subtype, tumor size, nodal status, and proliferation score, based on a subset of 11 proliferation genes [48]. The test has been validated in 2 large independent datasets from the TransATAC [50] and ABCSG-8 [51] trials.

## *Endopredict®*

Endopredict (EP) is a multigene signature based on RNA expression of 8 cancer related genes and 3 housekeeping genes using RT-qPCR [52]. It predicts the likelihood of distant recurrence in patients with HR positive, HER2-negative breast

**Table 2.4** Phase III clinical trials prospectively evaluating the intermediate risk patient

| Trial | Study population | n | Test | Comparison | Results? |
|---|---|---|---|---|---|
| TailorX | Phase III trial<br>ER + ve, node negative BC; | 11000 | RS | Randomization of intermediate risk RS (defined as 11–25) patients to chemo vs. no chemo | Recruitment completed, results early 2016 (low risk published) |
| MINDACT | Phase III trial, ER + ve node negative and positive BC | 6600 | Mamma-print | Randomized study comparing Mammaprint with clinicopathological criteria for chemo | Expected 2015 (pilot phase published) |
| RxPONDER | Phase III trial, ER + ve node positive BC | 9400 | RS; also comparison with PAM 50 | RS $\leq$ 25 randomized to chemo vs. no chemo | Recruiting |
| OPTIMA | Adaptive design, ER + ve, node positive and node negative BC, | 1860 | Multiple platforms compared | (i) To determine best test for chemo selection;<br>(ii) To establish the cost-effectiveness of test-guided treatment strategies | Recruiting (preliminary study presented) |

cancer treated with adjuvant endocrine therapy with prespecified cut-offs for low (<10 % risk of distant recurrence at 10 years) and high risk (>10 % risk). It was developed using 964 ER-positive, HER2-negative tumors from patients treated with adjuvant tamoxifen only. EP has been validated in two large trials from ABCSG-6 (n = 378) and ABCSG-8 (n = 1324) showing continuous EP was an independent predictor of distant recurrence in multivariate analysis (ABCSG-6: $P = 0.010$, ABCSG-8: $P < 0.001$) [52].

### *Mammaprint*

Mammaprint is a 70-gene profile using microarray developed originally from 78 patients with predominantly HR positive, node negative breast cancer, stratifying into low-risk or high-risk prognostic groups [53]. It has been independently validated in 307 node negative patients from five European centers [54] as well as in a larger series on younger woman with node positive and node negative disease [55]. Whilst originally developed on microarrays using RNA from freshly frozen tissues, in an independent validation study, Mammaprint has been shown to be high reproducible using FFPE, with an overall equivalence of 91.5 % (CI 86.9–94.5) between the 211 independent matched FFPE and fresh tumor samples [56].

### *Breast Cancer Index*

Breast Cancer Index (BCI) is a prognostic assay based on qRT-PCR and has been developed from the combination of two gene signatures: HOXB13:IL17BR, a two gene ratio that predicts recurrence in tamoxifen treated patients [57], and the molecular grade index (MGI), consisting of five cell cycle-related genes [58]. BCI has been shown to significantly predict 10 year risk of breast cancer of recurrence beyond standard clinicopathological factors [59].

## Other Biomarkers for Predicting Risk of Recurrence

Achieving a pathological complete response (pCR) after neoadjuvant therapy is significantly associated with improved overall survival [60] and it is currently approved as surrogate endpoint to accelerate drug development and licensing [61]. Alternatively, identifying residual disease after pre-surgical treatment has become a way of identifying a higher risk population who may then be targeted for novel adjuvant therapies. However it is recognized that in HR positive disease, not achieving a pCR doesn't necessarily portend a poor prognosis, given many of these patients do very well. Both the baseline and residual Ki67 values after exposure to pre-surgical therapies have been shown to be prognostic [62, 63]. A combined score using the residual cancer burden, Ki67 and ER has been shown predict long term outcome after neoadjuvant chemotherapy [64].

The identification of micrometastatic disease either in the form of circulating tumor cells or tumor DNA may provide a method of tracking patients in follow up to identify those at future risk of clinical relapse [65, 66]. If preclinical relapse can be reliably identified by such techniques, it is also necessary to show that intervening before clinical relapse (whilst the patient is asymptomatic and without measurable disease) improves survival.

## What Are the Timeframes for Relapse?

Breast cancer relapse can occur at any time, even decades after the original diagnosis. There are more typical patterns for the timing of relapse depending on the breast cancer subtype. Triple negative and HER2 positive breast cancers tend to relapse early, in the first few years whereas the risk for HR positive breast cancers continues up to 10 years and even beyond [67, 68]. It is this ongoing risk that has become a major focus of research to identify those patients at risk for late relapse, in order to better tailor extended adjuvant endocrine therapy. The existing genomic assays have been interrogated for their ability to predict late relapse [69–72]. Whilst none of these have been originally designed for this purpose, currently the ROR and BCI outperform the other signatures in their ability to predict distant recurrence after 5 years [69, 70].

Obtaining a metastatic biopsy at the point of first (or indeed subsequent) relapse is now recognized as an important consideration, provided the site is safely accessible with a core needle. It is important to reassess ER, PgR and HER2 on the metastatic relapse, particularly if there has been a long disease-free interval, as these may change in up to 15 % of patients [73]. This also provides an opportunity to molecularly profile the tumor at the time of relapse, which may guide further therapy and/or clinical trial eligibility.

## What Are the Patterns of Relapse?

Breast cancer can relapse at virtually any site. In Kennecke's historical series, bone was the most common site of distant metastases in all subtypes except basal-like [24]. Triple negative breast cancers are more likely to present with visceral metastases [74]. Local recurrence should be treated with curative intent if feasible and radiotherapy should be considered, pending prior treatment [75]. Primary systemic therapy to achieve operability may also be used.

Cerebral metastases are more common in triple negative and HER2 positive disease. With improvements in effective systemic therapies to control extracranial disease, the treatment of brain metastases has become more aggressive as patients' outcomes improve. In a more modern series, the median overall survival after the development of brain metastases was longest for HER2 positive disease [76].

Oligometastatic disease describes very limited metastatic spread, ether as a single lesion or a single site with only a few metastatic lesions identified. This select group of metastatic patients has been identified as a possible target for more aggressive local therapies using either modern ablative or surgical techniques. Further prospective studies are needed and patient selection is obviously critical to best select those who are likely to achieve long term survival.

## Conclusion

The majority of patients diagnosed with early breast cancer are cured with multimodality therapy. There are multiple decision aids and molecular assays to help stratify patients so that we can better tailor systemic therapies accordingly with particular emphasis on later relapse risk in HR positive disease. It is likely as modern adjuvant therapies improve, the typical patterns of relapse as described in historical series may also change the natural history of recurrent disease.

## References

1. Gourgou-Bourgade S, Cameron D, Poortmans P, Asselain B, Azria D, Cardoso F, et al. Guidelines for time-to-event end point definitions in breast cancer trials: results of the DATECAN initiative (Definition for the Assessment of Time-to-event Endpoints in CANcer trials). Ann Oncol Off J Eur Soc Med Oncol/ESMO. 2015;26(5):873–9.
2. Cossetti RJ, Tyldesley SK, Speers CH, Zheng Y, Gelmon KA. Comparison of breast cancer recurrence and outcome patterns between patients treated from 1986 to 1992 and from 2004 to 2008. J Clin Oncol Off J Am Soc Clin Oncol. 2015;33(1):65–73.
3. Howlader N, Noone A, Krapcho M, Garshell J, Miller D, Altekruse SF, Kosary CL, Yu M, Ruhl J, Tatalovich Z,Mariotto A, Lewis DR, Chen HS, Feuer EJ, Cronin KA, editors. SEER cancer statistics review. Bethesda: National Cancer Institute; 1975–2012. http://seer.cancer.gov/csr/1975_2012/. Based on November 2014 SEER data submission, posted to the SEER web site, April 2015.
4. Miller AB, Wall C, Baines CJ, Sun P, To T, Narod SA. Twenty five year follow-up for breast cancer incidence and mortality of the Canadian National Breast Screening Study: randomised screening trial. BMJ. 2014;348:g366.
5. Bleyer A, Welch HG. Effect of three decades of screening mammography on breast-cancer incidence. N Engl J Med. 2012;367(21):1998–2005.
6. Marmot MG, Altman DG, Cameron DA, Dewar JA, Thompson SG, Wilcox M. The benefits and harms of breast cancer screening: an independent review. Br J Cancer. 2013;108(11): 2205–40.
7. Early Breast Cancer Trialists' Collaborative Group (EBCTCG). Effects of chemotherapy and hormonal therapy for early breast cancer on recurrence and 15-year survival: an overview of the randomised trials. Lancet. 2005;365(9472):1687–717.
8. Early Breast Cancer Trialists' Collaborative Group, Dowsett M, Forbes JF, Bradley R, Ingle J, Aihara T, et al. Aromatase inhibitors versus tamoxifen in early breast cancer: patient-level meta-analysis of the randomised trials. Lancet. 2015;386(10001):1341–52.

9. Early Breast Cancer Trialists' Collaborative Group, Clarke M, Coates AS, Darby SC, Davies C, Gelber RD, et al. Adjuvant chemotherapy in oestrogen-receptor-poor breast cancer: patient-level meta-analysis of randomised trials. Lancet. 2008;371(9606):29–40.
10. Piccart-Gebhart MJ, Procter M, Leyland-Jones B, Goldhirsch A, Untch M, Smith I, et al. Trastuzumab after adjuvant chemotherapy in HER2-positive breast cancer. N Engl J Med. 2005;353(16):1659–72.
11. Smith I, Procter M, Gelber RD, Guillaume S, Feyereislova A, Dowsett M, et al. 2-year follow-up of trastuzumab after adjuvant chemotherapy in HER2-positive breast cancer: a randomised controlled trial. Lancet. 2007;369(9555):29–36.
12. Early Breast Cancer Trialists' Collaborative Group, Darby S, McGale P, Correa C, Taylor C, Arriagada R, et al. Effect of radiotherapy after breast-conserving surgery on 10-year recurrence and 15-year breast cancer death: meta-analysis of individual patient data for 10,801 women in 17 randomised trials. Lancet. 2011;378(9804):1707–16.
13. Ebctcg MG. P, Taylor C, Correa C, Cutter D, Duane F, et al. Effect of radiotherapy after mastectomy and axillary surgery on 10-year recurrence and 20-year breast cancer mortality: meta-analysis of individual patient data for 8135 women in 22 randomised trials. Lancet. 2014;383(9935):2127–35.
14. Goss PE, Ingle JN, Martino S, Robert NJ, Muss HB, Piccart MJ, et al. Randomized trial of letrozole following tamoxifen as extended adjuvant therapy in receptor-positive breast cancer: updated findings from NCIC CTG MA.17. J Natl Cancer Inst. 2005;97(17):1262–71.
15. Gray RG, Rea D, Handley K, et al. ATTom: long-term effects of continuing adjuvant tamoxifen to 10 years versus stopping at 5 years in 6953 women with early breast cancer. J Clin Oncol. 2013;31(Suppl 31, abstr 5).
16. Davies C, Pan H, Godwin J, Gray R, Arriagada R, Raina V, et al. Long-term effects of continuing adjuvant tamoxifen to 10 years versus stopping at 5 years after diagnosis of oestrogen receptor-positive breast cancer: ATLAS, a randomised trial. Lancet. 2013;381(9869):805–16.
17. Francis PA, Regan MM, Fleming GF, Lang I, Ciruelos E, Bellet M, et al. Adjuvant ovarian suppression in premenopausal breast cancer. N Engl J Med. 2015;372(5):436–46.
18. Pagani O, Regan MM, Walley BA, Fleming GF, Colleoni M, Lang I, et al. Adjuvant exemestane with ovarian suppression in premenopausal breast cancer. N Engl J Med. 2014;371(2):107–18.
19. Hershman DL. Perfecting breast-cancer treatment--incremental gains and musculoskeletal pains. N Engl J Med. 2015;372(5):477–8.
20. Sorlie T, Perou CM, Tibshirani R, Aas T, Geisler S, Johnsen H, et al. Gene expression patterns of breast carcinomas distinguish tumor subclasses with clinical implications. Proc Natl Acad Sci U S A. 2001;98(19):10869–74.
21. Parker JS, Mullins M, Cheang MC, Leung S, Voduc D, Vickery T, et al. Supervised risk predictor of breast cancer based on intrinsic subtypes. J Clin Oncol: Off J Am Soc Clin Oncol. 2009;27(8):1160–7.
22. Ades F, Zardavas D, Bozovic-Spasojevic I, Pugliano L, Fumagalli D, de Azambuja E, et al. Luminal B breast cancer: molecular characterization, clinical management, and future perspectives. J Clin Oncol Off J Am Soc Clin Oncol. 2014;32(25):2794–803.
23. Perou CM, Parker JS, Prat A, Ellis MJ, Bernard PS. Clinical implementation of the intrinsic subtypes of breast cancer. Lancet Oncol. 2010;11(8):718–9. author reply 20-1.
24. Kennecke H, Yerushalmi R, Woods R, Cheang MC, Voduc D, Speers CH, et al. Metastatic behavior of breast cancer subtypes. J Clin Oncol Off J Am Soc Clin Oncol. 2010;28(20):3271–7.
25. Goldhirsch A, Gelber RD, Piccart-Gebhart MJ, de Azambuja E, Procter M, Suter TM, et al. 2 years versus 1 year of adjuvant trastuzumab for HER2-positive breast cancer (HERA): an open-label, randomised controlled trial. Lancet. 2013;382(9897):1021–8.
26. Haybittle JL, Blamey RW, Elston CW, Johnson J, Doyle PJ, Campbell FC, et al. A prognostic index in primary breast cancer. Br J Cancer. 1982;45(3):361–6.
27. Galea MH, Blamey RW, Elston CE, Ellis IO. The Nottingham Prognostic Index in primary breast cancer. Breast Cancer Res Treat. 1992;22(3):207–19.
28. Ravdin PM, Siminoff LA, Davis GJ, Mercer MB, Hewlett J, Gerson N, et al. Computer program to assist in making decisions about adjuvant therapy for women with early breast cancer. J Clinical Oncol Off J Am Soc Clin Oncol. 2001;19(4):980–91.

29. Olivotto IA, Bajdik CD, Ravdin PM, Speers CH, Coldman AJ, Norris BD, et al. Population-based validation of the prognostic model ADJUVANT! for early breast cancer. J Clin Oncol Off J Am Soc Clin Oncol. 2005;23(12):2716–25.
30. Early Breast Cancer Trialists' Collaborative Group. Effects of chemotherapy and hormonal therapy for early breast cancer on recurrence and 15-year survival: an overview of the randomised trials. Lancet. 2005;365(9472):1687–717.
31. Wishart GC, Azzato EM, Greenberg DC, Rashbass J, Kearins O, Lawrence G, et al. PREDICT: a new UK prognostic model that predicts survival following surgery for invasive breast cancer. Breast Cancer Res. 2010;12(1):R1.
32. Wishart GC, Bajdik CD, Azzato EM, Dicks E, Greenberg DC, Rashbass J, et al. A population-based validation of the prognostic model PREDICT for early breast cancer. Eur J Surg Oncol. 2011;37(5):411–7.
33. Wishart GC, Bajdik CD, Dicks E, Provenzano E, Schmidt MK, Sherman M, et al. PREDICT Plus: development and validation of a prognostic model for early breast cancer that includes HER2. Br J Cancer. 2012;107(5):800–7.
34. Wishart GC, Greenberg DC, Britton PD, Chou P, Brown CH, Purushotham AD, et al. Screen-detected vs symptomatic breast cancer: is improved survival due to stage migration alone? Br J Cancer. 2008;98(11):1741–4.
35. Cuzick J, Dowsett M, Pineda S, Wale C, Salter J, Quinn E, et al. Prognostic value of a combined estrogen receptor, progesterone receptor, Ki-67, and human epidermal growth factor receptor 2 immunohistochemical score and comparison with the Genomic Health recurrence score in early breast cancer. J Clin Oncol Off J Am Soc Clin Oncol. 2011;29(32): 4273–8.
36. Yeo B, Zabaglo L, Hills M, Dodson A, Smith I, Dowsett M. Clinical utility of the IHC4+C score in oestrogen receptor-positive early breast cancer: a prospective decision impact study. Br J Cancer. 2015;113(3):390–5.
37. Dodson A, Zabaglo L, Yeo B, Miller K, Smith I, Dowsett M. Risk of recurrence estimates with IHC4+C are tolerant of variations in staining and scoring: an analytical validity study. J Clin Pathol. 2015.
38. Sestak I, Cuzick J. Markers for the identification of late breast cancer recurrence. Breast Cancer Res. 2015;17:10.
39. Fisher B, Dignam J, Wolmark N, DeCillis A, Emir B, Wickerham DL, et al. Tamoxifen and chemotherapy for lymph node-negative, estrogen receptor-positive breast cancer. J Natl Cancer Inst. 1997;89(22):1673–82.
40. Prat A, Ellis MJ, Perou CM. Practical implications of gene-expression-based assays for breast oncologists. Nat Rev Clin Oncol. 2012;9(1):48–57.
41. Dowsett M, Cuzick J, Wale C, Forbes J, Mallon EA, Salter J, et al. Prediction of risk of distant recurrence using the 21-gene recurrence score in node-negative and node-positive postmenopausal patients with breast cancer treated with anastrozole or tamoxifen: a TransATAC study. J Clin Oncol Off J Am Soc Clin Oncol. 2010;28(11):1829–34.
42. Harris L, Fritsche H, Mennel R, Norton L, Ravdin P, Taube S, et al. American Society of Clinical Oncology 2007 update of recommendations for the use of tumor markers in breast cancer. J Clin Oncol Off J Am Soc Clin Oncol. 2007;25(33):5287–312.
43. Coates AS, Winer EP, Goldhirsch A, Gelber RD, Gnant M, Piccart-Gebhart M, et al. Tailoring therapies-improving the management of early breast cancer: St Gallen International Expert Consensus on the Primary Therapy of Early Breast Cancer 2015. Ann Oncol Off J Eur Soc Med Oncol ESMO. 2015;26(8):1533–46.
44. NICE diagnostic guidance 10. Gene expression profiling and expanded immunohistochemistry tests for guiding adjuvant chemotherapy decisions in early breast cancer management: MammaPrint OD, IHC4 and Mammostrat. September 2013. ISBN: 978-1-4731-0296-5.
45. Paik S, Tang G, Shak S, Kim C, Baker J, Kim W, et al. Gene expression and benefit of chemotherapy in women with node-negative, estrogen receptor-positive breast cancer. J Clin Oncol Off J Am Soc Clin Oncol. 2006;24(23):3726–34.
46. Albain KS, Barlow WE, Shak S, Hortobagyi GN, Livingston RB, Yeh IT, et al. Prognostic and predictive value of the 21-gene recurrence score assay in postmenopausal women with

node-positive, oestrogen-receptor-positive breast cancer on chemotherapy: a retrospective analysis of a randomised trial. Lancet Oncol. 2010;11(1):55–65.
47. Perou CM, Sorlie T, Eisen MB, van de Rijn M, Jeffrey SS, Rees CA, et al. Molecular portraits of human breast tumours. Nature. 2000;406(6797):747–52.
48. Nielsen TO, Parker JS, Leung S, Voduc D, Ebbert M, Vickery T, et al. A comparison of PAM50 intrinsic subtyping with immunohistochemistry and clinical prognostic factors in tamoxifen-treated estrogen receptor-positive breast cancer. Clin Cancer Res Off J Am Assoc Cancer Res. 2010;16(21):5222–32.
49. Chia SK, Bramwell VH, Tu D, Shepherd LE, Jiang S, Vickery T, et al. A 50-gene intrinsic subtype classifier for prognosis and prediction of benefit from adjuvant tamoxifen. Clin Cancer Res Off J Am Assoc Cancer Res. 2012;18(16):4465–72.
50. Dowsett M, Sestak I, Lopez-Knowles E, Sidhu K, Dunbier AK, Cowens JW, et al. Comparison of PAM50 risk of recurrence score with oncotype DX and IHC4 for predicting risk of distant recurrence after endocrine therapy. J Clin Oncol Off J Am Soc Clin Oncol. 2013;31(22):2783–90.
51. Gnant M, Filipits M, Greil R, Stoeger H, Rudas M, Bago-Horvath Z, et al. Predicting distant recurrence in receptor-positive breast cancer patients with limited clinicopathological risk: using the PAM50 Risk of Recurrence score in 1478 postmenopausal patients of the ABCSG-8 trial treated with adjuvant endocrine therapy alone. Ann Oncol Off J Eur Soc Med Oncol ESMO. 2014;25(2):339–45.
52. Filipits M, Rudas M, Jakesz R, Dubsky P, Fitzal F, Singer CF, et al. A new molecular predictor of distant recurrence in ER-positive, HER2-negative breast cancer adds independent information to conventional clinical risk factors. Clin Cancer Res Off J Am Assoc Cancer Res. 2011;17(18):6012–20.
53. Van't Veer LJ, Dai H, van de Vijver MJ, He YD, Hart AA, Mao M, et al. Gene expression profiling predicts clinical outcome of breast cancer. Nature. 2002;415(6871):530–6.
54. Buyse M, Loi S, van't Veer L, Viale G, Delorenzi M, Glas AM, et al. Validation and clinical utility of a 70-gene prognostic signature for women with node-negative breast cancer. J Natl Cancer Inst. 2006;98(17):1183–92.
55. van de Vijver MJ, He YD, van't Veer LJ, Dai H, Hart AA, Voskuil DW, et al. A gene-expression signature as a predictor of survival in breast cancer. N Engl J Med. 2002;347(25):1999–2009.
56. Sapino A, Roepman P, Linn SC, Snel MH, Delahaye LJ, van den Akker J, et al. MammaPrint molecular diagnostics on formalin-fixed, paraffin-embedded tissue. J Mol Diagn. 2014;16(2):190–7.
57. Ma XJ, Wang Z, Ryan PD, Isakoff SJ, Barmettler A, Fuller A, et al. A two-gene expression ratio predicts clinical outcome in breast cancer patients treated with tamoxifen. Cancer Cell. 2004;5(6):607–16.
58. Ma XJ, Salunga R, Dahiya S, Wang W, Carney E, Durbecq V, et al. A five-gene molecular grade index and HOXB13:IL17BR are complementary prognostic factors in early stage breast cancer. Clin Cancer Res Off J Am Assoc Cancer Res. 2008;14(9):2601–8.
59. Jerevall PL, Ma XJ, Li H, Salunga R, Kesty NC, Erlander MG, et al. Prognostic utility of HOXB13:IL17BR and molecular grade index in early-stage breast cancer patients from the Stockholm trial. Br J Cancer. 2011;104(11):1762–9.
60. Mieog JS, van der Hage JA, van de Velde CJ. Preoperative chemotherapy for women with operable breast cancer. Cochrane Database Syst Rev. 2007;(2):CD005002.
61. Prowell TM, Pazdur R. Pathological complete response and accelerated drug approval in early breast cancer. N Engl J Med. 2012;366(26):2438–41.
62. Urruticoechea A, Smith IE, Dowsett M. Proliferation marker Ki-67 in early breast cancer. J Clin Oncol Off J Am Soc Clin Oncol. 2005;23(28):7212–20.
63. Dowsett M, Smith IE, Ebbs SR, Dixon JM, Skene A, A'Hern R, et al. Prognostic value of Ki67 expression after short-term presurgical endocrine therapy for primary breast cancer. J Natl Cancer Inst. 2007;99(2):167–70.
64. Sheri A, Smith IE, Johnston SR, A'Hern R, Nerurkar A, Jones RL, et al. Residual proliferative cancer burden to predict long-term outcome following neoadjuvant chemotherapy. Ann Oncol Off J Eur Soc Med Oncol ESMO. 2015;26(1):75–80.

65. Garcia-Murillas I, Schiavon G, Weigelt B, Ng C, Hrebien S, Cutts RJ, et al. Mutation tracking in circulating tumor DNA predicts relapse in early breast cancer. Sci Transl Med. 2015;7(302):302ra133.
66. Lucci A, Hall CS, Lodhi AK, Bhattacharyya A, Anderson AE, Xiao L, et al. Circulating tumour cells in non-metastatic breast cancer: a prospective study. Lancet Oncol. 2012;13(7):688–95.
67. Pagani O, Price KN, Gelber RD, Castiglione-Gertsch M, Holmberg SB, Lindtner J, et al. Patterns of recurrence of early breast cancer according to estrogen receptor status: a therapeutic target for a quarter of a century. Breast Cancer Res Treat. 2009;117(2):319–24.
68. Kast K, Link T, Friedrich K, Petzold A, Niedostatek A, Schoffer O, et al. Impact of breast cancer subtypes and patterns of metastasis on outcome. Breast Cancer Res Treat. 2015;150(3):621–9.
69. Sgroi DC, Sestak I, Cuzick J, Zhang Y, Schnabel CA, Schroeder B, et al. Prediction of late distant recurrence in patients with oestrogen-receptor-positive breast cancer: a prospective comparison of the breast-cancer index (BCI) assay, 21-gene recurrence score, and IHC4 in the TransATAC study population. Lancet Oncol. 2013;14(11):1067–76.
70. Sestak I, Cuzick J, Dowsett M, Lopez-Knowles E, Filipits M, Dubsky P, et al. Prediction of late distant recurrence after 5 years of endocrine treatment: a combined analysis of patients from the Austrian breast and colorectal cancer study group 8 and arimidex, tamoxifen alone or in combination randomized trials using the PAM50 risk of recurrence score. J Clin Oncol Off J Am Soc Clin Oncol. 2015;33(8):916–22.
71. Filipits M, Nielsen TO, Rudas M, Greil R, Stoger H, Jakesz R, et al. The PAM50 risk-of-recurrence score predicts risk for late distant recurrence after endocrine therapy in postmenopausal women with endocrine-responsive early breast cancer. Clin Cancer Res Off J Am Assoc Cancer Res. 2014;20(5):1298–305.
72. Dubsky P, Brase JC, Jakesz R, Rudas M, Singer CF, Greil R, et al. The EndoPredict score provides prognostic information on late distant metastases in ER+/HER2- breast cancer patients. Br J Cancer. 2013;109(12):2959–64.
73. Houssami N, Macaskill P, Balleine RL, Bilous M, Pegram MD. HER2 discordance between primary breast cancer and its paired metastasis: tumor biology or test artefact? Insights through meta-analysis. Breast Cancer Res Treat. 2011;129(3):659–74.
74. Rodriguez-Pinilla SM, Sarrio D, Honrado E, Hardisson D, Calero F, Benitez J, et al. Prognostic significance of basal-like phenotype and fascin expression in node-negative invasive breast carcinomas. Clin Cancer Res Off J Am Assoc Cancer Res. 2006;12(5):1533–9.
75. Cardoso F, Harbeck N, Fallowfield L, Kyriakides S, Senkus E, Group EGW. Locally recurrent or metastatic breast cancer: ESMO Clinical Practice Guidelines for diagnosis, treatment and follow-up. Ann Oncol Off J Eur Soc Med Oncol ESMO. 2012;(23 Suppl 7):vii11–9.
76. Niikura N, Hayashi N, Masuda N, Takashima S, Nakamura R, Watanabe K, et al. Treatment outcomes and prognostic factors for patients with brain metastases from breast cancer of each subtype: a multicenter retrospective analysis. Breast Cancer Res Treat. 2014;147(1):103–12.

# Chapter 3
# Detection of Recurrence: Clinical Follow-Up

**Anne Mc Loughlin and Nicola Roche**

**Abstract** Breast cancer follow up after treatment of early disease has evolved in recent years to allow for a more patient centered approach. Various models of follow up successfully exist, aiming to provide early detection of treatable local recurrence in the ipsilateral or contra-lateral breast, identify symptoms suggestive of secondary breast cancer and to support patients who may have treatment related sequelae, albeit physical or emotional. A novel model for a patient-led approach is outlined in detail.

**Keywords** Clinical follow up • Early detection • Psychological support

With improvements in early cancer detection, novel and expanding treatment options and the growing elderly population the number of cancer survivors is burgeoning. Worldwide it is estimated that over 25 million people are living with a history of cancer [1]. Within the UK, over two thirds of women diagnosed with breast cancer now survive more than 20 years [2]. The growth in cancer survivorship has led to a substantial increase in the number of people requiring follow up care. Because of the complexity of problems faced by people with cancer appropriate and acceptable follow up care is important. Whilst many enjoy a good quality of life, some survivors sustain treatment or disease related health problems that persist for many years. Along with the on-going risk of recurrence, potential long term and late effects of cancer treatment include neuropathy, fatigue, pain, cardiovascular compromise, lymphedema, depression, sexual dysfunction, cognitive and functional decline, as well as secondary malignancy. This chapter aims to assess the evidence for the benefits of clinical follow up following a breast cancer diagnosis and discuss how recent changes in follow up care may help to meet the ongoing physical and emotional needs of survivors, ensuring that those living with and beyond their cancer diagnosis receive the information and support they need to lead healthy and active lives following completion of treatment.

A. Mc Loughlin, BSc (Hons), MSc • N. Roche, MB, BCh, BAO, MCh, FRCS (✉)
The Breast Unit, The Royal Marsden NHS Foundation Trust, London, UK
e-mail: anne.mcloughlin@rmh.nhs.uk; nicky.roche@rmh.nhs.uk



A. Ring, M. Parton (eds.), *Breast Cancer Survivorship*,
DOI 10.1007/978-3-319-41858-2_3

The aim of breast cancer follow up is:

1. The early detection of treatable local recurrence
2. Early detection of contralateral breast cancers
3. Identification of symptoms suggestive of secondary breast cancer
4. Management of treatment related sequelae and provision of psychological support.

## Guidelines

For many years the traditional model of follow up has been a series of clinical appointments at increasing intervals following initial treatment. Indeed the American Society for Clinical Oncology (ASCO) still recommends a physical examination every 3–6 months for the first 3 years, every 6–12 months for years 4 and 5, and annually thereafter [3]. On the other hand, in the UK, the National Institute for Clinical Excellence [4] focuses more on a more patient directed follow up and with agreed care plans.

## Clinical Examination and Routine Appointments

Intuitively more frequent clinic visits should lead to earlier detection of recurrence and improved survival. However there is no evidence to support this and several publications have questioned the effectiveness of outpatient appointments, highlighting that most recurrences or new breast cancers are detected either by a routine surveillance mammogram or as interval events with patients presenting with new symptoms in between appointments [5–7].

Regular clinical examination rarely detects local recurrence [8, 9] and is not known to confer any survival benefits. There is little evidence to support the role of clinical breast examination and breast self- examination; indeed some authors suggest that they may do more harm than good [10–12].

Whilst there is no evidence that routine follow up improves prognosis or reduces rates of recurrence, many women may value follow up for the reassurance it offers them, in particular the availability of specialist expertise as well as access to diagnostic tests [13]. However long waiting times, rushed consultations and lack of continuity [14] often result in consultations that frequently read fail to address the real concerns for patients, hence the current trend in breast cancer follow up towards patient directed follow up.

**Early detection of recurrence and contralateral breast cancers** The rates of in breast tumor recurrence (IBTR) have fallen with modern multi-modality treatment, with current IBTR rates of around 5 % at 10 years [15]. Non-gene carriers are also at a small increased risk of contralateral breast cancer (CBC) in comparison to the general population, the risk of CBC being in the region of 0.6 % per year [16].

The development of IBTR has an adverse impact on survival. The time from treatment of the primary to IBTR being significant with those occurring after a shorter interval having a worse prognosis. The early detection of IBTR and CBC confers a survival advantage [17]. Current UK practice is to perform a surveillance mammogram every 12–24 months for 5 years or till the patient reaches the age of routine breast screening through the NHS breast screening programme. The incidence of IBTR and CBC has been shown to be fairly constant over the first 10 years supporting a longer surveillance strategy. Optimal imaging strategies for detecting local recurrence are discussed further in Chap. 4.

## Identification of Early Secondary Disease

Multiple diagnostic investigations designed to detect metastatic (or secondary) disease are not recommended, as they have not been shown to prolong survival and may even have a detrimental effect on the quality of life [3]. Guidelines do not recommend the use of routine bloods and tumor markers in the follow up of asymptomatic patients [18]. Whilst a rise in tumor markers such as CA 15.3 may predict disease recurrence in advance of symptoms, there is currently no evidence that this translates to a survival advantage or improved quality of life. Advances in detection of circulating tumor cells [19] or more recently detection of circulating tumor DNA [20] may prove to be more sensitive predictors of recurrence but studies still need to demonstrate that a therapeutic intervention at an early stage translates to a better outcome in terms of survival and quality of life

## Models of Follow Up Care

No consensus exists as to where follow up should take place, within the hospital or primary care, and which type of health professional doctors or nurses, should provide follow up care [21, 22]. Alternative methods of follow up such as nurse led or follow up in primary care have demonstrated high levels of acceptability, with no reduction in the quality of life or increase in anxiety. Strategies focusing less on survival and more on patient's satisfaction have shown benefits to patients [6, 21]. However much of the research published to date is not powered sufficiently to establish safety.

Within the UK, work has been undertaken to improve the quality and effectiveness of care and support to those living with and beyond cancer. When the National cancer survivorship initiative set out its goals for cancer care in its vision document [23] it highlighted five key shifts, outlined in Table 3.1, necessary to deliver high quality care and support to people living with and beyond a cancer diagnosis. Current health policy advocates a move away from routine follow up to an approach based on individualized needs and preferences along with the promotion of recovery, health and well-being following completion of treatment, with an aim that by 2020

**Table 3.1** Five shifts in care and support for people living with and beyond cancer

| |
|---|
| A cultural shift in the approach to care and support for people affected by cancer to a greater focus on recovery, health and well-being after treatment |
| A shift towards holistic assessment, information provision and personalized care based on assessment of individual risk, needs and preferences. |
| A shift towards supported self-management, an approach which empowers individuals to take responsibility for their condition |
| A shift from a single model of follow up care to tailored support that enables early recognition of the consequences of treatment and the signs and symptoms of further disease |
| A shift from an emphasis on measuring clinical activity to a new emphasis on measuring experience and outcomes for cancer survivors through routine use of patient reported outcomes |

DH 2010 [23]

**Table 3.2** Addressing the holistic needs of the patient

| |
|---|
| Address physical and practical concerns |
| Signposting to national/local support groups |
| Support self- management courses |
| Refer to allied health care support |
| Advice related to lifestyle: stop smoking, weight loss |
| Information or referral to physical activity program |
| Information or referral on diet and nutrition |
| Referral for counseling/psychological support |
| Support related to work and financial concerns |

DH 2011 [25]

every person with cancer will have access to elements of this 'recovery package' [24]. Information should be provided on long term side effects alongside rapid access to specialist medical care if and when problems arise [25] and emphasis is placed upon addressing the holistic needs of patients as shown in Table 3.2.

This desire to improve the quality and effectiveness of services has been greeted with enthusiasm within many breast units who are keen to implement new models of survivorship care, so that follow up services are patient-led, enabling ongoing access to clinical teams as needed. These types of follow up are referred to as Patient led follow up or Open access follow up and are underpinned by an ethos of supported self-management. There is evidence to suggest that implementation of new models of care, for those living with and beyond their cancer diagnosis can improve the quality of life for people following treatment for cancer through addressing their needs, and helping them to return to living their lives as positively as possible [23, 25].

## Potential Model for Patient-Led Care

The key components to successful patient led care are listed in Table 3.3. Many models exist but a potential framework is outlined in this section.

**Table 3.3** Key components of supported self- management

| |
|---|
| Holistic Needs Assessments to identify and address any outstanding needs and to ensure patient has the knowledge and confidence to self-manage |
| End of Treatment Summaries and Survivorship Care Plans |
| Access to Health and Well-being events |
| A Remote Monitoring System to manage ongoing surveillance tests |
| Good communication between specialist and primary care teams |
| A system that allows rapid re -access to the specialist team if needed |

DH 2010 [23], 2011 [25]

**End of treatment consultation** Patient suitability should be confirmed at a multidisciplinary meeting (MDM). Patients who may be less suitable for entry in to a supported self-management program at the end of hospital based treatment may include patients with learning disabilities, very elderly patients, those with mental health problems or those who do not speak English as first language. At the end of treatment, patients are invited to attend a consultation with a specialist nurse or other member of the multidisciplinary team. It has long been recognized that the skills of specialist nurses could be harnessed to provide a quality service whilst reducing the burden on hospital clinics [26]. Breast care nurses are uniquely placed to address the information and psychosocial needs of affected women and to provide follow up services. Telephone follow up in particular by specialist breast care nurses has positive benefits for women with breast cancer and can provide a fast responsive system when patients really need it [26, 27].

**Holistic needs assessment (HNA)** Holistic needs assessment is a process of gathering and discussing information with the patient in order to develop an understanding of what the person living beyond their cancer knows, understands and needs [23, 25]. Patients are given a HNA form which they can complete before the end of treatment consultation. This is shown in http://www.londoncanceralliance.nhs.uk/media/60440/London%20Holistic%20Needs%20Assessment_print%20version_2013.pdf. The assessment results are used to inform a Survivorship care plan and can identify unmet needs and help address physical, practical and psychological concerns. It is recognized that treatment completion is a time of uncertainty for patients and some report a lack of support from health professionals. While many patients adapt well to the physical and psychological effects of breast cancer well after completing treatment, research has identified that up to 30 % of all patients had five or more unmet needs at the end of treatment. The most frequently reported are fear of recurrence, psychological needs, financial difficulties and altered relationships [28]. Patients can be referred to the appropriate rehabilitation or supportive services within the hospital, community or voluntary sector.

**End of treatment summary** The Survivorship care plan is a communication tool that empowers the user to self-manage and improve their quality of life. The plan for follow up care is confirmed including mammographic (or other) surveillance, duration of endocrine treatment and frequency of DEXA bone density scans. These

**Table 3.4** Signs and symptoms of a possible recurrence

| Changes to look and feel for | Signs and symptoms to report |
|---|---|
| A change in shape or size of the breast | Lymphedema or tingling in arm |
| A lump or thickening that feels different | Bone pain greater than 2 weeks |
| Change in skin texture such as puckering or dimpling | Pain beneath the rib cage or swelling |
| Swelling in the upper arm | Ongoing nausea |
| Pain | Persistent cough or breathlessness |
| Nipple discharge | Early morning headaches |
| Redness or a rash on the skin and or around the nipple | |
| An inverted nipple or changes in the position or shape of the nipple | |
| A swelling in the arm pit or around the collar bone | |

dates are recorded, along with the diagnosis and treatment summary on the patients end of treatment care plan. End of treatment summaries can help to support communication with primary care and any further reviews undertaken by the GP. Patients are given a Treatment Summary and a Survivorship care plan is developed, which can be shared with the General Practitioner (GP).

**Trigger symptoms and signs** Patients need to become breast aware. This involves getting used to what the treated breast looks and feels like, as well as noticing any new changes. Surgery and radiotherapy alter the appearance, feel and sensation of the breasts after treatment. For example, the area around the scar may feel lumpy, numb or sensitive. Breast awareness is important for patients who have had breast conserving surgery or a mastectomy (with or without a reconstruction) and should be undertaken in addition to receiving regular mammograms. Getting to know how it looks and feels so an individual knows what is normal will help them to feel more confident about noticing changes and reporting them. It is also important to be aware of any new changes in the other breast and report them as soon as possible. Signs and symptoms of secondary (metastatic disease) are discussed and appropriate written information is offered. See Table 3.4.

**Data management** Imaging surveillance is managed remotely; patients attend the hospital for annual mammograms and receive the results by post. A virtual clinic/ MDM runs each month to capture patents who may have: completed endocrine treatment, benefit from extended adjuvant therapy, benefit from switching endocrine treatment or have completed mammographic surveillance and should return to the NHS Breast Screening Programme. Key events such as mammogram appointments, completion or switch dates of endocrine treatment and dates of DEXA scans are flagged on a database. A robust data base with ability to flag key events and recall patients for investigations is essential and key to running a safe patient led follow up. It also allows for data collection and research. If patients develop local or metastatic recurrence, they receive appropriate treatment and are taken off the remote monitoring system.

**Access to specialist team** Once patients enter the program, access to the breast unit is through the specialist nursing team whom they can phone should problems or concerns arise. The specialist nurse can provide advice or organise a return to clinic on an as needs basis, depending on the significance of new symptoms, worries or concerns that they may have.

**Health and well-being promotion** Advice on health promotion and lifestyle issues such as smoking, diet and exercise, weight management and alcohol intake are also discussed. Studies indicate a higher prevalence of obesity and lower levels of physical activity among cancer survivors compared to the general population [29]. Life expectancy for breast cancer survivors has been generally increasing, however those with a higher BMI and low physical activity levels are not only at increased risk of cancer recurrence [30] but could develop co-morbidities such as hypertension, cardiovascular disease and osteoarthritis. Evidence is now growing to support the role of physical activity during and after cancer treatment. Discussions about diet and physical activity are likely to be well received by patients. Following a diagnosis of cancer many patients will be focused on their health and may be more receptive to messages around lifestyle risk factors. This represents a teachable moment [31] which could be used to help people modify aspects of their lifestyle to reduce a variety of health conditions. Breast Units should be encouraged to run or sign post patients to health and well-being events. However attendance at these events is often low, supporting the idea that may patients return to normal after cancer treatment with a smaller proportion needing more intensive support and help.

**The patient-led follow-up model; a potentially suitable model for future breast cancer services** The perceived benefits of this supported self-managed or patient led approach to follow up are that women who are well and have no concerns do not need to attend the hospital. The anxiety associated with clinic appointments is decreased and unnecessary appointments are reduced. Giving attention to survivorship issues enables health professionals to respond effectively to straightforward problems that patients identify. Patients have their needs met in a timely manner, are better informed about their disease, treatment and longer term effects. Equally, patients who have more complex difficulties can be identified and referred to the appropriate specialist services. The reduction in unnecessary outpatient appointments for those who no longer require face to face appointments in turn releases capacity for those with complex needs and helps improve access for new referrals. Patients will understandably enquire about the value of scans, tumor markers and other tests that might lead to either reassurance or early detection but at present more intensive surveillance has not been shown to promote clinically significant changes in the time to recurrence or to improve survival or quality of life. Most patients will accept this, once the rationale is explained to them [32]. Chapman et al. [33] undertook an audit to assess patient satisfaction and GP workload following the introduction of patient led breast cancer follow up. A questionnaire was sent to 217 patients at low risk of recurrence. There were 130 respondents (60 %) and of these 126 (97 %) patients had a clear idea of how to contact the breast unit. Only 10 of 277

GP respondents (3.7 %) referred a patient back to the breast unit. Shepherd et al. [27] examined a model of care for breast cancer patients based on the concept of point of need access and investigated the effectiveness of this model in comparison to routine 6 monthly reviews. Two hundred fourteen patients participated, overall there was no increased risk of psychological morbidity or decline in quality of life when routine review was discontinued, the recurrences observed were unlikely to have been detected at a routine visit. Point of need access is acceptable to the majority of patients; there is no evidence to support the view that that regular clinical review improves psychological morbidity or quality of life. Rechis et al. [34] highlights post treatment cancer survivors who received an End of Treatment Summary reported that their needs had been met, including receiving information about possible late effects.

## Conclusion

Breast cancer is a heterogeneous disease and it is unlikely one follow protocol will be suitable for all patients. It is clear that most retrospective reviews of routine clinic visits have not been helpful in establishing either the best schedule for such visits or indeed whether visits are necessary [5]. There is no evidence that routine clinical follow up improves survival. The majority of breast cancer patients have a favorable prognosis and will live for many years after diagnosis. Follow up care should focus on diagnosis and management of second primary cancer, management of long term hormonal therapies, evaluation and management of treatment complications and the provision of ongoing psycho social support. The continued development of patient led follow up is likely to mean that in the future primary care will have an increasingly important role to play in supporting patients in the self- management of their conditions. Brearley et al. [35] recognizes that there has been a substantial amount of research describing many of the problems experienced by cancer survivors; this is strongest in the periods soon after treatment. As the complexity of treatment increases many patients report on-going side effects and concerns as well as lack of self-confidence. There will need to be greater ability of health professionals to identify and treat survivorship issues, more data is needed to understand the needs of this group and the effectiveness of interventions for the problems they have.

## References

1. Bellury L, Pett M, Ellington L, Beck SL, Clark JC, Stein KD. The effect of aging and cancer on the symptom experience and physical function of elderly cancer survivors. Cancer. 2012;118(24):6171–8.
2. Cancer research UK. 2014. www.cancerresearch.org.prod.

3. Khatcheressian J, Hurley P, Bantug E, Esserman L, Grunfeld E, Halberg F, Hantel A, Henry L, Hyman B, Smith T, Vogel V, Wolff A, Somerfield M, Davidson N. Breast cancer follow up and management after primary treatment: American Society of Clinical Oncology Clinical practice guideline update. J Clin Oncol. 2013;31(7):961–5.
4. NICE. 2009. Early and locally advanced breast cancer: diagnosis and treatment. http://www.nice.org.uk/guidance/cg80/chapter/1-guidance#/followup. Accessed 20 April 16.
5. De Bock G, Bonema J, Van de Hage J, Kiewet J, Van de Velde C. Effectiveness of routine visits and tests in detecting isolates regional recurrences after treatment for early stage breast cancer: a meta-analysis and systematic review. J Clin Oncol. 2004;22(19):4010–8.
6. Montgomery D, Krupa K, Cooke T. Alternative methods of follow up in breast cancer: a systematic review of the literature. Br J Cancer. 2007;96:1625–32.
7. Geurts S, de vegt F, Siesling S, Flobbe K, Katja K, Aben H, Van der Heiden-van der loo, Verbeck, A, Jos A, Van Dijck A, Tjan-Heijnen C. Patterns of follow up care and early relapse detection in breast cancer patients. Breast Cancer Res Treat. 2012;136:859–68.
8. Donnelly PK, Hiller L, Dunn J. National randomised controlled trial is needed. BMJ. 2008;336:107–8.
9. Dixon M, Montgomery D. Extended follow up of breast cancer patients in clinic wastes time for both patients and doctors: the case for. Breast Cancer Res. 2008;10 Suppl 4:S7.
10. Roeke T, Van Brommel AC, Gaillard-Hemmink MP, Hartgrink HH, Mesker WE, Tollenaar RA. The additional cancer yield of clinical breast examination in screening of women at hereditary increased risk of breast cancer: a systematic review. Breast Cancer Res Treat. 2014;147(1): 15–23.
11. Spence, D. (2012). Bad medicine: clinical breast examination. BMJ. 2012;345:e6789. doi:10.1136/bmj.e6789.
12. McCready T, Littlewood D, Jenkinson J. Breast self-examination and breast awareness: a literature review. J Clin Nurs. 2005;5:570–8.
13. Vicary P, Johnson M, Maher J. To my oncologist- an open letter from a patient at the end of follow up. Clin Oncol (R Coll Radiol). 2007;19:746–7.
14. Pennery E, Mallet J. A preliminary study of patients' perceptions of routine follow up after treatment for breast cancer. Eur J Oncol Nurs. 2000;4(3):138–45.
15. Haviland J, Owen R, Dewar J, Agrawal R, Barrett J, Barrett-lee P, Dobbs J, Hopwood P, Lawton P, Magee B, Mills J, Simmons S, Sydenham M, Venables K, Bliss J, Yarnold J. The UK Standardisation of breast radiotherapy (START) trials of radiotherapy hypofractionation for treatment of early breast cancer: 10 year follow up results of two randomised controlled trials. Lancet Oncol. 2013;14:1086–94.
16. Taggart F, Donnelly P, Dunn J. Options for early breast cancer follow up in primary and secondary care- a systematic review. BMC Cancer. 2012;12:238.
17. Robertson C, Arcot Ragupathy SK, Boachie C, Dixon JM, Fraser C, Hernandez R, Heys S, Jack W, Kerr GR, Lawrence G, MacLennan G, Maxwell A, McGregor J, Mowatt G, Pinder S, Ternent L, Thomas RE, Vale L, Wilson R, Zhu S, and Gilbert FJ. The clinical effectiveness and cost effectiveness of different surveillance mammography regimens after the treatment for primary breast cancer: systematic reviews, registry database analyses and economic evaluation. Health Technol Assess. 2011;15(34): v–vi, 1–322.
18. Runowicz C, Leach C, Henry L, Henry K, Mackey H, Cowens-Alvarado, R, Cannady R, Pratt-Chapman M, Edge S, Jacobs L, Hurria A, Marks L, La Monte S, Warner E, Lyman G, Ganz P, et al. 2015. American Cancer Society/American Society of Clinical Oncology Breast Cancer Survivorship Care Guideline. http://www.asco.org/practice-guidelines/quality-guidelines/guidelines/breast-cancer#/9526. Accessed 20 Apr 16.
19. Lucci A, Hall CS, Lodhi AK, Bhattacharya A, Anderson AE, Xiao L, Bedrosian I, Kuerer HM, Krishnamurthy S. Circulating tumour cells in non-metastatic breast cancer: a prospective study. Lancet Oncol 2012;13(7):688–95. doi: 10.1016/S1470-2045(12)70209-7.
20. Garcia-Murillas I, Schaivon G, Weigelt B, Ng C, Hrebian S, Cutts RJ, Cheang M, Osin P, Nerurkar A, Kozarewa I, Garrido JA, Dowsett M, Reiss-Filho JS, Smith IE, Turner

NC. Mutation tracking in circulating tumour DNA predicts relapse in early breast cancer. Sci Transl Med. 2015;7(302):302ra133. doi:10.1126/scitranslmed.aab0021
21. Koinberg L, Fridlund B, Engholm G, Holmberg L. Nurse led follow up on demand or by a physician after breast cancer surgery: a randomised study. Eur J Oncol Nurs. 2004;8:109–17.
22. Grunfeld E, Levine A, Julian J, Coyle D, Szechtman B, Mirsky D, Verma S, Sawka C, Pritchard K, Ginsburg D, Wood M, Whelan T. Randomised trial of long term follow up for early stage breast cancer: a comparison of family physician versus specialist care. J Clin Oncol. 2006;24:848–54.
23. Department of Health. Macmillan Cancer Support and NHS Improvement. 2010. The National cancer survivorship initiative vision. London: NHS. Accessed via www.ncsi.org.uk/wp-content/uploads/NCSI-Vision-Document.pdf.
24. Department of Health. Achieving world class cancer outcomes. London: DH; 2015.
25. Department of Health. Improving outcomes: a strategy for cancer. London: DH; 2011.
26. Beaver K, Tysver-Robinson D, Campbell M, Twomey M, Williamson S, Hindley A, Susnerwala S, Dunn G, Luker K. Comparing hospital and telephone follow up after treatment for breast cancer: randomised equivalence trial. BMJ. 2009;338:a3147.
27. Shepherd C, Higgins B, Wise M, Yiangou C, Dubois D, Kilburn S. Breast cancer follow up: a randomised controlled trial comparing point of need access versus routine 6 monthly clinical review. Eur J Oncol Nurs. 2009;1:2–8. doi:10.1016/j.ejon.2008.11.005. Epub 2008 Dec 31.
28. Armes J, Crowe AM, Colbourne L. Patients supportive care needs beyond the end of cancer treatment: a prospective longitudinal survey. J Clin Oncol. 2009;27(36):6172–9.
29. Elliot J, Fallows A, Staetsky L, Smith P, Foster C, Maher E, Corner J. The health and well-being of cancer survivors in the UK: findings from a population based survey. Br J Cancer. 2011;105(Supp 1):S11–20.
30. Campbell A, Stevinson C, Crank H. The British association of sport and exercise sciences expert statement on exercise and cancer survivorship. Sport and Exerc Scient. 2011;28:16–7.
31. Danmark-Wahnefried W, Aziz N, Rowlam J, Pinto B. Riding the crest of the teachable moment: promoting long term health after the diagnosis of cancer. J Clin Oncol. 2005;23(24):5814–30.
32. Peppercorn J, Partridge A, Burstein E, Winer P. Standards of follow up care of patients with breast cancer. Breast. 2005;14:500–8.
33. Chapman D, Cox E, Britton P, Wishart G. Patient led breast cancer follow up. Breast. 2009;18:100–2.
34. Rechis R, Beckjord E, Nutt S. Potential benefits of treatment summaries for survivors' health and information needs. Results from a Live strong survey. J Oncol Pract. 2014;10(10):75–8.
35. Brearly A, Stamataki Z, Addington-Hall J, Foster C, Hodges L, Jarrett N, Richardson A, Scott I, Sharpe M, Stark D, Siller C, Ziegler L, Amir Z. The physical and practical problems experienced by cancer survivors, a rapid review and synthesis of the literature. Eur J Oncol Nurs. 2011;15:204–12.

# Chapter 4
# Detection of Recurrence: Imaging Strategies

**Kate Downey and Steven Allen**

**Abstract** Women who have undergone previous treatment for early breast cancer are at risk of recurrent disease at local or distant sites, as well as the development of new primary breast cancers. Breast imaging improves survival when compared to clinical examination alone. Annual mammography is the routine imaging modality of choice, with MRI and ultrasound reserved for specific populations and problem-solving. Some scenarios such as mammographically occult tumors, imaging the post-mastectomy breast and higher risk groups require specific consideration. Routine imaging to detect distant recurrence in asymptomatic patients is not performed, as this approach has not been shown to improve survival. Future directions, including the roles of tomosynthesis and new imaging strategies to detect distant recurrence and in particular oligometastatic disease are also discussed in this chapter.

**Keywords** Mammography • Recurrence • MRI • Ultrasound

## Introduction

Women who have been treated for early breast cancer are at risk of recurrent disease within the breast itself as well as at distant sites and also remain at risk of developing a second primary breast malignancy. Breast imaging improves survival when compared to clinical examination in women who have completed treatment for early breast cancer. It detects smaller, impalpable and less invasive tumors that have a much better prognosis than those that are clinically detectable [1–4]. Depending on the surgery performed, both the treated and contralateral breast are subject to imaging surveillance which is stratified according to risk and usually takes the

K. Downey, BSc, MBBS, MD, FRCR (✉) • S. Allen, MBBS, MRCS, FRCR
Imaging Department, The Royal Marsden NHS Foundation Trust,
Fulham Road, London SW3 6JJ, UK
e-mail: kate.downey@me.com; stevenallen@nhs.net



A. Ring, M. Parton (eds.), *Breast Cancer Survivorship*,
DOI 10.1007/978-3-319-41858-2_4

form of yearly mammography either in conjunction with a fixed routine outpatient appointment and clinical examination or as part of the 'Open Access Follow Up' system; a program advocated by the London Cancer Alliance and widely adopted in many cancer centers in the UK [5].

## Current Imaging Modalities Used in Breast Cancer Survivors

### *Mammography*

Mammography is the imaging modality of choice for imaging surveillance following treatment for early breast cancer for both invasive disease and ductal carcinoma in situ (DCIS). The sensitivity of routine surveillance mammography for detecting ipsilateral breast cancer recurrence has been reported in the literature as 64–67 % with a specificity of 85–97 % [6]. For detecting contralateral metachronous tumors, annual mammography has a reported sensitivity of 70.8 % [3] and up to 81–88 % if combined with clinical examination [7]. The National Institute for Clinical Excellence (NICE) recommends annual mammographic surveillance in all those treated for early breast cancer following diagnosis until entering the NHS British screening programme (NHSBSP) at 50 years of age. The first post-treatment mammogram appointment is advocated at 12 months following initial diagnosis to prevent false positive reports due to treatment effects especially following radiotherapy. Mammographic follow up at shorter intervals than 12 months following conservative treatment has not been shown to affect survival [8]. In those already 50, annual mammography is recommended for 5 years as most episodes of local recurrence occur within the first 5 years following treatment. The frequency of imaging surveillance following 5 years is unclear; however the Royal College of Radiologists does not advocate routine surveillance after 75 years of age [9]. The evidence for earlier detection definitively improving outcome in those over 75 is currently lacking; however in an aging population this is likely to change.

The mammographic appearance of recurrent disease is often very similar to the primary tumor [10] and most frequently occurs at the excision site or within the same quadrant [11] following wide local excision. Granular or pleomorphic calcification within the surgical bed at follow up mammography is suggestive of recurrent disease especially if DCIS was present within the original pathological specimen (Fig. 4.1). Benign dystrophic calcification relating to scar tissue often occurs within the surgical bed in the breast following surgery. This is usually coarse or curvilinear but can sometimes be difficult to distinguish from malignant calcification. A low threshold for biopsy is warranted in the investigation of post surgical calcification

**Fig. 4.1** Reconstructed medio-lateral oblique (MLO) and cranio-caudal (CC) 'c' views from two consecutive tomosynthesis studies following previous wide local excision for DCIS. Images 1 year following surgery (**a**, **b**) demonstrate normal post-operative appearances however 2 years following surgery (**c**, **d**) there is an area of pleomorphic calcification near the excision site in keeping with recurrent DCIS

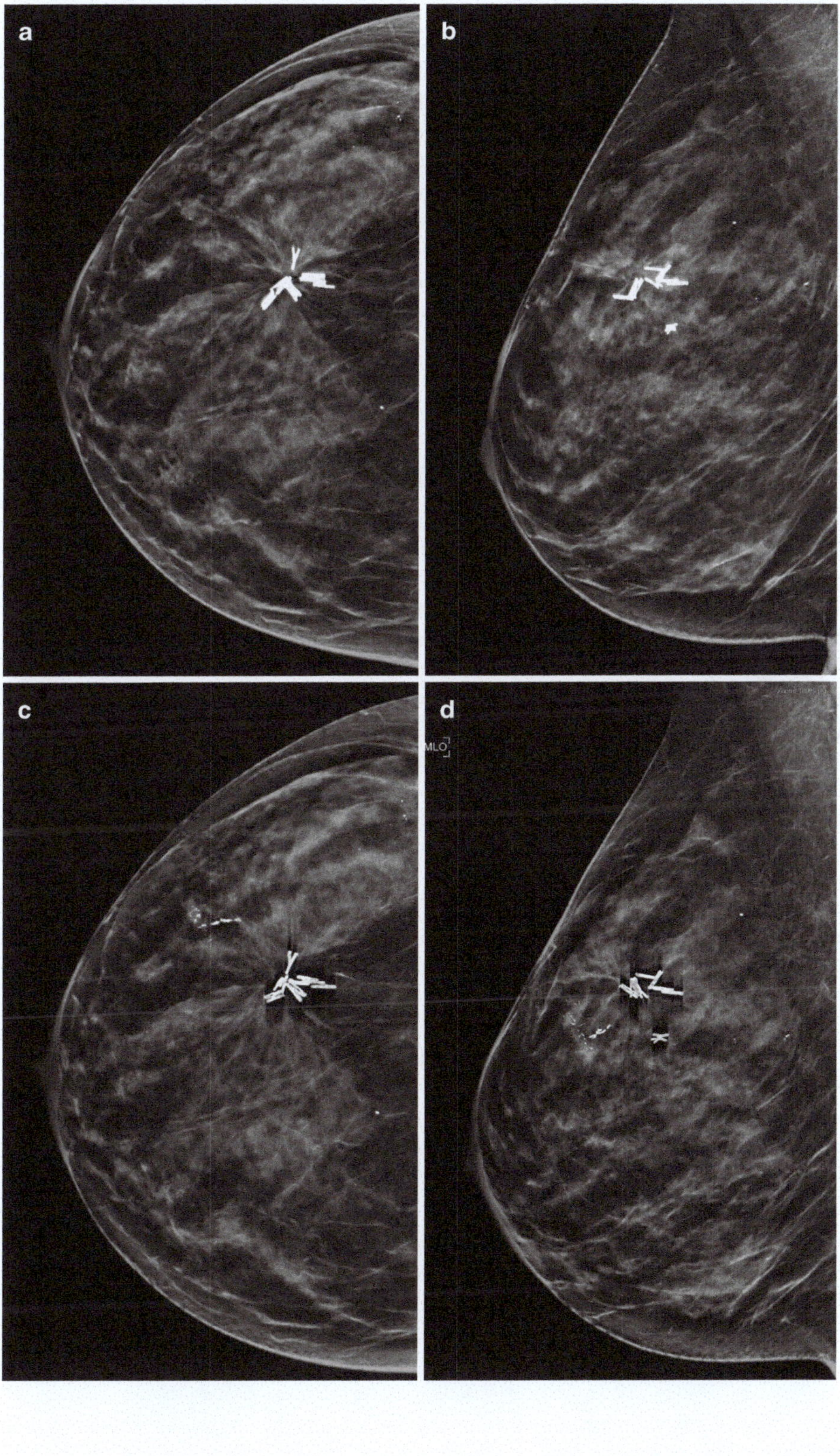
a
b
c
d
MLO

unless typically benign features are demonstrated. Survival benefit may not be associated with detecting low or even intermediate grade DCIS however it has been reported that up to approximately one third of cases of recurrence following surgery for DCIS contains invasive disease [12]. Optimal sampling of indeterminate calcification is performed under stereotactic guidance with either a stereo-core or stereo-vacuum technique. The sample obtained is imaged whilst the breast is still compressed to ensure representative calcification is present within the specimen and a marker clip is usually deployed at the site of biopsy to ensure the exact location of sampling is known.

Recurrent disease in men is usually clinically apparent and mammographic surveillance following treatment for male breast cancer is not routinely offered. An ultrasound is usually sufficient for diagnosis in men who present with symptoms of recurrent disease.

## *Magnetic Resonance Imaging and Ultrasound*

MRI has a higher sensitivity in comparison to mammography for differentiation of post-treatment changes from recurrent disease and reported as ranging from 86 to 100 % [13, 15]. There is however a significant false-positive rate especially when MRI is performed within 18 months of surgery [16].

The reported sensitivity and specificity of ultrasound ranges from 71 to 91 % and 82 to 98 % [17–20]. It has been shown that ultrasound in addition to mammography increases the diagnostic yield of recurrence detection in high risk women however a high false positive rate is also demonstrated [21].

There is currently insufficient evidence to advocate the routine use of MRI or ultrasound in the post-treatment breast. Under NICE guidelines, neither MRI nor ultrasound are currently offered for routine surveillance in patients who have been treated for DCIS or early invasive disease [22]. They are often however used as adjuncts to mammography in those patients who have mammographically occult primary tumors, as a problem solving tool when clinical and conventional imaging appearances are discordant and in those who have a genetic predisposition to breast cancer.

Appearances of recurrent disease on MRI are often similar to the primary tumor and both morphological and enhancement characteristics are assessed [13]. Tumor is usually demonstrated as a mass that is low signal on T1-weighted and intermediate to high signal on T2-weighted imaging with avid and early contrast enhancement. Enhancement can either be homogeneous, heterogeneous, rim or non-mass like. As for primary tumors, kinetic analysis of contrast enhancement characteristics can help to distinguish benign from malignant enhancement. Type I curves demonstrate progressive enhancement and are usually associated with benign lesions with a less than 10 % chance of malignancy [23]. The sensitivity and specificity for a benign lesion when associated with a type 1 curve is 53 and 71 % [24]. Type II curves demonstrate initial uptake followed by a plateau phase and type III curves demonstrate relatively rapid uptake followed by a washout phase. Both type II and III curves are more concerning for malignancy; up to 76 % of tumors with a type III curve are associated with malignant tumors [25]. The specificity of detecting malignancy with a type II curve is reported as 75 % with a sensitivity of 43 % and although specificity with a type III curve is high (up to 90 %), sensitivity is low (as low as 21 %) [24].

Appearances of recurrent disease on ultrasound may also be similar to the primary tumor; hypoechoic, irregular, associated posterior acoustic shadowing and increased vascularity. Ultrasound can be helpful to confirm the malignant nature of a clinically palpable or mammographically apparent mass and to assess the axilla or neck for associated lymphadenopathy. Ultrasound is also more sensitive than mammography when there is chest wall recurrence. Typically, once recurrence is suspected on mammography, ultrasound is used to confirm mammographic findings and guide percutaneous biopsy for histopathological confirmation.

Axillary recurrence following standard treatment of the axilla is rare and most cases following lymph node dissection are detected clinically [26]. Abnormal lymph nodes can be detected incidentally on mammographic MLO views but ultrasound of the axilla is performed when palpable lymph nodes are detected clinically or when recurrence occurs within the breast. If there are imaging findings of concern (rounded shape, loss of the fatty hilum, cortical thickening) a fine needle aspiration or core biopsy of the lymph node is performed for analysis.

## Mammographically Occult Tumors

Patients who are diagnosed with mammographically occult tumors, especially in those with dense breasts, are considered for ultrasound surveillance in addition to yearly mammogram. If a tumor is both mammographically and ultrasound occult, MRI is usually performed. The individual imaging pathway should be confirmed at a subspecialty breast multidisciplinary meeting or by the patient's consultant and documented in the patient notes/electronic patient record.

## Imaging the Post Mastectomy Breast

Under current guidelines, if there are no concerning features on clinical examination, routine imaging of the ipsilateral post mastectomy soft tissues is not recommended. Although recurrence rates following mastectomy are low, a small volume of breast tissue may remain especially after skin-sparing mastectomy within the anterolateral chest wall and axilla and within the posterior breast over the pectoralis muscle. Mammographic imaging of the mastectomy site does not increase the detection of recurrence [27]. Reconstruction post mastectomy is either implant-based or

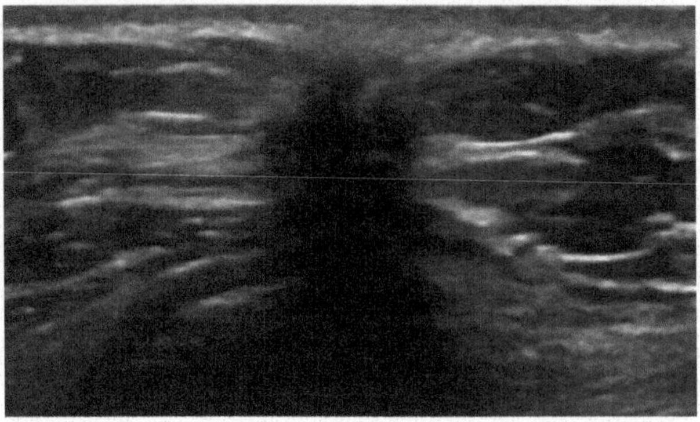

**Fig. 4.2** Ultrasound image of the chest wall demonstrating a palpable 12 mm hypoehoic irregular mass in keeping with a subcutaneous recurrence (histology: invasive ductal carcinoma) following previous mastectomy

comprised of autologous tissue (myocutaneous or free perforator flap) grafts. Free perforator flaps such as the deep inferior epigastric perforator (DIEP) flap reconstruction are gaining popularity in many institutions that can offer microsurgery; as well as improved cosmetic results, they are associated with fewer complications at the donor site, earlier mobilization post surgery and a shorter hospital stay than muscle-based reconstruction. Although rare, when ipsilateral recurrence occurs in the reconstructed breast, it is usually superficial in location within the skin envelope or within the subcutaneous fat and clinically detected as a palpable mass. Less than one third are posteriorly located at the chest wall [28]. If there is clinical concern, an ultrasound is most often performed which will help to confirm malignant appearances of a palpable mass and can guide biopsy if the lesion is located within the subcutaneous tissues (Fig. 4.2). Recurrent disease is often found medially within the breast due to lymphatic drainage to the internal mammary lymph node chain that is not dissected at mastectomy. Ultrasound appearances usually represent that of the primary tumor however occasionally recurrent disease within the reconstructed breast can be non-specific in appearance. Distinguishing recurrent disease from benign lesions such as fat necrosis can be sometimes be challenging and there should be a low threshold for image guided biopsy. A clinical punch biopsy is performed if the lesion is cutaneous. MRI may be used as a problem-solving tool when clinical and ultrasound findings are discordant or inconclusive however false positive cases may occur at the interface between the flap and the residual breast tissue where areas of post-surgical contrast enhancement may mimic recurrent disease [29].

## Higher Risk Groups

Women who are considered higher risk are those with BRCA 1, BRCA 2 or TP53 (Li Fraumeni syndrome) mutations or a significant family history. The London Cancer Alliance and NICE recommends that these patients should have annual imaging with either mammography alone, MRI alone or MRI with mammography depending on age and mutation type [5, 22]. Under these guidelines, BRCA1, BRCA 2 and TP53 mutation carriers or those at high risk of carrying BRCA1 or TP53 mutations from untested or inconclusively tested families are recommended to have annual MRI from 30 to 39 years (20–49 years in TP53 carriers or a risk of TP53 >30 %) and then annual MRI and mammography from 40 to 49 years. From 50 to 69 years, those who are BRCA carriers are offered annual mammography ± MRI.

## Staging in Recurrent Disease

Identification of asymptomatic metastases has not to date been shown to prolong survival and therefore cross-sectional and or nuclear medicine imaging studies do not form part of normal surveillance protocols after treatment for breast cancer [30, 31]. When locally recurrent disease is detected however all patients are restaged before a definitive treatment plan is confirmed to optimize patient outcome as a significant number will have systemic disease [32]. When recurrent disease is detected, those at particular risk of disseminated disease are those who initially had lymph node positive disease, skin involvement or lymphovascular space invasion [33]. Restaging is also performed when patients are symptomatic or rising tumor markers are detected suggesting recurrent disease. A CT of the chest abdomen and pelvis is usually performed with a high start to ensure the supraclavicular fossae are included. 100–150 ml of iodinated contrast medium is injected at 3–4 ml/s and images are acquired in the portal venous phase at 1 mm sections reconstructed for viewing at 3 and 5 mm slice thickness [34]. Multi-planar reformats are often helpful especially when assessing the skeleton for bone metastases. CT is usually sufficient for staging in the context of recurrent disease however a combination of CT, liver MRI, whole spine MRI and $^{18}$PET-CT may be required. Liver MRI with the use of contrast can help to distinguish benign from malignant liver lesions and PET-CT or Tc-99 m-MDP bone scans can define skeletal metastases and nodal involvement. In patients with elevated tumor markers or clinical or imaging findings in keeping with recurrent disease, FDG PET-CT has been found to have a sensitivity of between 91 and 97 % and a specificity between 76 and 92 % for detecting disease recurrence [35]. It is however costly and involves ionizing radiation. Specific symptoms may guide further investigations such as MRI of the brain and brachial plexus.

## Future Directions

### *Tomosynthesis*

Tomosynthesis is a mammographic technique which uses a digital detector and multiple x-rays that move in an arc around the breast to build a 3D image. It addresses the problem of soft tissue superimposition resembling pathology encountered with conventional 2D mammography and may help to detect recurrent disease earlier than mammography, especially within the dense breast. Digital Breast Tomosynthesis (DBT) has shown to improve cancer detection and reduce recall rates [36, 37] in the screening setting and some studies have suggested that DBT could be used as an alternative to additional views in the symptomatic/surveillance setting [38, 39]. More studies are warranted to establish DBT as a viable alternative to mammographic surveillance post treatment. In our institution, it is used as a problem-solving tool replacing conventional compression views when required and is recommended in younger patients aged 40–50 years who often have denser breasts or in patients of any age with a P4/5 examination. It can also be used to guide stereotactic biopsy in cases of suspected DCIS recurrence not visible on ultrasound.

### *Oligometastatic Disease*

Most work in the literature concentrates on loco-regional recurrent disease and there is limited data on oligometastatic recurrence. It is known that the survival rate for patients with metastatic disease is continuously improving aided not only by improvements in systemic therapies but also advancements in imaging techniques capable of diagnosing small volume disease at an earlier timepoint [40]. Certain patients with oligometastatic disease that are managed appropriately can attain long term survival [41]. In the near future detecting oligometastatic disease may have a survival benefit owing to advances in surgery for metastatic disease as well as focal therapies such as stereotactic radiotherapy, radiofrequency and microwave ablation techniques [42]. This could mean that we see an increase in the use of whole body imaging in the form of PET-CT, whole body MRI or indeed combined whole body PET-MRI [43].

### *Risk Stratified Surveillance*

Risk of recurrent disease is multifactorial and is not only linked to original stage but also the molecular identity of the tumor. Rather than adopting a standardized surveillance strategy, monitoring post treatment may increasingly be stratified with timing and modality of imaging linked to individual patient risk. This clearly involves a multidisciplinary team approach including oncologists, surgeons, pathologists and radiologists.

## Conclusion

At present imaging strategies to detect locoregional recurrent disease are centered on mammography. Ultrasound and MRI are reserved for guiding biopsies and problem solving or in those patients with dense breasts or those deemed at higher risk (genetic or family history). Patients who are symptomatic, have rising tumor markers or histopathologically proven locoregional recurrence undergo formal staging with cross sectional imaging to ascertain the presence of disseminated disease and to optimize treatment strategies.

## References

1. Ciatto S, Miccinesi G, Zappa M, Marco Z, Guido M. Prognostic impact of the early detection of metachronous contralateral breast cancer. Eur J Cancer. 2004;40(10):1496–501.
2. Houssami N, Ciatto S, Martinelli F, Bonardi R, Duffy SW. Early detection of second breast cancers improves prognosis in breast cancer survivors. Ann Oncol. 2009;20(9):1505–10.
3. Lu W, Schaapveld M, Jansen L, Bagherzadegan E, Sahinovic MM, Baas PC, Hanssen LM, van der Mijle HC, Brandenburg JD, Wiggers T, De Bock GH. The value of surveillance mammography of the contralateral breast in patients with a history of breast cancer. Eur J Cancer. 2009;45(17):3000–7.
4. Lu WL, Jansen L, Post WJ, Bonnema J, Van de Velde JC, De Bock GH. Impact on survival of early detection of isolated breast recurrences after the primary treatment for breast cancer: a meta-analysis. Breast Cancer Res Treat. 2009;114(3):403–12.
5. The London Cancer Alliance. LCA breast cancer clinical guidelines. 2013. Retrieved 12 March 2016. http://www.londoncanceralliance.nhs.uk/media/59178/FINAL%20LCA_Breast Guidelines_231013%20revised%20(3).pdf.
6. Robertson C, Ragupathy SK, Boachie C, Fraser C, Heys SD, Maclennan G, Mowatt G, Thomas RE, Gilbert FJ, M. S. H. T. A. Group. Surveillance mammography for detecting ipsilateral breast tumour recurrence and metachronous contralateral breast cancer: a systematic review. Eur Radiol. 2011;21(12):2484–91.
7. Temple LK, Wang EE, McLeod RS. Preventive health care, 1999 update: 3. Follow-up after breast cancer. Canadian Task Force on Preventive Health Care. CMAJ. 1999;161(8):1001–8.
8. Lewis JL, Tartter PI. The value of mammography within 1 year of conservative surgery for breast cancer. Ann Surg Oncol. 2012;19(10):3218–22.
9. The Royal College of Radiologists. Guidance on screening and symptomatic breast imaging. 3rd ed. 2013. Retrieved 12 March 2016. https://www.rcr.ac.uk/sites/default/files/publication/BFCR%2813%295_breast.pdf.
10. Orel SG, Troupin RH, Patterson EA, Fowble BL. Breast cancer recurrence after lumpectomy and irradiation: role of mammography in detection. Radiology. 1992;183(1):201–6.
11. Günhan-Bilgen I, Oktay A. Mammographic features of local recurrence after conservative surgery and radiation therapy: comparison with that of the primary tumor. Acta Radiol. 2007;48(4):390–7.
12. Liberman L, Van Zee KJ, Dershaw DD, Morris EA, Abramson AF, Samli B. Mammographic features of local recurrence in women who have undergone breast-conserving therapy for ductal carcinoma in situ. AJR Am J Roentgenol. 1997;168(2):489–93.
13. Belli P, Costantini M, Romani M, Marano P, Pastore G. Magnetic resonance imaging in breast cancer recurrence. Breast Cancer Res Treat. 2002;73(3):223–35.
14. Preda L, Villa G, Rizzo S, Bazzi L, Origgi D, Cassano E, Bellomi M. Magnetic resonance mammography in the evaluation of recurrence at the prior lumpectomy site after conservative surgery and radiotherapy. Breast Cancer Res. 2006;8(5):R53.
15. Robertson C, Arcot Ragupathy SK, Boachie C, Dixon JM, Fraser C, Hernández R, Heys S, Jack W, Kerr GR, Lawrence G, MacLennan G, Maxwell A, McGregor J, Mowatt G, Pinder S, Ternent L, Thomas RE, Vale L, Wilson R, Zhu S, Gilbert FJ. The clinical effectiveness and cost-effectiveness of different surveillance mammography regimens after the treatment for primary breast cancer: systematic reviews registry database analyses and economic evaluation. Health Technol Assess. 2011;15(34): v–vi, 1–322.

16. Heywang-Köbrunner SH, Schlegel A, Beck R, Wendt T, Kellner W, Lommatzsch B, Untch M, Nathrath WB. Contrast-enhanced MRI of the breast after limited surgery and radiation therapy. J Comput Assist Tomogr. 1993;17(6):891–900.
17. Balu-Maestro C, Bruneton JN, Geoffray A, Chauvel C, Rogopoulos A, Bittman O. Ultrasonographic posttreatment follow-up of breast cancer patients. J Ultrasound Med. 1991;10(1):1–7.
18. Ciatto S. Detection of breast cancer local recurrences. Ann Oncol. 1995;6 Suppl 2:23–6.
19. Aichinger U, Schulz-Wendtland R, Krämer S, Lell M, Bautz W. Scar or recurrence—comparison of MRI and color-coded ultrasound with echo signal amplifiers. Rofo. 2002; 174(11):1395–401.
20. Shin JH, Han BK, Choe YH, Nam SJ, Park W, Im YH. Ultrasonographic detection of occult cancer in patients after surgical therapy for breast cancer. J Ultrasound Med. 2005;24(5):643–9.
21. Berg WA, Blume JD, Cormack JB, Mendelson EB, Lehrer D, Böhm-Vélez M, Pisano ED, Jong RA, Evans WP, Morton MJ, Mahoney MC, Larsen LH, Barr RG, Farria DM, Marques HS, Boparai K, Investigators A. Combined screening with ultrasound and mammography vs mammography alone in women at elevated risk of breast cancer. JAMA. 2008;299(18):2151–63.
22. The National Institute for Health and Care Excellence (NICE). 2009. Early and locally advanced breast cancer: diagnosis and treatment. Retrieved 12 March 2016. https://www.nice.org.uk/guidance/cg80/evidence/full-guideline-242201629.
23. Kuhl CK, Mielcareck P, Klaschik S, Leutner C, Wardelmann E, Gieseke J, Schild HH. Dynamic breast MR imaging: are signal intensity time course data useful for differential diagnosis of enhancing lesions? Radiology. 1999;211(1):101–10.
24. Bluemke DA, Gatsonis CA, Chen MH, DeAngelis GA, DeBruhl N, Harms S, de Boer R, Hillen HF, Roumen RM, Rutten HJ, van der Sangen MJ, Voogd AC. Detection, treatment and outcome of axillary recurrence after axillary clearance for invasive breast cancer. Br J Surg. 2001;88(1):118–22.
25. Schnall MD, Blume J, Bluemke DA, DeAngelis GA, De Bruhl N, Harms S, Heywang-Köbrunner SH, Hylton N, Kuhl CK, Pisano ED, Causer P, Schnitt SJ, Thickman D, Stelling CB, Weatherall PT, Lehman C, Gatsonis CA. Diagnostic architectural and dynamic features at breast MR imaging: multicenter study. Radiology. 2006;238(1):42–53.
26. de Boer R, Hillen HF, Roumen RM, et al. *Detection, treatment and outcome* of axillary recurrence after axillary clearance for invasive breast cancer. Br J Surg. 2001;88:118.
27. Fajardo LL, Roberts CC, Hunt KR. Mammographic surveillance of breast cancer patients: should the mastectomy site be imaged? AJR Am J Roentgenol. 1993;161(5):953–5.
28. Pinel-Giroux FM, El Khoury MM, Trop I, Bernier C, David J, Lalonde L. Breast reconstruction: review of surgical methods and spectrum of imaging findings. Radiographics. 2013;33(2):435–53.
29. Rieber A, Schramm K, Helms G, von Pückler S, Nuessle K, Kreienberg R, Brambs HJ, Kuehn T. Breast-conserving surgery and autogenous tissue reconstruction in patients with breast cancer: efficacy of MRI of the breast in the detection of recurrent disease. Eur Radiol. 2003;13(4):780–7.
30. Rosselli Del Turco M, Palli D, Cariddi A, Ciatto S, Pacini P, Distante V. Intensive diagnostic follow-up after treatment of primary breast cancer. A randomized trial. National Research Council Project on Breast Cancer follow-up. JAMA. 1994;271(20):1593–7.
31. Khatcheressian JL, Hurley P, Bantug E, Esserman LJ, Grunfeld E, Halberg F, Hantel A, Henry NL, Muss HB, Smith TJ, Vogel VG, Wolff AC, Somerfield MR, Davidson NE, American Society of Clinical Oncology. Breast cancer follow-up and management after primary treatment: American Society of Clinical Oncology clinical practice guideline update. J Clin Oncol. 2013;31(7):961–5.
32. The Association of Breast Surgery (BASO). 2009 Surgical guidelines for the management of breast cancer. Retrieved 12 March 2016 http://www.associationofbreastsurgery.org.uk/media/4565/surgical_guidelines_for_the_management_of_breast_cancer.pdf.
33. Shen J, Hunt KK, Mirza NQ, Buchholz TA, Babiera GV, Kuerer HM, Bedrosian I, Ross MI, Ames FC, Feig BW, Singletary SE, Cristofanilli M, Meric-Bernstam F. Predictors of systemic

recurrence and disease-specific survival after ipsilateral breast tumor recurrence. Cancer. 2005;104(3):479–90.
34. The Royal College of Radiologists. 2014. Recommendations for cross-sectional imaging in cancer management. Breast cancer. 2nd ed. Retrieved 12 March 2016. https://www.rcr.ac.uk/sites/default/files/publication/BFCR%2814%292_25_Breast.pdf.
35. Groheux D, Espié M, Giacchetti S, Hindié E. Performance of FDG PET/CT in the clinical management of breast cancer. Radiology. 2013;266(2):388–405.
36. Skaane P, Gullien R, Bjørndal H, Eben EB, Ekseth U, Haakenaasen U, Jahr G, Jebsen IN, Krager M. Digital breast tomosynthesis (DBT): initial experience in a clinical setting. Acta Radiol. 2012;53(5):524–9.
37. Rafferty EA, Park JM, Philpotts LE, Poplack SP, Sumkin JH, Halpern EF, Niklason LT. Assessing radiologist performance using combined digital mammography and breast tomosynthesis compared with digital mammography alone: results of a multicenter, multireader trial. Radiology. 2013;266(1):104–13.
38. Hakim CM, Chough DM, Ganott MA, Sumkin JH, Zuley ML, Gur D. Digital breast tomosynthesis in the diagnostic environment: A subjective side-by-side review. AJR Am J Roentgenol. 2010;195(2):W172–6.
39. Zuley ML, Bandos AI, Ganott MA, Sumkin JH, Kelly AE, Catullo VJ, Rathfon GY, Lu AH, Gur D. Digital breast tomosynthesis versus supplemental diagnostic mammographic views for evaluation of noncalcified breast lesions. Radiology. 2013;266(1):89–95.
40. Andre F, Slimane K, Bachelot T, Dunant A, Namer M, Barrelier A, Kabbaj O, Spano JP, Marsiglia H, Rouzier R, Delaloge S, Spielmann M. Breast cancer with synchronous metastases: trends in survival during a 14-year period. J Clin Oncol. 2004;22(16):3302–8.
41. Pagani O, Senkus E, Wood W, Colleoni M, Cufer T, Kyriakides S, Costa A, Winer EP, Cardoso F, Force E-MT. International guidelines for management of metastatic breast cancer: can metastatic breast cancer be cured? J Natl Cancer Inst. 2010;102(7):456–63.
42. Giordano SH, Buzdar AU, Smith TL, Kau SW, Yang Y, Hortobagyi GN. Is breast cancer survival improving? Cancer. 2004;100(1):44–52.
43. Sawicki LM, Grueneisen J, Schaarschmidt BM, Buchbender C, Nagarajah J, Umutlu L, Antoch G, Kinner S. Evaluation of (18)F-FDG PET/MRI, (18)F-FDG PET/CT, MRI, and CT in whole-body staging of recurrent breast cancer. Eur J Radiol. 2016;85(2):459–65.

# Chapter 5
# Follow Up of Patients with Germline Mutations in High Risk Predisposition Genes

**Zoe Kemp**

**Abstract** Patients with germline mutations in high risk predisposition genes have significantly raised risks of certain cancers compared to those in the general population and may be affected at a young age. For a patient this can give an explanation as to why they have developed cancer but it can also indicate that they are at increased risk of further primaries.

This chapter will review the genetic architecture of breast cancer and will consider how knowledge of a germline mutation can translate into clinical practice. It will focus on how an understanding of the risks of cancer associated with *BRCA1* or *BRCA2* germline mutations can guide the follow up of those who have already been affected by breast cancer. Both the risk of contralateral breast cancer and of ovarian cancer will be considered and what measures can be taken to reduce these risks.

Finally we will also consider family issues related to germline mutations including fertility and preimplantation genetic diagnosis and cascade testing.

**Keywords** Predisposition genes • *BRCA1/BRCA2* • Contralateral mastectomy • Ovarian cancer • Ovarian screening • Risk reducing surgery

## The Genetic Architecture of Breast Cancer Susceptibility

Inherited susceptibility to breast cancer arises through germline mutations in predisposition genes. Three classes of susceptibility genes have been described, each distinctive in terms of prevalence in the population and the degree of risk of breast cancer conferred. Although this classification partly reflects the methodology employed to discover the genes, it also provides a useful framework for understanding the genetic architecture of breast cancer and its application to clinical practice [1, 2] (Table 5.1).

Z. Kemp, BSc, MBBS, PhD
Breast and Cancer Genetics Units, The Royal Marsden NHS Foundation Trust, London, UK
e-mail: zoe.kemp@rmh.nhs.uk

 
A. Ring, M. Parton (eds.), *Breast Cancer Survivorship*,
DOI 10.1007/978-3-319-41858-2_5

**Table 5.1** The genetic architecture of breast cancer

| Penetrance | Relative risk | UK population carrier frequency | Examples | Associated syndromes | Associated cancers in high penetrance genes |
|---|---|---|---|---|---|
| High | 10–20 fold | ≤0.1 % | *BRCA1* | | Ovarian |
| | | | *BRCA2* | | Ovarian, prostate, pancreas |
| | | | *TP53* | Li Fraumeni | Sarcoma, brain, adrenocortical, childhood cancers |
| | | | *PTEN* | Cowden's | Thyroid, endometrial |
| | | | *STK11* | Peutz-Jeghers | Colon, pancreas, ovarian sex cord-stromal tumors |
| | | | *CDH1* | | Diffuse-type gastric |
| Moderate | 2–4 fold | ≤0.6 % | *CHEK2* | | |
| | | | *ATM* | | |
| | | | *BRIP1* | | |
| | | | *PALB2* | | |
| Low | 1.25 fold | 5–50 % | Various single-nucleotide polymorphisms(SNPs) | | |

The three classes of predisposition alleles are:

- Rare, high-penetrance alleles
- Rare, moderate-penetrance alleles
- Common, low-penetrance alleles

## *Rare, High-Penetrance Predisposition Genes*

Mutations in these predisposition genes are rare (UK population carrier frequency ≤0.1 %) but heterozygous carriers have a 10–20 fold relative risk of developing breast cancer. This group is dominated by *BRCA1* and *BRCA2*, the protein products of which are integral to DNA double-strand break repair. Pathogenic mutations usually result in protein truncation and hence inactivation. Pathogenic germline mutations in *TP53*, *PTEN*, *STK11*, and *CDH1* also cause increased risk of breast cancer.

## *Rare, Moderate-Penetrance Predisposition Genes*

For other rare predisposition genes (UK population carrier frequency ≤0.6 %) penetrance is more moderate with a 2–4 fold relative risk of breast cancer. The lower level of risk means that most carriers will not develop the disease and the disease may not always segregate with the mutation within families.

Breast cancer predisposition genes residing in this category were identified through the examination of candidate genes, chosen because of their involvement in the *BRCA1/2* pathways. They include *CHEK2*, *ATM*, *BRIP1* and *PALB2*.

## *Common, Low-Penetrance Predisposition Genes*

These are common variants that confer very little risk alone but may act multiplicatively thus generating larger risk. Predisposition variants are identified through breast cancer case-control series but very large numbers of samples are required to generate robust results.

## *Clinical Utility*

The advent of next generation sequencing has revolutionized the capacity and speed of genetic testing. However, the clinical utility of the information generated is dependent on being able to determine whether an identified variant is pathogenic [3]. Even then substantial evidence is required to generate risk estimates of breast cancer.

For these reasons the main focus of this chapter will be on *BRCA1* and *BRCA2*. Here knowledge of variants and risk is most advanced though continues to mature. Evidence regarding breast cancer predisposition genes will be accelerated through new technology and may blur the distinction between high, moderate and low penetrance groups in the future.

## Germline *BRCA1* and *BRCA2* Mutations and Risks of Cancer

The relative risk of breast cancer associated with rare, high penetrance genes is described above but for the purpose of counseling and consideration of management options absolute risks are more helpful. Reliable risk estimates are difficult to obtain since figures will vary depending on whether they are derived from population-based studies unselected for family history or family-based studies. For example risks estimates based on families ascertained because of multiple affected individuals will be much higher. It is therefore important to know the population from which the estimates are derived [4–6].

A useful approach is to use a range of risk as in the Cancer Genetics Clinical Protocols developed by the Institute of Cancer Research and the Royal Marsden Hospital. These protocols describe the lifetime risk of developing breast cancer for *BRCA1* carriers as between 60 and 90 % and for *BRCA2* 45–85 %. The lifetime risks of developing ovarian cancer are described as 40–60 % and 10–30 % for *BRCA1* and *BRCA2* respectively [7].

Given these risks there are a number of areas that should be discussed with carriers following a breast cancer diagnosis (Box 5.1).

**Box 5.1. Important Discussion Points for *BRCA1/2* Carriers Following a Primary Diagnosis of Breast Cancer**

- Risk of contralateral breast cancer versus risk of recurrent disease
- Risk of ovarian cancer
- Fertility
- Cascade testing

### *Contralateral Breast Cancer in BRCA Carriers*

For *BRCA* carriers who are undergoing or have completed treatment for unilateral breast cancer, the risk of subsequent contralateral primary is of understandable concern. Increasing requests for bilateral mastectomy have been observed both in *BRCA* mutation carriers and those with negative or unknown *BRCA* status [8]. This may in part be attributable to the trend in earlier genetic diagnosis as testing becomes more widely available and can be carried out during neoadjuvant therapy thus potentially influencing surgery and chemotherapy decision making.

It is therefore essential that reliable risk estimates of contralateral disease are communicated to patients and that these are balanced with the risk of recurrence from any current or previous breast cancer, the risks and efficacy of the procedure, and the affects of adjuvant treatment and risk reducing bilateral salpingo-oophorectomy [9].

## Risk of Contralateral Breast Disease in *BRCA* Carriers

The annual risk of contralateral disease is approximately 0.5 % in the general population but rises to 2.5–3 % in *BRCA* carriers [6, 10]. For carriers risk is also increased by young age at diagnosis of first breast cancer and family history of breast cancer. In a retrospective study Graeser et al. report a cumulative risk for contralateral breast cancer 25 years after first breast cancer of 47.4 % (95 % CI, 38.8–56.0 %). For *BRCA1* patients with an initial diagnosis of breast cancer under the age of 40, the 25 year cumulative risk was 62.9 % (95 % CI, 50.4–75.4 %) compared to 19.6 % (95 % CI, 5.3–33.9 %) for those diagnosed after the age of 50. A similar but not statistically significant trend was also observed in *BRCA2* carriers [11]. In addition to age, Metcalfe et al. report an effect of family history with carriers under 50 years with 2 or more first-degree relatives with early onset breast cancer being at increased risk compared to those with no first-degree relatives with breast cancer (50 vs. 36 %, $P = 0.005$) [10].

## Impact of Contralateral Prophylactic Mastectomy

When considering contralateral prophylactic mastectomy (CPM) it is important to consider what the procedure achieves. It is clear that it reduces the risk of contralateral breast cancer and therefore reduces the likelihood of a woman needing to undergo breast cancer treatment again. It also negates the need for surveillance imaging which in itself can be a source of great anxiety for some women. However, whether CPM conveys an overall survival benefit in *BRCA* carriers remains controversial.

There are limitations to the available published data. For example Metcalfe et al. performed an observational study in 390 *BRCA* carriers with stage I or II breast cancer. A 48 % (HR 0.52, 95 % CI 0.29–0.93; P=0.03) reduction in death from breast cancer was observed in those who underwent mastectomy of the contralateral breast. However, the findings were only statistically significant in the second decade post surgery and only 20 deaths occurred in this time compared to 59 in the first decade. It should also be noted that information on receptor status was not available for many participants and was therefore not included in the analysis [12].

In Heemskerk-Gerritsen et al. a prospective study of *BRCA* carriers with a history of primary breast cancer, a reduction in mortality was observed in those carriers who underwent CPM compared to those who remained under surveillance (HR 0.49, 95 % CI 0.29–0.82). This advantage persisted when patients who had died within 2 years of primary diagnosis, and therefore might not have had the opportunity for CPM, were excluded (HR 0.55, 95 % CI 0.32–0.95). The greatest survival benefit was observed when primary diagnosis occurred before 40 years, was grade I or II, not triple negative disease and in patients who had not received adjuvant chemotherapy. Therefore the advantage was seen in those with the highest risk of contralateral disease and the lowest risk of primary breast cancer specific mortality and emphases the need to take both factors into consideration [13].

This is not an area where randomized clinical trials are feasible or appropriate but the move towards more routine genetic testing at the point of diagnosis to aid treatment decisions may allow a more straightforward comparison of surgical approaches. Long term follow up will remain a necessity.

Overall contralateral prophylactic mastectomy remains a very personal decision. It is a decision that needs to be informed regarding risks of current and potential new primaries and efficacy of surgery. However, it is also a decision about body image, sexuality and managing anxiety, and a comprehensive multidisciplinary approach to address these facets of care needs to be used.

### Breast Screening in *BRCA* Carriers

There is a consensus that women who carry *BRCA* mutations should be screened annually for breast cancer using a combination of magnetic resonance imaging (MRI) and mammography. In the UK the National Institute for Clinical Excellence recommends MRI from ages 30–49 and mammography from 40 to 69 whereas in the United States the National Comprehensive Cancer Network advises MRI from 25 to 75 years and mammography from 30 to 75 years [14, 15]. No specific guidance exists for the follow up of those who have been diagnosed with breast cancer but annual screening for those who have not had bilateral mastectomy should continue after routine follow up has finished.

## Ovarian Cancer in *BRCA* Carriers

As alluded to above the risk of ovarian cancer in *BRCA1* carriers is 40–60 % over the course of a lifetime and in *BRCA2* carriers 10–30 %. For *BRCA1* carriers most of this risk is conferred after the age of 40 and for *BRCA2* carriers after the age of 50 [16]. It is therefore generally recommended that carriers should have risk reducing bilateral salpingo-oophorectomy from the age of 40 onwards and once childbearing is complete.

## *Ovarian Screening*

Many patients enquire about screening for ovarian cancer, either as a tool prior to risk reducing surgery or as an alternative to surgery. The majority of women with ovarian cancer present with advanced disease (FIGO stage III-IV). Outlook for these women is poor with the probability of surviving 5 years being less than 30 % [17].

For a screening test to be effective is must therefore be able to demonstrate a clinically meaningful stage shift, with patients being diagnosed at an earlier stage of ovarian cancer resulting in improved overall survival. It is also important to evaluate the number of surgeries performed due to false positive screening tests for each case of invasive cancer diagnosed. Whilst the tumor marker CA-125 and transvaginal ultrasound (TVUS) are both highly sensitive in the diagnosis of late stage disease their value as screening tools is far less certain.

The Prostate, Lung, Colorectal and Ovarian (PLCO) cancer screening randomized controlled trial and the United Kingdom Collaborative Trial of Ovarian Cancer Screening (UKCTOCS) have both evaluated annual CA-125 and TVUS use in post menopausal women. The PLCO study did not demonstrate a stage shift or an improvement in mortality [18]. Mortality data is still awaited from the UKCTOCS study but they have reported 4.8 surgeries per invasive disease diagnosis [19].

In the initial phase of the United Kingdom Familial Ovarian Cancer Screening Study (UKFOCSS), women with a >10 % lifetime risk of ovarian cancer were screened prospectively with annual CA-125 and TVUS. Although sensitivity was >80 % the proportion of early stage disease diagnosed was disappointing although a trend towards optimal cytoreduction was noted. Four surgeries were reported for each invasive cancer diagnosed.

Work continues both in UKFOCSS with the evaluation of more frequent screening and in other studies (Gynecologic Oncology Group Trial 0199 study) but at the current time ovarian cancer screening cannot be considered a safe alternative to risk reducing surgery [20, 21].

## *Risk Reducing Bilateral Salpingo-Oophorectomy*

The prophylactic removal of both ovaries and fallopian tubes reduces the risk of ovarian cancer by approximately 80 % [16, 22]. The fallopian tubes are removed in addition to the ovaries as a significant proportion of ovarian cancer is thought to derive from the fallopian tubes. The risk of primary peritoneal cancer remains and occult primaries may be discovered at the time of surgery.

Most authors suggest surgery from 40 years onwards although some have recommended intervention as early as 35 years. Decision making in these pre-menopausal women needs to balance age-related risks of cancer with the long term effects of premature menopause such as cardiovascular disease and bone health [23]. This has generated research into the idea of a two-stage procedure where the fallopian tubes are removed first and the ovaries nearer the natural age of menopause [24, 25].

### *Impact of Oophorectomy After Breast Cancer Diagnosis*

For carriers of germline *BRCA1* and *BRCA2* mutations without a prior breast cancer diagnosis who undergo RRBSO there is a reduction in their subsequent breast cancer risk. This is most marked in women who have surgery whilst premenopausal but is also seen in the post-menopausal group [26, 27].

The question as to whether risk reducing bilateral salphingo-oophorectomy (RRBSO) impacts survival in those who have already had a breast cancer diagnosis is more contentious. Finch et al. reported a reduction in all cause mortality including those carriers with a history of breast cancer and Domchek et al. reported a decreased risk of breast cancer disease-specific mortality [16, 27]. However, suggestions that *BRCA1* carriers with estrogen receptor negative disease would benefit from early oophorectomy have been met with more skepticism [28, 29].

## Other High-Risk Predisposition Genes

Germline mutations in the *TP53* gene are associated with a spectrum of cancers including breast cancer, sarcomas, brain tumors, adrenocortical carcinoma and childhood cancers. When this pattern is seen within a family it is known as Li Fraumeni syndrome. However mutations may be identified in families without classic histories. Lifetime risks of cancer are high and are influenced both by family history and the position and type of mutation.

Other genes where mutations confer a high risk of breast cancer are *PTEN* (Cowden's syndrome), *STK11* (Peutz-Jeghers syndrome) and *CDH1* (diffuse-type gastric cancer and lobular breast cancer). Although the risk of breast cancer with these syndromes is not disputed, robust risk estimates are lacking due to ascertainment bias in studies.

## Implications for Family Members

### *Fertility and Preimplantation Genetic Diagnosis (PGD)*

Fertility is an important issue for many young breast cancer patients and for carriers of mutations in high penetrance disposition genes there is the additional concern of whether their future offspring will inherit their germline mutation.

Preimplantation Genetic Diagnosis (PGD) involves the testing of genetic material from an embryo to determine whether it has inherited a specific germline mutation from one of the parents. Assisted reproductive techniques are used to obtain and fertilize eggs with subsequent testing of the embryo.

### *Cascade Testing*

Cascade testing is the testing of relatives of known carriers. It is an important mechanism of identifying those at risk of disease.

Breast cancer and genetics teams will help patients to convey information to family members so that they can chose whether or not they wish to be tested to see if they also carry the mutation. For first degree relatives the risk will be 50:50. For *BRCA1* or *BRCA2* families, children should not be tested since there is no risk of childhood cancers but should wait until adulthood when they can make their own choice about testing.

## The Future

The integration of germline information into clinical decision-making requires a foundation of meticulous data collation to enable accurate determination of which variants are pathogenic and robust estimates of the risks of cancer associated with them.

For genes such as *BRCA1* and *BRCA2* this process is well underway and initiatives such as BRCA Challenge, a collaboration between the Global Alliance for Genomics and Health and the Human Variome Project, will drive forward improved data sharing. For other genes, such as the moderate penetrance gene *PALB2*, data is only just beginning to emerge making its use in a clinical setting challenging [30, 31].

Both scientists and the clinician in the clinic must strive to translate this complexity into understandable risks and choices of risk-reducing strategies.

## References

1. Stratton MR, Rahman N. The emerging landscape of breast cancer susceptibility. Nat Genet. 2008;40(1):17–22.
2. Rahman N. Realizing the promise of cancer predisposition genes. Nature. 2014;505(7483):302–8.
3. Easton DF, Pharoah PD, Antoniou AC, Tischkowitz M, Tavtigian SV, Nathanson KL, et al. Gene-panel sequencing and the prediction of breast-cancer risk. N Engl J Med. 2015; 372(23):2243–57.

4. Antoniou A, Pharoah PD, Narod S, Risch HA, Eyfjord JE, Hopper JL, et al. Average risks of breast and ovarian cancer associated with BRCA1 or BRCA2 mutations detected in case Series unselected for family history: a combined analysis of 22 studies. Am J Hum Genet. 2003;72(5):1117–30.
5. Chen S, Parmigiani G. Meta-analysis of BRCA1 and BRCA2 penetrance. J Clin Oncol. 2007;25(11):1329–33.
6. Mavaddat N, Peock S, Frost D, Ellis S, Platte R, Fineberg E, et al. Cancer risks for BRCA1 and BRCA2 mutation carriers: results from prospective analysis of EMBRACE. J Natl Cancer Inst. 2013;105(11):812–22.
7. Hanson H, Rahman N. http://www.icr.ac.uk/our-research/research-divisions/division-of-genetics-and-epidemiology/genetic-susceptibility/research-projects/cancer-genetic-clinical-protocols. 2015.
8. Tracy MS, Rosenberg SM, Dominici L, Partridge AH. Contralateral prophylactic mastectomy in women with breast cancer: trends, predictors, and areas for future research. Breast Cancer Res Treat. 2013;140(3):447–52.
9. Valachis A, Nearchou AD, Lind P. Surgical management of breast cancer in BRCA-mutation carriers: a systematic review and meta-analysis. Breast Cancer Res Treat. 2014;144(3):443–55.
10. Metcalfe K, Gershman S, Lynch HT, Ghadirian P, Tung N, Kim-Sing C, et al. Predictors of contralateral breast cancer in BRCA1 and BRCA2 mutation carriers. Br J Cancer. 2011;104(9):1384–92.
11. Graeser MK, Engel C, Rhiem K, Gadzicki D, Bick U, Kast K, et al. Contralateral breast cancer risk in BRCA1 and BRCA2 mutation carriers. J Clin Oncol. 2009;27(35):5887–92.
12. Metcalfe K, Gershman S, Ghadirian P, Lynch HT, Snyder C, Tung N, et al. Contralateral mastectomy and survival after breast cancer in carriers of BRCA1 and BRCA2 mutations: retrospective analysis. BMJ. 2014;348:g226.
13. Heemskerk-Gerritsen BA, Rookus MA, Aalfs CM, Ausems MG, Collee JM, Jansen L, et al. Improved overall survival after contralateral risk-reducing mastectomy in BRCA1/2 mutation carriers with a history of unilateral breast cancer: a prospective analysis. Int J Cancer. 2015;136(3):668–77.
14. Excellence NIfHaC. Familial breast cancer: classification, care and managing breast cancer and related risks in people with a family history of breast cancer. [CG164]. 2013. https://www.niceorguk/guidance/cg164.
15. Network NCC. NCCN guidelines: hereditary breast and/or ovarian cancer. http://www.nccnorg.
16. Finch AP, Lubinski J, Moller P, Singer CF, Karlan B, Senter L, et al. Impact of oophorectomy on cancer incidence and mortality in women with a BRCA1 or BRCA2 mutation. J Clin Oncol. 2014;32(15):1547–53.
17. Jemal A, Siegel R, Ward E, Hao Y, Xu J, Thun MJ. Cancer statistics, 2009. CA Cancer J Clin. 2009;59(4):225–49.
18. Buys SS, Partridge E, Black A, Johnson CC, Lamerato L, Isaacs C, et al. Effect of screening on ovarian cancer mortality: the Prostate, Lung, Colorectal and Ovarian (PLCO) Cancer Screening Randomized Controlled Trial. JAMA. 2011;305(22):2295–303.
19. Menon U, Ryan A, Kalsi J, Gentry-Maharaj A, Dawnay A, Habib M, et al. Risk algorithm using serial biomarker measurements doubles the number of screen-detected cancers compared with a single-threshold rule in the united kingdom collaborative trial of ovarian cancer screening. J Clin Oncol. 2015;33(18):2062–71.
20. Rosenthal ANFL, Philpott S, Manchanda R, Badman P, Hadwin R, Evans G, Eccles DM, Skates SJ, Mackay J, Menon U, Jacobs IJ. on behalf of the UK FOCSS collaborators. Results of 4-monthly screening in the UK Familial Ovarian Cancer Screening Study (UK FOCSS Phase 2). ASCO Abstract no 5507. 2013.
21. Sherman ME, Piedmonte M, Mai PL, Ioffe OB, Ronnett BM, Van Le L, et al. Pathologic findings at risk-reducing salpingo-oophorectomy: primary results from Gynecologic Oncology Group Trial GOG-0199. J Clin Oncol. 2014;32(29):3275–83.

22. Kauff ND, Domchek SM, Friebel TM, Robson ME, Lee J, Garber JE, et al. Risk-reducing salpingo-oophorectomy for the prevention of BRCA1- and BRCA2-associated breast and gynecologic cancer: a multicenter, prospective study. J Clin Oncol. 2008;26(8):1331–7.
23. Rocca WA, Grossardt BR, de Andrade M, Malkasian GD, Melton 3rd LJ. Survival patterns after oophorectomy in premenopausal women: a population-based cohort study. Lancet Oncol. 2006;7(10):821–8.
24. Kwon JS, Tinker A, Pansegrau G, McAlpine J, Housty M, McCullum M, et al. Prophylactic salpingectomy and delayed oophorectomy as an alternative for BRCA mutation carriers. Obstet Gynecol. 2013;121(1):14–24.
25. Narod SA. Salpingectomy to prevent ovarian cancer: a countercurrents series. Curr Oncol. 2013;20(3):145–7.
26. Eisen A, Lubinski J, Klijn J, Moller P, Lynch HT, Offit K, et al. Breast cancer risk following bilateral oophorectomy in BRCA1 and BRCA2 mutation carriers: an international case–control study. J Clin Oncol. 2005;23(30):7491–6.
27. Domchek SM, Friebel TM, Singer CF, Evans DG, Lynch HT, Isaacs C, et al. Association of risk-reducing surgery in BRCA1 or BRCA2 mutation carriers with cancer risk and mortality. JAMA. 2010;304(9):967–75.
28. Metcalfe K, Lynch HT, Foulkes WD, Tung N, Kim-Sing C, Olopade OI, et al. Effect of oophorectomy on survival after breast cancer in BRCA1 and BRCA2 mutation carriers. JAMA Oncol. 2015;1(3):306–13.
29. Kauff N, Robson M. Breast cancer: oophorectomy for BRCA1 ER-negative disease-an open debate. Nat Rev Clin Oncol. 2015;12(9):505–6.
30. Health GAfGa. BRCA challenge. http://www.genomicsandhealthorg/our-work/current-initiatives/brca-challenge.
31. Antoniou AC, Foulkes WD, Tischkowitz M. Breast-cancer risk in families with mutations in PALB2. N Engl J Med. 2014;371(17):1651–2.

# Part II
# Interventions to Reduce Risk of Recurrence

# Chapter 6
# Endocrine Therapy

**Stefania Redana**

**Abstract** Adjuvant endocrine therapy reduces breast cancer recurrences and deaths in women with hormone receptor positive breast cancer. Tamoxifen has been the standard of care for the past 30 years, until aromatase inhibitors (AIs) proved to be superior in preventing disease recurrence and improving breast cancer mortality in post-menopausal women. Nevertheless, women with early breast cancer remain at risk of relapse for at least 15 years after diagnosis, despite 5 years of adjuvant endocrine therapy. Extended adjuvant therapy with an AI after 5 years of tamoxifen and, more recently ten consecutive years of tamoxifen, have proven to further reduce the risk of recurrence in women who remained disease free after completion of 5 years of tamoxifen. Whether extended endocrine therapy with an AI leads to further benefit for patients treated with adjuvant AI for 5 years, is being investigated in several ongoing trials. In pre-menopausal women, where AIs are contraindicated, tamoxifen has been the standard of care. However recently, the role of ovarian function suppression/ablation in combination with tamoxifen or exemestane has been shown to be superior to tamoxifen alone in selected pre-menopausal patients, at the expense of increased toxicities. A challenge for clinicians is now selection of patients most likely to benefit from extended adjuvant therapy and the management of side effects to maximize adherence.

**Keywords** Endocrine therapy • Tamoxifen • Anastrazole • Letrozole • Exemestane

## Introduction

Endocrine therapy is the oldest form of targeted therapy, and dates back to 1880s when Thomas Nunn described a case of regression of breast cancer in a pre-menopausal woman, after her menstruation ceased [1]. Adjuvant endocrine therapy

S. Redana, MD, PhD
Breast Unit, The Royal Marsden NHS Foundation Trust, Surrey, UK
e-mail: stefania.redana@rmh.nhs.uk



A. Ring, M. Parton (eds.), *Breast Cancer Survivorship*,
DOI 10.1007/978-3-319-41858-2_6

following surgery is the mainstay treatment for women with hormone receptor positive (ER positive) early breast cancer (EBC), and leads to a reductions in both recurrence rates and mortality, irrespective of age, menopausal status, or use of adjuvant chemotherapy. The first widely available anti-hormonal treatment was the selective estrogen-receptor modulator – tamoxifen – which has been used for more than four decades and continues being a valid treatment option.

## Endocrine Therapy for the First 5 Years

### *Tamoxifen*

The first adjuvant tamoxifen trial randomized 1285 stage II pre-menopausal or stage I and II post-menopausal patients with breast cancer to receive tamoxifen for 2 years or no further treatment [2, 3]. At a median follow-up of 66 months, patients on tamoxifen had a significant 36 % reduction (95 % CI 23–47 %) in the risk of recurrence and a significant 29 % reduction (95 % CI 12–42 %) in the risk of death. The benefit was independent of menopausal, nodal and ER status [3]. Long term follow-up of this study suggested tamoxifen to have immediate effects on events, but also delayed effects on survival. Since this study, numerous adjuvant systemic therapy studies have been conducted and have collectively been analyzed by the Early Breast Cancer Trialists's Collaborative Group (EBCTCG) in a series of meta-analyses. The first meta-analysis of adjuvant tamoxifen included approximately 30,000 women randomized to receive adjuvant tamoxifen for 1, 2 or 5 years or no endocrine therapy, as part of clinical trials. Allocation to tamoxifen significantly reduced mortality amongst women ≥50 years of age, with a 20 % reduction in the annual odds of death during the first 5 years [4]. Subsequent updates of this analysis clearly demonstrated superiority of 5 years of tamoxifen over shorter duration [5]. With a median follow-up of 13 years, the most recent meta-analysis shows that 5 years of tamoxifen reduces 15-years risks of breast cancer recurrence and death in ER positive breast cancer. A 39 % reduction in recurrence rate was observed over all time periods (RR 0.61, $p<0.00001$). Breast cancer mortality was reduced by about a third throughout the first 15 years after randomization (rate ratio (RR) 0.70 $p<0.00001$). The RRs were 0.71 in years 0–4, 0.66 in years 5–9 and 0.68 in years 10–14, all significant. The absolute mortality difference tripled from year 5 to year 15, indicating a carryover effect for many years after treatment discontinuation.

Despite the obvious benefits of adjuvant tamoxifen, some patients are primarily resistant to tamoxifen or will develop resistance after an initial benefit. Moreover, prolonged use of tamoxifen increases the risk of life threatening conditions such as thromboembolic events and uterine cancer, in particular in women aged ≥55 years [6]. This has stimulated interest in alternative endocrine therapies, including the use of ovarian function suppression or ablation in pre-menopausal women and aromatase inhibitors in post-menopausal women.

## *Ovarian Function Suppression in Pre-menopausal Women*

Ovarian ablation was one of the first available treatments for breast cancer [7] and its effectiveness was confirmed by a 1996 EBCTCG meta-analysis [8]. However, with the availability of several other endocrine therapies, the role of ovarian ablation (usually by bilateral oophorectomy) or ovarian suppression (through use of LHRH analogs) remained controversial. Several trials addressed this topic and a comprehensive systematic review published in 2007 included almost 12,000 pre-menopausal women with EBC receiving standard of care treatment who were randomized to receive luteinizing hormone releasing hormone (LHRH) or not [9]. LHRH in combination with tamoxifen or chemotherapy significantly reduced the risks of recurrence by 13 % ($p=0.02$) and the risk of death after recurrence by 15 % ($p=0.03$). This improvement was not significant when LHRH was used as the only adjuvant therapy.

Recently, results of two large randomized phase III studies (the TEXT and SOFT trials) evaluating ovarian suppression with adjuvant endocrine therapy for pre-menopausal women with ER positive EBC became available [10, 11]. These studies were designed not only to investigate the benefit of adding ovarian suppression to tamoxifen, but also to investigate the role of adjuvant aromatase inhibitor (exemestane) in combination with ovarian suppression in pre-menopausal patients. (Aromatase inhibitors are only indicated in pre-menopausal patients if they have undergone ovarian ablation or are receiving ovarian function suppression, to render them post-menopausal). A pre-planned combined analysis was carried out. Eligible patients were pre-menopausal women with ER positive breast cancer who had undergone complete surgical excision of primary breast cancer and radiotherapy when deemed necessary.

In the TEXT trial all patients received the LHRH analog triptorelin 3.75 mg every 28 days and were randomized to receive either tamoxifen or exemestane. If chemotherapy was administered, triptorelin was started concomitantly to chemotherapy, if not patients started endocrine therapy 6–8 weeks after commencing triptorelin [10]. At a median follow-up of 68 months a significant 28 % reduction in the risk of recurrence was observed favoring exemestane (HR 0.72, $p>0.001$) and 5 years DFS was 91.1 % in the exemestane arm compared to 87.3 % in the tamoxifen arm. The rate of freedom from breast cancer was also improved for patients receiving exemestane with HR 0.66, $p>0.001$. OS did not significantly differ between the two treatment groups [10].

In the SOFT trial patients who remained pre-menopausal after completion of adjuvant or neoadjuvant chemotherapy were randomized to receive tamoxifen for 5 years, ovarian suppression plus tamoxifen or ovarian suppression plus exemestane in a 1:1:1 ratio [11].

Results of comparison between tamoxifen and tamoxifen + ovarian suppression in 3066 patients in the SOFT trial became available in January 2015 [11] showing no significant benefit from adding ovarian suppression to tamoxifen in the whole population (HR for DFS 0.83, $p=0.10$). However, for women whose cancer was deemed at sufficient risk to warrant adjuvant chemotherapy, 5 years freedom from breast cancer was 82.5 % amongst those assigned ovarian suppression plus tamoxifen and 78 % for those receiving tamoxifen alone. In the small subgroup of patients younger than 35 years of age (350 patients), of whom 94 % received adjuvant chemotherapy, 5 years freedom from breast cancer was 67.7 % (95 % CI 57.3–76.0) in the tamoxifen group, 78.9 % (95 % CI 69.8–85.5) in the ovarian suppression + tamoxifen and 83.4 % (95 % CI 74.9–89.3) in the ovarian suppression plus exemestane group.

In conclusion, ovarian suppression in combination with tamoxifen or exemestane should be considered for pre-menopausal patients with EBC at sufficient risk to warrant adjuvant chemotherapy. However, the side effects of this treatment and impact on quality of life should not be underestimated. (These are discussed in Chaps. 13 and 14).

## Aromatase Inhibitors (AIs)

Aromatase is the enzyme catalyzing the conversion of endogenous androgens to estrogens in post-menopausal women or in pre-menopausal women whose ovarian function has been suppressed or whose ovaries have been removed [12]. Development of third generation AIs (letrozole, anastrozole and exemestane) provided a method of estrogen deprivation without a significant effect on other endocrine pathways. These drugs were found to almost completely inhibit aromatase activity [13, 14]; and proved to be superior to tamoxifen as first line therapy in patients with metastatic breast cancer [15–17].

Third generation AIs have been studied as adjuvant endocrine therapy for post-menopausal women with EBC in several randomized trials, both as upfront treatment in comparison with tamoxifen and after an initial 2–3 years of tamoxifen (Table 6.1). Endocrine therapy containing an AI is now recommended as standard of care adjuvant treatment for post-menopausal women with EBC.

## Up-Front Trials

### *ATAC Trial*

The ATAC trial was the first trial to be published which presented data directly comparing tamoxifen and an AI in the adjuvant treatment of EBC [26]. A total of 9366 post-menopausal women with early invasive breast cancer were randomized 1:1:1 to receive anastrozole or tamoxifen or the combination of anastrozole plus tamoxifen for a total of 5 years after completion of their loco-regional treatment, and chemotherapy when appropriate. At the time the trial was started, patients with

**Table 6.1** Clinical trials comparing tamoxifen and aromatase inhibitors as adjuvant therapy for early breast cancer (EBC)

| Trial | Patient population | Treatment arms | Number of patients | Primary end point | Primary Outcome results HR (95 % CI) | OS HR (95 % CI) | References |
|---|---|---|---|---|---|---|---|
| *Up-front comparison of AIs vs T* | | | | | | | |
| ATAC<br>10 yrs follow-up | ER+ or – or unk EBC | A vs T vs A + T for 5 yrs | 9366 | DFS, safety | 0.91 (0.83–0.99) $p = 0.04$<br>ER+ 0.86 (0.78–0.95) $p = 0.003$ | 0.97 (0.88–1.08) $p = 0.6$<br>ER+ 0.95 (0.84–1.06) $p = 0.4$ | Cuzick et al. [18] |
| BIG 1–98<br>8.7 yrs follow-up | ER+ EBC | L vs T vs L → T vs T → L for 5 yrs | 8010 | DFS | IPCW 0.82 (0.74–0.92) $p < 0.0002$ | IPCW 0.79 (0.69–0.90) $p < 0.0006$ | Regan et al. [19] |
| TEAM<br>2.75 yrs follow-up | ER+ EBC | Up-front T vs E (2.5–3 yrs), Sequential T (2.5–3 yrs) → E vs E for 5 yrs | 9766 | DFS | 0.89 (0.77–1.03) $p = 0.12$ | NA | Coombes et al. [20] |
| *Switch strategy* | | | | | | | |
| ITA<br>128 months follow-up | ER+ or unk, node +, EBC. Prior 2–3 yrs of T | T for 5 yrs vs T for 2–3 yrs → A for 3–2 yrs | 448 (planned 996) | RFS | 0.64 (0.44–0.94) $p = 0.02$ | 0.79 (0.52–1.21) $p = 0.3$ | Boccardo et al. [21] |
| ARNO 95<br>30.1 months follow-up | ER+ EBC. Prior 2 yrs of T | T for 5 yrs vs T for 2 yrs → A for 3 yrs | 979 | DFS | 0.66 (0.44–1.00) $p = 0.049$ | 0.53 (0.28–0.99) $p = 0.045$ | Kaufmann et al. [22] |
| ABCSG-8<br>5 yrs follow-up | ER+ EBC. Prior 2–3 yrs of T | T for 5 yrs vs T for 2 yrs → A for 3 yrs | 3714 | RFS | 0.80 (0.631– 1.013) $p = 0.06$ | 0.87 (0.64–1.16) $p = 0.33$ | Dubsky et al. [23] |

(continued)

**Table 6.1** (continued)

| Trial | Patient population | Treatment arms | Number of patients | Primary end point | Primary Outcome results HR (95 % CI) | OS HR (95 % CI) | References |
|---|---|---|---|---|---|---|---|
| IES<br>91 months follow-up | ER+ EBC | T for 5 yrs vs T for 2–3 yrs → E for 3–2 yrs | 4742 | DFS | 0.81 (0.72–0.91) $p<0.001$ | 0.53 (0.75–0.99) $p<0.04$ | Bliss et al. [24] |
| BIG 1–98<br>8 yrs follow-up | ER+ EBC | L vs T vs L → T vs T → L for 5 yrs | 8010 | DFS | 1.06 (0.91–1.23) $p=0.48$ | 0.97 (0.80–1.19) $p=0.79$ | Regan et al. [19] |
| TEAM<br>5.1 yrs follow-up | ER+ EBC | Up-front T vs E (2.5–3 yrs), Sequential T (2.5–3 yrs) → E vs E for 5 yrs | 9766 | DFS | 1.06 (0.91–1.24) $p=0.42$ | 1.00 (0.89–1.14) $p>0.99$ | Van de Velde et al. [25] |

*ER* hormone receptor, *unk* unknown, *EBC* early breast cancer, *A* anastrozole, *T* tamoxifen, *yrs* years, *DFS* disease-free survival, *RFS* recurrence-free survival, *IPCW* Inverse Probability Censoring Weighted, *L* letrozole, *E* exemestane, *RFS* recurrence-free survival, *NA* not available, *ATAC* Arimidex, Tamoxifen, Alone or in Combination, *BIG* Breast International Group, *TEAM* Tamoxifen Exemestane Adjuvant Multinational, *ITA* Italian Tamoxifen Anastrozole (trial), *ARNO 95* Arimidex-Nolvadex 95, *ABCSG* Austrian Breast and Colorectal Cancer Study Group, *IES* Intergroup Exemestane Study

ER negative or unknown status were allowed to enter the study and 84 % of enrolled patients had known ER positive breast cancer. The first results were released after a median follow-up of 33.3 months. Patients receiving anastrozole had significantly improved disease free survival (DFS) compared to patients randomized to either tamoxifen (HR 0.83, p=0.013) or the combination (HR 0.81, p=0.006). Results with the combination treatment were not significantly different from those with tamoxifen alone. DFS improvement was evident for women with ER positive breast cancer but not for those with ER negative disease. With longer follow up of 10 years, long term superior efficacy of anastrozole over tamoxifen was confirmed [18]. Treatment with anastrozole led to improved DFS, time to recurrence (TTR) and time to distant recurrence (TTDR). In women with ER positive breast cancer, the absolute reduction in recurrence was 2.7 % at 5 years and 4.3 % at 10 years with HR 0.86 (p=0.003) for DFS. The greatest benefits were seen during the first 2 years of active treatment, but differences remained significant throughout the entire follow-up and after treatment completion. With longer follow-up, evidence of a non significant reduction in mortality became evident.

## *BIG 1–98 Trial*

This trial involved 8010 post-menopausal women with ER positive breast cancer who were randomized to receive letrozole or tamoxifen for 5 years or the sequence of tamoxifen for 2 years followed by letrozole for 3 years or letrozole for 2 years followed by tamoxifen for 3 years. The primary analysis published in 2005 [27], compared the two groups assigned to receive letrozole or tamoxifen initially. The primary end point was DFS defined as time from randomization to local, regional or distant recurrence, new invasive contralateral breast cancer, any second non breast cancer or death without breast cancer recurrence. At a median follow-up of 25.8 months patients randomized to letrozole had a significant 19 % (HR 0.81, p=0.003) reduction in the risk of a DFS event compared to patients on tamoxifen, similarly the risk of distant disease progression was reduced in patients receiving letrozole (HR 0.78, p=0.001) [27]. With longer (median 8.7 years) follow-up letrozole continued to significantly improve distant recurrence free interval, breast cancer free interval, DFS (HR 0.82 (95 % CI, 0.74–0.92)) and OS (HR 0.79 (95 % CI, 0.69–0.90)) when compared with tamoxifen monotherapy [19].

In the sequential treatment comparison, at a median follow-up of 8.0 years after randomization, non-significant differences in any of the four endpoints was observed, for any sequences. However, letrozole monotherapy tended to be better than tamoxifen followed by letrozole, especially in controlling distant recurrences in patients at higher risk of early relapse. Nonetheless switching to tamoxifen *after* an initial 2 years of letrozole, would seem to be a reasonable option for patients who require letrozole cessation for any reason [19].

## TEAM Trial

The tamoxifen and exemestane adjuvant multinational (TEAM) trial was initially designed to compare head to head 5 years of exemestane with 5 years of adjuvant tamoxifen in post-menopausal women with ER positive EBC. However, after report of initial results of the IES [28], the protocol was amended to compare 5 years of exemestane monotherapy with sequence of tamoxifen for 2.5–3 years followed by exemestane to complete 5 years of adjuvant treatment. At a median follow-up of 5.1 years, DFS at 5 years was not significantly different in the two treatment groups: 86 % vs 85 % in the monotherapy group and sequential group, respectively. No difference was observed in term of OS, RFS and DDFS between patients on monotherapy or sequential treatment [25].

## Switch Strategy Trials

Several trials have addressed the topic of switching to an AI after initial 2–3 years of tamoxifen in post-menopausal women with ER+ BC (Table 6.1), including the Italian Tamoxifen Anastrozole (ITA) trial, the Arimidex-Nolvadex 95 (ARNO 95) trial, the Austrian Breast and Colorectal Cancer Study Group −8 (ABCSG-8), the Intergroup Exemestane Study (IES). Results of all these trials were consistent in showing benefit favoring the switch to an AI after initial treatment with tamoxifen for 2–3 years.

## Meta-analysis of Aromatase Inhibitors Versus Tamoxifen in Early Breast Cancer

Recently, the Early Breast Cancer Trialists' Collaborative Group published a patient-level meta-analysis of randomized trials of AIs versus tamoxifen [20]. This meta-analysis addressed three different comparisons in almost 32,000 post-menopausal women with ER positive EBC randomized in trials of AIs versus tamoxifen (either upfront or sequential strategies). Primary outcomes were any recurrence of breast cancer (distant, loco-regional, new primary contralateral breast cancer), breast cancer mortality, death without recurrence and all-cause mortality.

In trials comparing 5 years of an AI versus 5 years of tamoxifen, both recurrence and mortality were significantly reduced for patients treated with AI. Significant reduction in recurrence rates was noted during years 0–1 and 2–4 after surgery, but not thereafter. The absolute difference in 10 years recurrence risk was 3.6 % (95 % CI, 1.7–5.4 %) being 19.1 % in the AI group and 22.7 % in the tamoxifen group. Allocation to AI significantly reduced the rate of local recurrence, contralateral recurrence and distant recurrence. Patients treated with AI had 15 % reduced risk of breast cancer death and 11 % reduced risk of all cause mortality compared to patients treated with tamoxifen.

Comparison of 5 years of AI versus 2–3 years of tamoxifen followed by an AI to complete 5 years, showed a significant reduction in recurrence was observed only during the time period when treatment differed (RR 0.74, 95 % CI 0.62–0.89; 2p = 0.002) and was similar when both groups were receiving an AI. A non significant reduction in breast cancer mortality was noted favoring patients on AI monotherapy (RR 0.89, 95 % CI 0.78–1.03; 2p = 0.11).

Finally, comparison of 2–3 years of tamoxifen followed by an AI to complete 5 years versus 5 years of tamoxifen demonstrated a significant improvement in both recurrences and mortality in favor of AI containing therapy. This difference was significant during years 2–4 after randomization, but not after treatment completion. The absolute difference in 10 years recurrence risk was 2 % (95 % CI, 0.2–3.8 %): 17 % in the AI group and 19 % in the tamoxifen group. Similar to the head to head comparison, allocation to an AI significantly reduced distant recurrence, contralateral recurrence, breast cancer mortality and all-cause mortality.

Overall, risk ratios favored AIs during the periods when treatment differed, the recurrence rate was about 30 % lower in patients receiving an AI during year 0–1 (RR 0.70, 95 % CI 0.61–0.81; 2p = <0.0001) and during years 2–4 (RR 0.71, 95 % CI 0.62–0.80; $p < 0.0001$), with little and non significant further effect after year 5.

In conclusion, adjuvant AI for post-menopausal EBC reduces recurrence rates by about 30 %, compared to tamoxifen, while treatment differs, but not thereafter. Five years of AI treatment reduces 10 years breast cancer mortality by about 15 % compared to tamoxifen. This benefit is independent from age, nodal status and progesterone receptor status. In two of these trials crossover from tamoxifen to an AI was allowed after results of other trials were released. Therefore, the real benefit of AIs in this setting, with full compliance, may be larger. Adjuvant AIs for post-menopausal women with ER positive breast cancer, upfront or after a few years of tamoxifen, is now considered a standard of care. Whether one AI is better than another remains an unresolved issue. Head to head comparison between anastrozole and exemestane for 5 years failed to show any superiority of the steroidal AI compared to non-steroidal [29]. The Gruppo Italiano Mammella 3 (GIM3) study is a 6 arms study in which ER+ HER2- post-menopausal patients are randomized to receive anastrozole or letrozole or exemestane for 5 years or tamoxifen for 2 years followed by each of the AIs for 3 years [30]. Results will hopefully be available soon and might add some clarity to this issue.

## Endocrine Therapy Beyond 5 Years

ER positive breast cancer is characterized by a long term risk of relapse. The Oxford Overview shows that about 50 % of breast cancer recurrences occur more than 5 years after diagnosis [5, 31]. Despite adjuvant tamoxifen for 5 years some patients have an annual rate of relapse in excess of 2 % for about 15 years [32]; and a similar risk remains for at least 10 years after adjuvant AIs [18]. On the basis of these observations, there is a rationale to extend hormonal therapy beyond 5 years.

## *Extended Tamoxifen Beyond 5 Years*

Several small studies in the mid 1990s explored prolonged tamoxifen beyond 5 years, but the results were inconclusive [33, 34]. In both studies a non-statistically significant benefit in favor of 5 years of tamoxifen was observed, and in fact suggested a potential detrimental effect of continuing tamoxifen for longer than 5 years. However in 2013 the results of two much larger trials addressing the question of tamoxifen beyond 5 years became available.

The Adjuvant Tamoxifen: Longer Against Shorter (ATLAS) trial [35] included 12,894 women with EBC who remained disease free after completion of 5 years of adjuvant tamoxifen. Patients were randomized to receive tamoxifen for an additional 5 years or no further treatment. Among 6846 women with ER positive breast cancer, continuing tamoxifen significantly reduced breast cancer recurrences ($p=0.002$), breast cancer mortality ($p=0.01$) and overall mortality ($p=0.01$). The benefit became evident after 10 years of treatment with only modest reduction of recurrences during the 5 additional years (years 5–10). Likewise, mortality was significantly reduced only after 10 years of tamoxifen and no effects were seen during active treatment. The apparent benefit of continuing tamoxifen for a total of 10 years is the combined effect of two factors: the carryover effect of the first 5 years of treatment and the additional therapeutic benefit of the second 5 years of treatment. These results suggested that 10 years of tamoxifen treatment can approximately halve breast cancer mortality during the second decade after diagnosis, at the expenses of side effects that normally occur during the active treatment period.

A UK trial with similar design (Adjuvant Tamoxifen: To offer More?) included 6953 women with ER positive or unknown breast cancer who were disease free after 5 years of tamoxifen and were randomized to continue tamoxifen for a total of 10 years or stop after 5. Similarly to the ATLAS trial, 10 years of tamoxifen reduced breast cancer recurrence ($p=0.003$) in a time dependent manner. RR was 0.99 during years 5–6, 0.84 in years 7–9 and 0.75 later. Likewise, breast cancer mortality was reduced ($p=0.05$) with evident benefit accruing only after year 9 RR 0.86. The authors concluded that 10 years of adjuvant tamoxifen compared to none, reduces breast cancer mortality by about a third in the first decade after diagnosis and by half afterwards [36].

A combined analysis of these two trials enhanced statistical significance of extended tamoxifen on recurrence ($p<0.0001$), breast cancer mortality ($p=0.002$) and overall survival ($p=0.005$) benefits [36].

## *Extended AI After 5 Years of Tamoxifen*

In post-menopausal women, the alternative to further tamoxifen after an initial 5 years, is an AI. A seminal trial, NCIC-CTG MA.17/BIG 1–97 (MA.17 hereafter) assessed efficacy of 5 years of letrozole after 5 years of adjuvant tamoxifen in this population of patients [37]. At a median follow-up of 2.4 years, patients receiving letrozole had a significant 43 % reduction in the risk of recurrence (p=0.00008) and a non significant reduction in all cause mortality. As a consequence, the trial was unblinded and patients on placebo were offered selective crossover to letrozole. Several further analysis followed, including an ITT analysis at 64 months follow-up showing a persistent 32 % benefit in DFS despite 66 % of patients on tamoxifen crossing-over to letrozole [38]. A more recent analysis has confirmed that patients initially assigned to receive letrozole had significantly better DFS (HR 0.52), distant DFS (HR 0.51) and better OS (HR 0.61), compared to control patients [39]. Amongst patients who were pre-menopausal when starting tamoxifen and became post-menopausal during treatment, the reduction in DFS events was about 75 % (HR 0.26, p=0.03), suggesting this strategy should be adopted for all pre-menopausal patients who become post-menopausal during tamoxifen treatment [40].

The 66 % of patients crossing over in MA.17, provided the opportunity of analyzing whether starting an AI a considerable time after stopping tamoxifen is still beneficial [41]. In this sub-population, with a median follow up of 5.3 years, there was a significant reduction in the risk of recurrence (HR 0.37, p<0.0001) and a significant reduction in distant DFS (HR 0.39, p=0.004). These results suggest that starting letrozole up to 7 years after initial diagnosis, can still improve prognosis for post-menopausal women with ER positive EBC patients who have completed 5 years of tamoxifen.

Subsequently, a number of other trials have investigated the role of AIs following completion of 5 years of tamoxifen. In the Austrian Breast and Colorectal Cancer Study Group (ABCSG) 6a trial, 856 ER+ patients who were disease free after 5 years of adjuvant tamoxifen (± aminoglutethimide) were randomized to receive an additional 3 years of anastrozole or no further treatment. At a median follow-up of 62.3 months, women who received anastrozole had a significant 38 % reduction in the risk of recurrence (p=0.31), and no significant difference in OS [42]. In the NSABP B-33 trial, 1598 post-menopausal patients with clinical T1-3, N0, M0 ER and/or PR+ BC, disease free after completion of adjuvant tamoxifen, were randomized to receive exemestane for 5 years or placebo. The study was discontinued early after results of the MA.17 were released and 44 % of patients on placebo crossed over to exemestane. At a median follow-up of 30 months, original assignment to exemestane led to a non significant 32 % reduction in the risk of recurrence (HR 0.68, p=0.07) but a significant improvement in 4 years RFS (96 % vs 94 %, RR 0.44, p=0.004) [43].

An EBCTCG meta-analysis of these trials showed AI therapy was associated with an absolute 2.9 % decrease in BC recurrence (relative decrease, 43 %,

**Table 6.2** Ongoing clinical trials of extended aromatase inhibitor endocrine therapy for early breast cancer

| Clinical trial | Clinical trial number | Patients population | Treatment | Number of patients | Primary end point (s) |
|---|---|---|---|---|---|
| MA.17R | NCT00754845 | Completed 4.5–6 yrs of AI, with or without prior T[a]<br>AI completed ≤2 yrs prior treatment assignment | L vs Placebo for 5 yrs | 1918 | DFS |
| DATA | NCT00301457 | T for 2–3 yrs | A for 6 yrs vs A for 3 yrs | 1900 | DFS |
| SALSA | NCT00295620 | Any prior endocrine therapy for 5 yrs | A for 2 yrs vs A for 5 yrs | 3500 | DFS |
| NSABP-B42 | NCT00382070 | AI or T→AI[b] | L vs Placebo for 5 yrs | 3966 | DFS |
| LEAD | NCT01064635 | T for 2–3 yrs and 3 months | L for 2–3 yrs vs L for 5 yrs | 4050 | DFS |
| SOLE | NCT00553410 | Any prior endocrine therapy[c] for 4–6 yrs | Continuous L for 5 yrs vs Intermittent L[d] | 4800 | DFS |

[a]Including patients previously enrolled in MA.17
[b]Prior endocrine therapy must have consisted of an AI or a combination of up to 3 years of T followed by an AI. T may not have been given during years 4 and 5 of the 5 years of adjuvant endocrine therapy
[c]Must have completed 4–6 years of prior adjuvant T, AI or a sequential combination of both. When calculating 4–6 years, neoadjuvant endocrine therapy should not be included
[d]48 months over 5 years: 4×9 months (9 months followed by 3 months treatment-free interval in years 1–4, → 36 months) plus 1×12 months in year 5→48 months
*Yrs* years, *AI* aromatase inhibitor, *T* tamoxifen, *L* letrozole, *DFS* disease free survival, *A* anastrozole, *DATA* Different Durations of Anastrozole after Tamoxifen trial, *SALSA* Secondary Adjuvant Long-term Study with Arimidex trial, *LEAD* Letrozole Adjuvant Therapy Duration trial, *SOLE* Study of Letrozole Extension trial

$p<0.0000$) and an absolute 0.5 % decrease in BC mortality (relative decrease 27 %, $2p=0.11$) at a median follow-up of 2.5 years [44].

## *Extended AIs Beyond 5 Years of Adjuvant AIs*

Up-front AIs are now considered standard of care for post-menopausal women with ER positive EBC rendering results of the above mentioned trials not applicable to women who are post-menopausal at diagnosis (and who will start an AI rather than tamoxifen). Whether continuing AIs beyond 5 years in these women can further improve these patients prognosis is being investigated in several ongoing trials (Table 6.2).

## Conclusions

Several treatment options are now available for women with ER positive early breast cancer. For post-menopausal patients AIs given for 5 years have replaced tamoxifen. For pre-menopausal women, tamoxifen remains the standard therapy for many patients, however in those at high risk of recurrence ovarian function suppression and an aromatase inhibitor should be considered. The role of extended adjuvant endocrine therapy beyond 5 years is well established, with the use of tamoxifen (in pre-menopausal women) and the option of (switching to or continuing) an AI in post-menopausal women. With so many options available, the challenge will now be to identify those patients who benefit most from extended adjuvant therapy, and to manage the side-effects of treatment to maximize adherence (Chaps. 13 and 14).

## References

1. Nunn TW. On cancer of the breast. London: J & A Churchill. Ref Type: Report; 1882.
2. Controlled trial of tamoxifen as adjuvant agent in management of early breast cancer. Interim analysis at four years by Nolvadex Adjuvant Trial Organisation. Lancet. 1983;1(8319): 257–61. doi:S0140-6736(83)91683-5 [pii].
3. Controlled trial of tamoxifen as a single adjuvant agent in the management of early breast cancer. 'Nolvadex' Adjuvant Trial Organisation. Br J Cancer. 1988;57(6):608–11.
4. Effects of adjuvant tamoxifen and of cytotoxic therapy on mortality in early breast cancer. An overview of 61 randomized trials among 28,896 women. Early Breast Cancer Trialists' Collaborative Group. N Engl J Med. 1988;319(26):1681–92. doi:10.1056/NEJM198812293192601.
5. Early Breast Cancer Trialists' Collaborative Group (EBCTCG). Effects of chemotherapy and hormonal therapy for early breast cancer on recurrence and 15-year survival: an overview of the randomised trials. Lancet. 2005;365(9472):1687–717. doi:10.1016/S0140-6736(05)66544-0. S0140-6736(05)66544-0 [pii].
6. Fisher B, Costantino JP, Wickerham DL, Cecchini RS, Cronin WM, Robidoux A, Bevers TB, Kavanah MT, Atkins JN, Margolese RG, Runowicz CD, James JM, Ford LG, Wolmark N. Tamoxifen for the prevention of breast cancer: current status of the National Surgical Adjuvant Breast and Bowel Project P-1 study. J Natl Cancer Inst. 2005;97(22):1652–62. doi:10.1093/jnci/dji372. 97/22/1652 [pii].
7. Love RR, Philips J. Oophorectomy for breast cancer: history revisited. J Natl Cancer Inst. 2002;94(19):1433–4.
8. Ovarian ablation in early breast cancer: overview of the randomised trials. Early Breast Cancer Trialists' Collaborative Group. Lancet. 1996;348(9036): 1189–96. doi:S0140673696050234 [pii].
9. Cuzick J, Ambroisine L, Davidson N, Jakesz R, Kaufmann M, Regan M, Sainsbury R. Use of luteinising-hormone-releasing hormone agonists as adjuvant treatment in premenopausal patients with hormone-receptor-positive breast cancer: a meta-analysis of individual patient data from randomised adjuvant trials. Lancet. 2007;369(9574):1711–23. doi:10.1016/S0140-6736(07)60778-8. S0140-6736(07)60778-8 [pii].
10. Pagani O, Regan MM, Walley BA, Fleming GF, Colleoni M, Lang I, Gomez HL, Tondini C, Burstein HJ, Perez EA, Ciruelos E, Stearns V, Bonnefoi HR, Martino S, Geyer Jr CE, Pinotti G, Puglisi F, Crivellari D, Ruhstaller T, Winer EP, Rabaglio-Poretti M, Maibach R, Ruepp B, Giobbie-Hurder A, Price KN, Bernhard J, Luo W, Ribi K, Viale G, Coates AS, Gelber RD,

Goldhirsch A, Francis PA. Adjuvant exemestane with ovarian suppression in premenopausal breast cancer. N Engl J Med. 2014;371(2):107–18. doi:10.1056/NEJMoa1404037.
11. Francis PA, Regan MM, Fleming GF, Lang I, Ciruelos E, Bellet M, Bonnefoi HR, Climent MA, Da Prada GA, Burstein HJ, Martino S, Davidson NE, Geyer Jr CE, Walley BA, Coleman R, Kerbrat P, Buchholz S, Ingle JN, Winer EP, Rabaglio-Poretti M, Maibach R, Ruepp B, Giobbie-Hurder A, Price KN, Colleoni M, Viale G, Coates AS, Goldhirsch A, Gelber RD. Adjuvant ovarian suppression in premenopausal breast cancer. N Engl J Med. 2015;372(5):436–46. doi:10.1056/NEJMoa1412379.
12. Smith IE, Dowsett M. Aromatase inhibitors in breast cancer. N Engl J Med. 2003;348(24):2431–42. doi:10.1056/NEJMra023246. 348/24/2431 [pii].
13. Geisler J, King N, Dowsett M, Ottestad L, Lundgren S, Walton P, Kormeset PO, Lonning PE. Influence of anastrozole (Arimidex), a selective, non-steroidal aromatase inhibitor, on in vivo aromatisation and plasma oestrogen levels in postmenopausal women with breast cancer. Br J Cancer. 1996;74(8):1286–91.
14. Geisler J, King N, Anker G, Ornati G, di Salle E, Lonning PE, Dowsett M. In vivo inhibition of aromatization by exemestane, a novel irreversible aromatase inhibitor, in postmenopausal breast cancer patients. Clin Cancer Res. 1998;4(9):2089–93.
15. Paridaens R, Dirix L, Lohrisch C, Beex L, Nooij M, Cameron D, Biganzoli L, Cufer T, Duchateau L, Hamilton A, Lobelle JP, Piccart M. Mature results of a randomized phase II multicenter study of exemestane versus tamoxifen as first-line hormone therapy for postmenopausal women with metastatic breast cancer. Ann Oncol. 2003;14(9):1391–8.
16. Bonneterre J, Buzdar A, Nabholtz JM, Robertson JF, Thurlimann B, von Euler M, Sahmoud T, Webster A, Steinberg M. Anastrozole is superior to tamoxifen as first-line therapy in hormone receptor positive advanced breast carcinoma. Cancer. 2001;92(9):2247–58. doi:10.1002/1097-0142(20011101)92:9<2247::AID-CNCR1570>3.0.CO;2-Y.
17. Mouridsen H, Gershanovich M, Sun Y, Perez-Carrion R, Boni C, Monnier A, Apffelstaedt J, Smith R, Sleeboom HP, Janicke F, Pluzanska A, Dank M, Becquart D, Bapsy PP, Salminen E, Snyder R, Lassus M, Verbeek JA, Staffler B, Chaudri-Ross HA, Dugan M. Superior efficacy of letrozole versus tamoxifen as first-line therapy for postmenopausal women with advanced breast cancer: results of a phase III study of the International Letrozole Breast Cancer Group. J Clin Oncol. 2001;19(10):2596–606.
18. Cuzick J, Sestak I, Baum M, Buzdar A, Howell A, Dowsett M, Forbes JF. Effect of anastrozole and tamoxifen as adjuvant treatment for early-stage breast cancer: 10-year analysis of the ATAC trial. Lancet Oncol. 2010;11(12):1135–41. doi:10.1016/S1470-2045(10)70257-6. S1470-2045(10)70257-6 [pii].
19. Regan MM, Neven P, Giobbie-Hurder A, Goldhirsch A, Ejlertsen B, Mauriac L, Forbes JF, Smith I, Lang I, Wardley A, Rabaglio M, Price KN, Gelber RD, Coates AS, Thurlimann B. Assessment of letrozole and tamoxifen alone and in sequence for postmenopausal women with steroid hormone receptor-positive breast cancer: the BIG 1–98 randomised clinical trial at 8.1 years median follow-up. Lancet Oncol. 2011;12(12):1101–8. doi:10.1016/S1470-2045(11)70270-4. S1470-2045(11)70270-4 [pii].
20. Dowsett M, Forbes JF, Bradley R, Ingle J, Aihara T, Bliss J, Boccardo F, Coates A, Coombes RC, Cuzick J, Dubsky P, Gnant M, Kaufmann M, Kilburn L, Perrone F, Rea D, Thurlimann B, van de Velde V, Pan H, Peto R, Davies C, Gray R. Aromatase inhibitors versus tamoxifen in early breast cancer: patient-level meta-analysis of the randomised trials. Lancet. 2015;386(10001):1341–52. doi:10.1016/S0140-6736(15)61074-1. S0140-6736(15)61074-1 [pii].
21. Boccardo F, Guglielmini P, Bordonaro R, Fini A, Massidda B, Porpiglia M, Roagna R, Serra P, Orzalesi L, Ucci G, Rubagotti A. Switching to anastrozole versus continued tamoxifen treatment of early breast cancer: long term results of the Italian Tamoxifen Anastrozole trial. Eur J Cancer. 2013;49(7):1546–54. doi:10.1016/j.ejca.2012.12.025. S0959-8049(13)00003-8 [pii].
22. Kaufmann M, Jonat W, Hilfrich J, Eidtmann H, Gademann G. Zuna I, von MG Improved overall survival in postmenopausal women with early breast cancer after anastrozole initiated after treatment with tamoxifen compared with continued tamoxifen: the ARNO 95 Study. J Clin Oncol. 2007;25(19):2664–70. doi:10.1200/JCO.2006.08.8054. JCO.2006.08.8054 [pii].

23. Dubsky PC, Jakesz R, Mlineritsch B, Postlberger S, Samonigg H, Kwasny W, Tausch C, Stoger H, Haider K, Fitzal F, Singer CF, Stierer M, Sevelda P, Luschin-Ebengreuth G, Taucher S, Rudas M, Bartsch R, Steger GG, Greil R, Filipcic L, Gnant M. Tamoxifen and anastrozole as a sequencing strategy: a randomized controlled trial in postmenopausal patients with endocrine-responsive early breast cancer from the Austrian Breast and Colorectal Cancer Study Group. J Clin Oncol. 2012;30(7):722–8. doi:10.1200/JCO.2011.36.8993. JCO.2011.36.8993 [pii].
24. Bliss JM, Kilburn LS, Coleman RE, Forbes JF, Coates AS, Jones SE, Jassem J, Delozier T, Andersen J, Paridaens R, Van de Velde CJ, Lonning PE, Morden J, Reise J, Cisar L, Menschik T, Coombes RC. Disease-related outcomes with long-term follow-up: an updated analysis of the intergroup exemestane study. J Clin Oncol. 2012;30(7):709–17. doi:10.1200/JCO.2010.33.7899. JCO.2010.33.7899 [pii].
25. Van de Velde CJ, Rea D, Seynaeve C, Putter H, Hasenburg A, Vannetzel JM, Paridaens R, Markopoulos C, Hozumi Y, Hille ET, Kieback DG, Asmar L, Smeets J, Nortier JW, Hadji P, Bartlett JM, Jones SE. Adjuvant tamoxifen and exemestane in early breast cancer (TEAM): a randomised phase 3 trial. Lancet. 2011;377(9762):321–31. doi:10.1016/S0140-6736(10)62312-4. S0140-6736(10)62312-4 [pii].
26. Baum M, Budzar AU, Cuzick J, Forbes J, Houghton JH, Klijn JG, Sahmoud T. Anastrozole alone or in combination with tamoxifen versus tamoxifen alone for adjuvant treatment of postmenopausal women with early breast cancer: first results of the ATAC randomised trial. Lancet. 2002;359(9324):2131–9. doi:S0140673602090888 [pii].
27. Thurlimann B, Keshaviah A, Coates AS, Mouridsen H, Mauriac L, Forbes JF, Paridaens R, Castiglione-Gertsch M, Gelber RD, Rabaglio M, Smith I, Wardley A, Price KN, Goldhirsch A. A comparison of letrozole and tamoxifen in postmenopausal women with early breast cancer. N Engl J Med. 2005;353(26):2747–57. doi:10.1056/NEJMoa052258. 353/26/2747 [pii].
28. Coombes RC, Hall E, Gibson LJ, Paridaens R, Jassem J, Delozier T, Jones SE, Alvarez I, Bertelli G, Ortmann O, Coates AS, Bajetta E, Dodwell D, Coleman RE, Fallowfield LJ, Mickiewicz E, Andersen J, Lonning PE, Cocconi G, Stewart A, Stuart N, Snowdon CF, Carpentieri M, Massimini G, Bliss JM, van de Velde C. A randomized trial of exemestane after two to three years of tamoxifen therapy in postmenopausal women with primary breast cancer. N Engl J Med. 2004;350(11):1081–92. doi:10.1056/NEJMoa040331. 350/11/1081 [pii].
29. Goss PE, Ingle JN, Pritchard KI, Ellis MJ, Sledge GW, Budd GT, Rabaglio M, Ansari RH, Johnson DB, Tozer R, D'Souza DP, Chalchal H, Spadafora S, Stearns V, Perez EA, Liedke PE, Lang I, Elliott C, Gelmon KA, Chapman JA, Shepherd LE. Exemestane versus anastrozole in postmenopausal women with early breast cancer: NCIC CTG MA.27 – a randomized controlled phase III trial. J Clin Oncol. 2013;31(11):1398–404. doi:10.1200/JCO.2012.44.7805. JCO.2012.44.7805 [pii].
30. NCT00541086. Study of anastrozole, letrozole or exemestane with or without tamoxifen in treating postmenopausal women with hormone-responsive breast cancer that has been completely removed by surgery. 2016. Ref Type: Online Source.
31. Davies C, Godwin J, Gray R, Clarke M, Cutter D, Darby S, McGale P, Pan HC, Taylor C, Wang YC, Dowsett M, Ingle J, Peto R. Relevance of breast cancer hormone receptors and other factors to the efficacy of adjuvant tamoxifen: patient-level meta-analysis of randomised trials. Lancet. 2011;378(9793):771–84. doi:10.1016/S0140-6736(11)60993-8. S0140-6736(11)60993-8 [pii].
32. Saphner T, Tormey DC, Gray R. Annual hazard rates of recurrence for breast cancer after primary therapy. J Clin Oncol. 1996;14(10):2738–46.
33. Fisher B, Dignam J, Bryant J, Wolmark N. Five versus more than five years of tamoxifen for lymph node-negative breast cancer: updated findings from the National Surgical Adjuvant Breast and Bowel Project B-14 randomized trial. J Natl Cancer Inst. 2001;93(9):684–90.
34. Tormey DC, Gray R, Falkson HC. Postchemotherapy adjuvant tamoxifen therapy beyond five years in patients with lymph node-positive breast cancer. Eastern Cooperative Oncology Group. J Natl Cancer Inst. 1996;88(24):1828–33.
35. Davies C, Pan H, Godwin J, Gray R, Arriagada R, Raina V, Abraham M, Medeiros Alencar VH, Badran A, Bonfill X, Bradbury J, Clarke M, Collins R, Davis SR, Delmestri A, Forbes JF, Haddad P, Hou MF, Inbar M, Khaled H, Kielanowska J, Kwan WH, Mathew BS, Mittra I,

Muller B, Nicolucci A, Peralta O, Pernas F, Petruzelka L, Pienkowski T, Radhika R, Rajan B, Rubach MT, Tort S, Urrutia G, Valentini M, Wang Y, Peto R. Long-term effects of continuing adjuvant tamoxifen to 10 years versus stopping at 5 years after diagnosis of oestrogen receptor-positive breast cancer: ATLAS, a randomised trial. Lancet. 2013;381(9869):805–16. doi:10.1016/S0140-6736(12)61963-1. S0140-6736(12)61963-1 [pii].

36. Gray RG, Rea D, Handley K, Bowden SJ, Perry P, Earl HM, Poole CJ, Bates T, Chetiyawardana S, Dewar JA, Fernando IN, Grieve R, Nicoll J, Rayter Z, Robinson A, Salman A, Yarnold J, Bathers S, Marshal A, Lee M. aTTom: long-term effects of continuing adjuvant tamoxifen to 10 years versus stopping at 5 years in 6,953 women with early breast cancer. J Clin Oncol. 2013;31(15_Suppl (Abs.5)).
37. Goss PE, Ingle JN, Martino S, Robert NJ, Muss HB, Piccart MJ, Castiglione M, Tu D, Shepherd LE, Pritchard KI, Livingston RB, Davidson NE, Norton L, Perez EA, Abrams JS, Therasse P, Palmer MJ, Pater JL. A randomized trial of letrozole in postmenopausal women after five years of tamoxifen therapy for early-stage breast cancer. N Engl J Med. 2003;349(19):1793–802. doi:10.1056/NEJMoa032312. NEJMoa032312 [pii].
38. Ingle JN, Tu D, Pater JL, Muss HB, Martino S, Robert NJ, Piccart MJ, Castiglione M, Shepherd LE, Pritchard KI, Livingston RB, Davidson NE, Norton L, Perez EA, Abrams JS, Cameron DA, Palmer MJ, Goss PE. Intent-to-treat analysis of the placebo-controlled trial of letrozole for extended adjuvant therapy in early breast cancer: NCIC CTG MA.17. Ann Oncol. 2008;19(5):877–82. doi:10.1093/annonc/mdm566. mdm566 [pii].
39. Jin H, Tu D, Zhao N, Shepherd LE, Goss PE. Longer-term outcomes of letrozole versus placebo after 5 years of tamoxifen in the NCIC CTG MA.17 trial: analyses adjusting for treatment crossover. J Clin Oncol. 2012;30(7):718–21. doi:10.1200/JCO.2010.34.4010. JCO.2010.34.4010 [pii].
40. Goss PE, Ingle JN, Martino S, Robert NJ, Muss HB, Livingston RB, Davidson NE, Perez EA, Chavarri-Guerra Y, Cameron DA, Pritchard KI, Whelan T, Shepherd LE, Tu D. Impact of premenopausal status at breast cancer diagnosis in women entered on the placebo-controlled NCIC CTG MA17 trial of extended adjuvant letrozole. Ann Oncol. 2013;24(2):355–61. doi:10.1093/annonc/mds330. mds330 [pii].
41. Goss PE, Ingle JN, Pater JL, Martino S, Robert NJ, Muss HB, Piccart MJ, Castiglione M, Shepherd LE, Pritchard KI, Livingston RB, Davidson NE, Norton L, Perez EA, Abrams JS, Cameron DA, Palmer MJ, Tu D. Late extended adjuvant treatment with letrozole improves outcome in women with early-stage breast cancer who complete 5 years of tamoxifen. J Clin Oncol. 2008;26(12):1948–55. doi:10.1200/JCO.2007.11.6798. JCO.2007.11.6798 [pii].
42. Jakesz R, Greil R, Gnant M, Schmid M, Kwasny W, Kubista E, Mlineritsch B, Tausch C, Stierer M, Hofbauer F, Renner K, Dadak C, Rucklinger E, Samonigg H. Extended adjuvant therapy with anastrozole among postmenopausal breast cancer patients: results from the randomized Austrian Breast and Colorectal Cancer Study Group Trial 6a. J Natl Cancer Inst. 2007;99(24):1845–53. doi:10.1093/jnci/djm246. djm246 [pii].
43. Mamounas EP, Jeong JH, Wickerham DL, Smith RE, Ganz PA, Land SR, Eisen A, Fehrenbacher L, Farrar WB, Atkins JN, Pajon ER, Vogel VG, Kroener JF, Hutchins LF, Robidoux A, Hoehn JL, Ingle JN, Geyer Jr CE, Costantino JP, Wolmark N. Benefit from exemestane as extended adjuvant therapy after 5 years of adjuvant tamoxifen: intention-to-treat analysis of the National Surgical Adjuvant Breast And Bowel Project B-33 trial. J Clin Oncol. 2008;26(12):1965–71. doi:10.1200/JCO.2007.14.0228. JCO.2007.14.0228 [pii].
44. Goss P, Mamounas E, Jakesz R, Markopoulos C, Dowsett M, Peto R, Godwin J, Davies C. Aromatase Inhibitors (AIs) Versus Not (Placebo/Observation) as Late Extended Adjuvant Therapy for Postmenopausal Women with Early Stage Breast Cancer (BC): Overviews of Randomized Trials of AIs after Γê+5 Years of Tamoxifen. Cancer Res. 2009; 69(24 Suppl):4081.

# Chapter 7
# Systemic Therapies to Reduce the Risk of Recurrence in Early Breast Cancer: New Strategies

**Narda Chaabouni, Christos Nikolaou, and Mark Harries**

**Abstract** The systemic adjuvant treatment of early breast cancer (EBC) has benefited from a multifaceted approach. Generic cytotoxic approaches, as well as a more targeted approach to the estrogen receptor or HER2 receptor are now established standards of care. Decades of innovative trials exploring bisphosphonates in breast cancer prevention and EBC for bone protection, as well as large prospective randomized trials have resulted in an overwhelming case for benefit in post menopausal women. Therapies such as everolimus and the PARP inhibitors, established in the secondary breast cancer setting, are being explored in the adjuvant setting for utility. Similarly, observational and retrospective studies have demonstrated a strong reduction in breast cancer risk with the use of metformin and aspirin, and hence large prospective randomized trials are underway.

**Keywords** Bisphosphonates • Aspirin • Cyclooxygenase • Add- aspirin • Metformin • Everolimus • PARP inhibitors

## Introduction

Breast cancer related outcomes have improved dramatically over the last few decades due in large part to earlier diagnosis through screening and progress in adjuvant treatments including chemotherapy, hormone therapy and targeted therapy such as Trastuzumab. Bisphosphonates, traditionally used to prevent skeletal related events in metastatic breast cancer and anti-estrogen therapy induced bone loss have

N. Chaabouni
The Breast Unit, The Royal Marsden NHS Foundation Trust, Surrey, UK

C. Nikolaou • M. Harries, MA, FRCP, PhD (✉)
Department of Medical Oncology, Guy's and St Thomas' Hospital, London, UK
e-mail: mark.harries@gstt.nhs.uk

 
A. Ring, M. Parton (eds.), *Breast Cancer Survivorship*,
DOI 10.1007/978-3-319-41858-2_7

been evaluated in several randomized clinical trials in the adjuvant setting and have shown a beneficial effect in a selected subset of patients as evidenced from the results of a recent meta-analysis. This chapter aims to review the results of trials evaluating the role of adjuvant bisphosphonates in early breast cancer as well discussing current studies exploring other systemic therapies such as aspirin, metformin and other targeted therapies.

## Bisphosphonates

Bisphosphonates are synthetic analogs of pyrophosphate that strongly bind to the hydroxyapatite crystals of bone and are released from the bone surface during bone resorption [1]. Bisphosphonates are then internalized by osteoclasts and produce cellular changes which eventually result in apoptosis of these cells [2]. Bisphosphonates are classified into non-nitrogen containing (clodronate and etidronate) and nitrogen containing compounds or aminobisphosphonates (alendronate, risedronate, pamidronate, and zoledronate) [3].

Initially used in patients with osteoporosis, bisphosphonates now are approved for use for the prevention of skeletal-related events in patients with bone metastatic disease, the treatment of hypercalcemia of malignancy, and to prevent bone loss associated with anti-estrogen therapy using aromatase inhibitors [2].

Bone is the most common site of distant metastasis in breast cancer [4]. It is thought that the bone microenvironment plays a major role in the development and growth of disseminated tumor cells (DTC). DTC have been found in the bone marrow in up to 30–40 % of patients with early breast cancer and are thought to be a source for subsequent distant metastases seeding at other secondary sites. The presence of such cells in the bone marrow at diagnosis is a strong negative prognostic factor for risk of recurrence [5]. DTC may remain dormant for many years in "pre-metastatic bone niches" where they are able to evade systemic chemotherapy [6]. Bisphosphonates are thought to alter the bone microenvironment by reducing the release of bone-derived growth factors and other modulators making the bone environment less favorable for dormant tumor cells to survive [6].

Data from preclinical studies prompted adjuvant studies of oral and intravenous bisphosphonates. The first study to report a benefit on breast cancer outcomes was a trial of oral clodronate in a cohort of 302 breast cancer patients with micrometastatic disease in bone marrow. Patients in this study were randomized to receive daily clodronate for 2 years or standard of care follow-up. At a median follow-up of 3 years, there was a significant reduction in the incidence of distant metastases, bone and visceral metastases as well as a significant survival advantage in patients in the clodronate arm [7].

Subsequently, results from a large double-blind multicenter trial of 1069 patients with EBC showed that patients treated with 2 years of clodronate had a 41 % reduction in the risk of developing bone metastases at 5 years ($P=0.043$) and a 23 % reduction in death with a median follow-up of 5.6 years ($P=0.048$). Interestingly the majority of patients enrolled in this trial were postmenopausal (61–64 %) [8].

However, results from these 2 early studies were contradicted by a Finnish study which enrolled 299 women with axillary node positive breast cancer and randomized them to either adjuvant clodronate for 3 years or control. At 10 years follow-up, Disease-free survival (DFS) was significantly lower in the clodronate arm (50 %) versus patients in the control arm (64 %; P = 0.004). Postmenopausal, ER positive women were the only subgroup not to have a negative effect from 3 years of clodronate treatment [9].

Data from the National Surgical Adjuvant Breast and Bowel Project protocol B-34 (NSABP-34) showed no DFS or overall survival (OS) benefit in patients treated with clodronate for 3 years, however subgroup analyses showed women 50 years or older treated in the clodronate arm had superior recurrence-free interval (P = 0.045), bone metastasis-free interval (P = 0.027) and non-bone metastasis-free interval (P = 0.014) compared to placebo [10].

Oral ibandronate was explored in the German adjuvant intergroup node-positive (GAIN) study: 3023 in which patients with early stage node positive breast cancer considered suitable for dose-dense chemotherapy were randomly assigned 1:1 to oral ibandronate 50 mg per day for 2 years versus observation. Similarly to the NSABP-34 results, patients on the ibandronate arm did not have a DFS or OS benefit compared to the observation arm. However, a trend towards improved DFS was observed in younger patients (<40) who had chemotherapy induced menopause or who had received ovarian suppression with LHRH treatment, and in postmenopausal patients (>60) [11].

Findings suggesting adjuvant bisphosphonates are beneficial in a "low estrogen" environment were strengthened by the ABCSG-12 trial, which showed that twice yearly intravenous zoledronate (ZA) in premenopausal women receiving ovarian suppression with LHRH treatment resulted in a 32 % improvement in DFS (P = 0.009) [12]. Similarly, the AZURE trial showed ZA reduced the risk of developing bone metastases and improved disease outcomes in women with established menopause (more than 5 years postmenopausal) [13]. Although designed to investigate the efficacy of ZA in preventing therapy-induced bone loss in postmenopausal women with hormone receptor positive EBC, the ZO-FAST trial showed an improvement in DFS and OS rates with up-front therapy in patients older than 60 years or more than 5 years post-menopausal [14].

These results suggest adjuvant bisphosphonates may be of clinical benefit and led The Early Breast Cancer Trialists' Collaborative Group (EBCTCG) to conduct a meta-analysis to clarify whether adjuvant bisphosphonates reduced the risk of bone and other metastases, and whether menopausal status affected efficacy. The study analyzed individual patient data from 26 trials including 18,766 women (11,767 of whom were post-menopausal) with early breast cancer who were randomized to bisphosphonates or a control group with no bisphosphonate. Taking all women together, regardless of menopausal status, the meta-analyses found a highly significant reduction only in bone recurrence, and not in other breast cancer outcomes. However subset analysis showed that the absolute reduction with bisphosphonate use in postmenopausal women at 10 years was 3.0 % for breast cancer recurrence, 3.4 % for distant recurrence, 2.2 % for bone recurrence and 3.3 % for breast cancer related mortality [15].

## Aspirin

Aspirin inhibits the enzyme cyclooxygenase (COX) that is responsible for the formation of prostanoids which are involved in the inflammatory response. Aspirin inhibits both isoforms of enzyme cyclooxygenase COX 1 and COX 2, although it preferentially inhibits COX 2 [16]. COX 2 synthesizes large amounts of prostaglandin E2 which stimulates tumor angiogenesis and proliferation, promotes inflammation and thrombosis and inhibits apoptosis and immune response [16, 17]. High concentrations of prostaglandins have been found in cancers compared with the surrounding normal tissues, supporting the hypothesis that prostaglandins might promote tumor growth and invasion [18]. As well as inhibiting COX, aspirin may act directly with other molecules and pathways implicated in tumor genesis [19, 20].

Individual patient data meta-analyses of randomized controlled trials primarily designed to assess the cardiovascular benefits of aspirin showed significant reductions in cancer incidence and cancer mortality associated with regular aspirin use (>3 years) in both the short and long term [21–23]. In addition, an updated analysis of observational studies on aspirin and cancer risk showed that the relative risk of developing breast cancer in aspirin users was 0.83 (95 % CI 0.76–0.91) in 10 case-control studies, and 0.93 (95 % CI 0.87–1.00) in 22 cohort studies [24].

ADD-ASPIRIN a phase III, multi-center, double-blind, placebo-controlled randomized trial will assess the effects of aspirin on disease recurrence and survival after primary therapy in common non-metastatic solid tumors. This study is currently recruiting patients in four tumor site specific cohorts: breast, colorectal, gastro esophageal and prostate cancer. Patients will be randomized after a run-in period in a 1:1:1 ratio to either 100 mg aspirin, 300 mg aspirin or a matched placebo orally for 5 years. The co primary endpoint will be overall survival and invasive disease-free survival for the breast cohort. The secondary endpoints in all patients will include adherence, toxicity including hemorrhage, cardiovascular events and some tumor site-specific secondary outcome measures. (www.Add-aspirintrial.org).

## Metformin

In recent years, there has been a growing interest in examining the role of metformin as an anti-cancer drug. Preclinical studies show that metformin can inhibit the growth of cancer cells by modulating several molecular pathways either directly or through downstream targets [25]. The key mechanism of action of metformin is thought to be mediated via activation of adenosine monophosphate-activated protein kinase (AMPK) which inhibits the mammalian target of rapamycin (mTOR) pathway responsible for cell growth and proliferation. Metformin may also act indirectly through inhibition of the insulin/IGF-1 signaling pathway resulting in reduced tumor cell growth. In addition, metformin may have immune modulatory properties enhancing T cell mediated immune response to tumor antigens [24, 26].

Data from observational studies has shown that diabetic patients treated with metformin have reduced breast cancer risk and better cancer related outcomes [27, 28]. A retrospective study of patients who received neoadjuvant chemotherapy for breast cancer showed that diabetic cancer patients receiving metformin during their chemotherapy had a higher pathological complete response rate than diabetic patients not receiving metformin (24 % versus 8 %, P = 0.007) [29]. Results from a recent meta-analysis performed on 37 studies, with a total of 1,535,636 patients comparing metformin users and non-users reported overall cancer incidence summary relative risk (SRR) as 0.73 and a 6 % reduction in breast cancer incidence [30].

So far, no trial has provided any data on survival benefit with the use of metformin in breast cancer but the phase III Randomized double-blind Trial of Metformin versus Placebo in Early stage Breast cancer MA-32 trial is addressing this question and results are expected in a few years' time (https://clinicaltrial.gov/ct2/show/NCT01101438).

## Everolimus

The phosphatidylinositol-3-kinase/protein kinase B/mammalian target of rapamycin (PI3K-AKT-mTOR) pathway is one of the main pathways that regulates cell regulation, growth and metabolism [31]. Dysregulation of this pathway is frequently observed in tumors and hyperactivation has been linked with disease progression and treatment resistance. In breast cancer the PI3K/Akt/mTOR pathway is important in the sensitivity of breast cancer cells to endocrine therapy [32]. Resistance of cancer cells to endocrine, cytotoxic and HER-2 targeted therapy can be developed through activation of the PI3K/Akt/mTOR pathway [33, 34]. Everolimus is an oral mTOR inhibitor with antitumor activity in preclinical models [35] and subsequent efficacy in clinical trials. It is approved both in Europe and USA for the treatment of ER positive HER-2 negative advanced breast cancer in combination with exemestane in patients resistant to non-steroidal aromatase inhibitors, based on the BOLERO-2 trial results [36].

Two large phase III trials will evaluate the role of everolimus in the adjuvant setting. In the **UNIRAD** trial premenopausal and postmenopausal women with ER positive HER-2 negative disease and at least 4 lymph nodes at diagnosis will receive routine adjuvant endocrine therapy. Patients still disease-free at 2 years will be then randomized to everolimus or placebo for 2 years in addition to hormone therapy. The primary endpoint is disease-free survival at 2 years post-randomization, and secondary endpoints include overall survival and biomarker assessments. In the United States, the SWOG trial S1207 will evaluate the addition of 1 year of everolimus to standard endocrine therapy in high risk patients (https://clinicaltrial.gov/ct2/show/NCT01805271).

## PARP Inhibitors

The poly (ADP-ribose) polymerases (PARPs) are a family of enzymes involved in various cellular processes. The most abundant of these multifunctional enzymes, PARP1 plays a key role in the repair of DNA single-strand breaks through the repair of base excisions [37]. When PARP is inhibited, double strand DNA breaks (DSBs) accumulate and under normal conditions are repaired via the BRCA pathway-dependent homologous recombination (HR) mechanism [38]. The simultaneous inhibition of these two major repair pathways, HR and PARP, causes loss of DNA integrity and cell death whereas inhibition of either one of the two pathways alone does not, due to adequate function of the alternative repair mechanism [38]. The dysfunction of BRCA1 or BRCA2 tumor suppressor proteins results in lack of homologous recombination and sensitization of cancer cells to PARP inhibition [39, 40]. In addition, inhibition of PARP acts synergistically with DNA damaging chemotherapeutics and many trials have tested this hypothesis in preclinical and clinical setting [41].

In Breast cancer, PARP inhibitors have been tested in BRCA mutated tumors as well as in triple negative breast cancer (TNBC) subtype where molecular and pathologic features resemble BRCA1 related breast cancers [42]. In a phase II trial olaparib was administered to women with BRCA1 and/or BRCA2 deficient advanced breast cancer with overall response rate of 41 % and Progression Free Survival (PFS) of 5.7 months [43]. Toxicities were mainly of low grade with the most frequent adverse events being fatigue, mild to moderate nausea, vomiting and anemia.

A few phase II and phase III trials are currently investigating the efficacy of PARP inhibitors in earlier stages [44]. The randomized, double-blind placebo controlled multicenter, phase III **Olympia** trial will assess the efficacy and safety of adjuvant therapy with olaparib versus placebo in patients with high-risk HER2-negative primary breast cancer and germ line *BRCA*-mutations, who have completed definitive local and systemic neoadjuvant (without pcR) or adjuvant treatment. The primary end point of the trial will be invasive disease free survival, and the secondary end points are overall survival, distant-disease-free survival and the development of new primary invasive cancers [43]. Recruitment began in April 2014 and the results are eagerly awaited.

## Conclusion

Compelling evidence from the Early Breast Cancer Trialists' Collaborative Group meta-analyses shows that adjuvant bisphosphonate use for 2–5 years in postmenopausal women significantly reduces the risk of bone recurrence and significantly improves overall survival. Given the favorable toxicity profile of these drugs, a change of standard practice has been advocated and efforts are currently underway to commission the use of adjuvant bisphosphonates in the UK. Future research should aim to define whether late intervention of adjuvant bisphosphonates would be of benefit.

Aspirin and metformin may prove to be effective adjuvant therapies which could benefit patients worldwide and have a huge impact on global cancer burden. However, until the results of the prospective randomized trials of these agents are known the drugs remain experimental for this indication.

Targeted therapies such as Evorilimus and PARP inhibitors are also being testing in randomized trials in early breast cancer the results are eagerly awaited.

The treatment landscape in early breast cancer is evolving beyond standard cytotoxic and hormone therapies. The history of adjuvant therapy in breast cancer has been one of small incremental gains and the agents discussed in this chapter are part of this evolving story.

## References


1. Mathew A, Brufsky A. Decreased risk of breast cancer associated with oral bisphosphonate therapy. Breast Cancer (Dove Med Press). 2012;4:75–81.
2. Mathew A, Brufsky A. Bisphosphonates in breast cancer. Int J Cancer. 2015;137(4):753–64.
3. Tabane K, Vorobiof DA. Bone targeted therapies in early breast cancer. Curr Treat Options Oncol. 2011;12(4):412–23.
4. Coleman RE. Skeletal complications of malignancy. Cancer. 1997;80(8 Suppl):1588–94.
5. Bidard FC, et al. Disseminated tumor cells of breast cancer patients: a strong prognostic factor for distant and local relapse. Clin Cancer Res. 2008;14(11):3306–11.
6. Santini D, et al. Bisphosphonates as anticancer agents in early breast cancer: preclinical and clinical evidence. Breast Cancer Res. 2015;17(1):121.
7. Diel IJ, et al. Adjuvant oral clodronate improves the overall survival of primary breast cancer patients with micrometastases to the bone marrow: a long-term follow-up. Ann Oncol. 2008;19(12):2007–11.
8. Powles T, et al. Randomized, placebo-controlled trial of clodronate in patients with primary operable breast cancer. J Clin Oncol. 2002;20(15):3219–24.
9. Saarto T, et al. Ten-year follow-up of a randomized controlled trial of adjuvant clodronate treatment in node-positive breast cancer patients. Acta Oncol. 2004;43(7):650–6.
10. Paterson AH, et al. Oral clodronate for adjuvant treatment of operable breast cancer (National Surgical Adjuvant Breast and Bowel Project protocol B-34): a multicentre, placebo-controlled, randomised trial. Lancet Oncol. 2012;13(7):734–42.
11. von Minckwitz G, et al. German adjuvant intergroup node-positive study: a phase III trial to compare oral ibandronate versus observation in patients with high-risk early breast cancer. J Clin Oncol. 2013;31(28):3531–9.
12. Gnant M, et al. Zoledronic acid combined with adjuvant endocrine therapy of tamoxifen versus anastrozol plus ovarian function suppression in premenopausal early breast cancer: final analysis of the Austrian Breast and Colorectal Cancer Study Group Trial 12. Ann Oncol. 2015;26(2):313–20.
13. Coleman R, et al. Adjuvant zoledronic acid in patients with early breast cancer: final efficacy analysis of the AZURE (BIG 01/04) randomised open-label phase 3 trial. Lancet Oncol. 2014;15(9):997–1006.
14. Coleman R, et al. Zoledronic acid (zoledronate) for postmenopausal women with early breast cancer receiving adjuvant letrozole (ZO-FAST study): final 60-month results. Ann Oncol. 2013;24(2):398–405.
15. Early Breast Cancer Trialists' Collaborative G, et al. Adjuvant bisphosphonate treatment in early breast cancer: meta-analyses of individual patient data from randomised trials. Lancet. 2015;386(10001):1353–61.

16. Simmons DL, Botting RM, Hla T. Cyclooxygenase isozymes: the biology of prostaglandin synthesis and inhibition. Pharmacol Rev. 2004;56(3):387–437.
17. Ulrich CM, Bigler J, Potter JD. Non-steroidal anti-inflammatory drugs for cancer prevention: promise, perils and pharmacogenetics. Nat Rev Cancer. 2006;6(2):130–40.
18. Easty GC, Easty DM. Prostaglandins and cancer. Cancer Treat Rev. 1976;3(4):217–25.
19. Martinez ME, et al. Pronounced reduction in adenoma recurrence associated with aspirin use and a polymorphism in the ornithine decarboxylase gene. Proc Natl Acad Sci U S A. 2003;100(13):7859–64.
20. Jankowski JA, Anderson M. Review article: management of oesophageal adenocarcinoma – control of acid, bile and inflammation in intervention strategies for Barrett's oesophagus. Aliment Pharmacol Ther. 2004;20 Suppl 5:71–80; discussion 95–6.
21. Rothwell PM, et al. Long-term effect of aspirin on colorectal cancer incidence and mortality: 20-year follow-up of five randomised trials. Lancet. 2010;376(9754):1741–50.
22. Rothwell PM, et al. Effect of daily aspirin on long-term risk of death due to cancer: analysis of individual patient data from randomised trials. Lancet. 2011;377(9759):31–41.
23. Rothwell PM, et al. Short-term effects of daily aspirin on cancer incidence, mortality, and non-vascular death: analysis of the time course of risks and benefits in 51 randomised controlled trials. Lancet. 2012;379(9826):1602–12.
24. Eikawa S, et al. Immune-mediated antitumor effect by type 2 diabetes drug, metformin. Proc Natl Acad Sci U S A. 2015;112(6):1809–14.
25. Ben Sahra I, et al. The antidiabetic drug metformin exerts an antitumoral effect in vitro and in vivo through a decrease of cyclin D1 level. Oncogene. 2008;27(25):3576–86.
26. Pearce EL, et al. Enhancing CD8 T-cell memory by modulating fatty acid metabolism. Nature. 2009;460(7251):103–7.
27. Noto H, et al. Cancer risk in diabetic patients treated with metformin: a systematic review and meta-analysis. PLoS One. 2012;7(3):e33411.
28. Col NF, et al. Metformin and breast cancer risk: a meta-analysis and critical literature review. Breast Cancer Res Treat. 2012;135(3):639–46.
29. Jiralerspong S, et al. Metformin and pathologic complete responses to neoadjuvant chemotherapy in diabetic patients with breast cancer. J Clin Oncol. 2009;27(20):3297–302.
30. Zhang P, et al. Association of metformin use with cancer incidence and mortality: a meta-analysis. Cancer Epidemiol. 2013;37(3):207–18.
31. Shaw RJ, Cantley LC. Ras, PI(3)K and mTOR signalling controls tumour cell growth. Nature. 2006;441(7092):424–30.
32. Perez-Tenorio G, Stal O, Southeast Sweden Breast Cancer Group. Activation of AKT/PKB in breast cancer predicts a worse outcome among endocrine treated patients. Br J Cancer. 2002;86(4):540–5.
33. Beeram M, et al. Akt-induced endocrine therapy resistance is reversed by inhibition of mTOR signaling. Ann Oncol. 2007;18(8):1323–8.
34. Bender LM, Nahta R. Her2 cross talk and therapeutic resistance in breast cancer. Front Biosci. 2008;13:3906–12.
35. Tanaka C, et al. Identifying optimal biologic doses of everolimus (RAD001) in patients with cancer based on the modeling of preclinical and clinical pharmacokinetic and pharmacodynamic data. J Clin Oncol. 2008;26(10):1596–602.
36. Baselga J, et al. Everolimus in postmenopausal hormone-receptor-positive advanced breast cancer. N Engl J Med. 2012;366(6):520–9.
37. Ame JC, Spenlehauer C, de Murcia G. The PARP superfamily. Bioessays. 2004;26(8):882–93.
38. Tentori L, Graziani G. Chemopotentiation by PARP inhibitors in cancer therapy. Pharmacol Res. 2005;52(1):25–33.
39. Bryant HE, et al. Specific killing of BRCA2-deficient tumours with inhibitors of poly (ADP-ribose) polymerase. Nature. 2005;434(7035):913–7.
40. Farmer H, et al. Targeting the DNA repair defect in BRCA mutant cells as a therapeutic strategy. Nature. 2005;434(7035):917–21.

41. O'Shaughnessy J, et al. Phase III study of iniparib plus gemcitabine and carboplatin versus gemcitabine and carboplatin in patients with metastatic triple-negative breast cancer. J Clin Oncol. 2014;32(34):3840–7.
42. Lips EH, et al. Triple-negative breast cancer: BRCAness and concordance of clinical features with BRCA1-mutation carriers. Br J Cancer. 2013;108(10):2172–7.
43. Tutt A, et al. Oral poly(ADP-ribose) polymerase inhibitor olaparib in patients with BRCA1 or BRCA2 mutations and advanced breast cancer: a proof-of-concept trial. Lancet. 2010;376(9737):235–44.
44. Sonnenblick A, et al. An update on PARP inhibitors – moving to the adjuvant setting. Nat Rev Clin Oncol. 2015;12(1):27–41.

# Chapter 8
# Exercise in Breast Cancer Survivors

**Nawa Mustafa Amin and Alistair Ring**

**Abstract** Epidemiological studies have shown that regular exercise reduces the risks of cardiovascular and cerebrovascular disease. As a result the UK Chief Medical Officer recommends that the population aged between 19 and 64 years should take 150 min of moderate intensity exercise in bouts of 10 min or more every week. There are a number of biological mechanisms by which exercise might be expected to be particularly beneficial in women with breast cancer. These mechanisms suggest that physical activity might have the potential to prevent primary breast cancer, reduce the risk of recurrence in women with a prior diagnosis of early breast cancer, and improve overall survival following a breast cancer diagnosis. This chapter discusses the clinical evidence from non-randomized studies that exercise can improve survival outcomes in women with a prior diagnosis of early breast cancer. The other potential health benefits of exercise in breast cancer survivors are also discussed, including the impacts on bone health, cancer-related fatigue and adherence to endocrine therapy.

**Keywords** Physical activity • Exercise • Breast cancer

## Introduction

Epidemiological studies suggest that people who take regular exercise have a lower risk of developing type II diabetes, cardiovascular disease, and cerebrovascular disease, including vascular dementia [1]. Consequently, the UK Chief Medical Officer recommends that the UK population aged between 19 and 64 years should take 150 min of moderate intensity exercise in bouts of 10 min or more every week.

---

N.M. Amin, BSc (Hons), MSc, MBBS, MRCP (✉)
The Royal Marsden NHS Foundation Trust, Surrey, UK
e-mail: Nawa.amin@rmh.nhs.uk; noamin80@hotmail.com

A. Ring, MA, FRCP, MD
Breast Unit, Royal Marsden Hospital, London, UK



A. Ring, M. Parton (eds.), *Breast Cancer Survivorship*,
DOI 10.1007/978-3-319-41858-2_8

**Table 8.1** The recommendations for exercise in adults 19–64 and ≥65 years

| Regimen | Recommended activities |
|---|---|
| A | At least 150 min of moderate aerobic activity e.g. cycling or fast walking every week, **and**<br>Strength exercises on ≥2 days a week that work all the major muscles (legs, hips, back, abdomen, chest, shoulders and arms) |
| | **OR** |
| B | 75 min of vigorous aerobic activity e.g. running or a game of singles tennis every week, **and**<br>Strength exercises on ≥2 days a week that work all the major muscles (legs, hips, back, abdomen, chest, shoulders and arms). |
| | **OR** |
| C | A mix of moderate and vigorous aerobic activity every week e.g. two 30-min runs plus 30 min of fast walking equates to 150 min of moderate aerobic activity, **and**<br>Strength exercises on ≥2 days a week that work all the major muscles (legs, hips, back, abdomen, chest, shoulders and arms) |

One suggested approach is to carry out 30 min of moderate intensity activity per day, five days per week. Additionally, it is recommended that muscle strengthening activities are performed on two or more days per week. Similar guidelines are available for older adults (aged 65 and older) [1] (Tables 8.1 and 8.2). Whilst this is national guidance, it is evident that a significant proportion of the population do not take this level of exercise on a regular basis [2].

There are a number of biological mechanisms by which exercise might be expected to be beneficial in women with breast cancer including effects of physical activity on sex hormones, insulin and insulin-like growth factors (IGFs) as well as other obesity-related factors (e.g. adipokines, inflammation) and immune function [3, 4]. These mechanisms suggest that physical activity might have the potential to prevent primary breast cancer, reduce the risk of recurrence in women with a prior diagnosis of early breast cancer, and improve overall survival following a breast cancer diagnosis.

This chapter addresses whether women who have had a diagnosis of early breast cancer should specifically be encouraged to undertake physical exercise, and if they do, what benefits they might derive.

## Exercise and Breast Cancer Outcomes

In a 2014 meta-analysis of 16 prospective studies of breast cancer survivors it was found that physical activity was associated with lower risk of breast cancer mortality [5]. Amongst breast cancer survivors high versus low pre-diagnosis physical activity was associated with decreased risk of overall mortality and breast cancer mortality. The summary relative risks (RRs) of overall and breast cancer mortality were 0.77 [95% confidence interval (CI)=0.69–0.88] and 0.77 (95% CI=0.66–0.90, respectively). Furthermore, high versus low post-diagnosis physical activity was also associated with

**Table 8.2** Intensity in 19–64 years and ≥65 years

| Intensity | 19–64 years | ≥65 years |
|---|---|---|
| Moderate | Walking fast<br>Water aerobics<br>Riding a bike on level ground or with few hills<br>Doubles tennis<br>Pushing a lawn mower | Walking<br>Water aerobics<br>Riding a bike on level ground or with few hills<br>Doubles tennis<br>Pushing a lawn mower |
| | Hiking<br>Volleyball<br>Skateboarding<br>Rollerblading<br>Basketball | Ballroom and line dancing<br>Volleyball<br>Canoeing |
| Vigorous | Jogging or running<br>Swimming fast<br>Aerobics<br>Riding a bike fast or on hills<br>Singles tennis<br>Football<br>Martial arts | Jogging or running<br>Swimming fast<br>Aerobics<br>Riding a bike fast or on hills<br>Singles tennis<br>Football<br>Martial arts |
| | Rugby<br>Skipping rope<br>Hockey<br>Gymnastics | Hiking uphill<br>Energetic dancing |

Individual physical and mental capabilities should be considered when interpreting the guidelines. Daily chores such as shopping, cooking or housework do not count towards the recommended 150 min as the effort is not enough to raise heart rate. However, they are important as they break up periods of sitting with light activity which is important. Generally, 1 min of vigorous activity provides the same health benefits as 2 min of moderate activity. Seventy-five minutes of vigorous activity can give similar health benefits to 150 min of moderate activity

decreased overall and breast cancer mortality. For post-diagnosis physical activity, the summary RRs of overall and breast cancer mortality were 0.52 (95 % CI=0.42–0.64) and 0.72 (95 % CI=0.60–0.85), respectively. Each 10 metabolic equivalent task-hour/week increase in post-diagnosis physical activity (equivalent to current recommendations of 150 min/week of at least moderate intensity activity) was associated with 24 % (95 % CI=11–36 %) decreased total mortality risk among breast cancer survivors. Breast cancer survivors who increased their physical activity by any level from pre- to post-diagnosis showed decreased total mortality risk (RR=0.61; 95 % CI=0.46–0.80) compared with those who did not change their physical activity level or were inactive/insufficiently active before diagnosis. The authors concluded that physical activity following a diagnosis of breast cancer was associated with reduced mortality risk. A key question is whether this association is causative.

The Nurses' Health Study was a prospective observational study conducted in nearly 3000 female nurses in the US who were diagnosed with stage I-III breast cancer between 1984 and 1998 [6]. The women were followed up until death or June 2002. Nurses enrolled in this study answered a number of questions about lifestyle, diet, medication use and one item on the questionnaire regarded physical activity. In one analysis of the Nurses' Health Study, breast cancer mortality was analyzed with respect levels of physical activity. Weekly physical activity was converted into metabolic equivalent Task (MET). A MET is approximately equivalent to the energy cost of sitting at rest, and activities are assigned a MET score depending on their intensity. Participants were defined according to their physical activity category: <3, 3–8.9, 9–14.9, 15–23.9, or ≥24 MET hours per week [6]. Three MET-hours is equivalent to walking at average pace of 2–2.9 mph for 1 h.

Compared with women who engaged in less than 3 MET-hours per week of physical activity, the adjusted relative risk (RR) of death from breast cancer was 0.80 (95 % confidence interval [CI], 0.60–1.06) for 3–8.9 MET-hours per week; 0.50 (95 % CI, 0.31–0.82) for 9–14.9 MET-hours per week; 0.56 (95 % CI, 0.38–0.84) for 15–23.9 MET-hours per week; and 0.60 (95 % CI, 0.40–0.89) for 24 or more MET-hours per week (P for trend = .004). The benefit of physical activity was particularly apparent among women with hormone-receptor positive tumors. The RR of breast cancer death for women with hormone-receptor positive tumors who engaged in 9 or more MET-hours per week of activity compared with women with hormone-receptor positive tumors who engaged in less than 9 MET-hours per week was 0.50 (95 % CI, 0.34–0.74). Compared with women who engaged in less than 3 MET-hours per week of activity, the absolute unadjusted mortality risk reduction was 6 % at 10 years for women who engaged in 9 or more MET-hours per week [6]. This apparent benefit of physical activity remained significant when adjusted for age, body mass index, menopausal status, hormone receptor status, disease stage and chemotherapy use.

These data from the meta-analysis including the Nurses' Health Study are from un-randomized observational studies and it is possible that some of the findings are confounded by factors which have not been taken into consideration. The question as to whether exercise definitively improves breast cancer outcomes would require a randomized trial and it seems unlikely that such a trial would be undertaken given the obvious population health benefits of the intervention under consideration (such that all women should be recommended to take exercise anyway regardless of breast cancer benefits) and of course the complexity of delivering and ethically controlling such a trial. Furthermore the benefits of exercise even in breast cancer survivors may not be restricted to benefits in terms of breast cancer recurrence.

## Exercise and Additional Health Benefits in Breast Cancer Survivors

### *Depression and Mood*

Depression and other mood disorders are not uncommonly associated with a diagnosis of early breast cancer (Chap. 19) and given the potential positive effects of physical activity on depression in the general population, the additional benefits in breast cancer survivors are an attractive concept. In a 2011 systematic review and meta-analysis of fifteen RCTs, it was found that exercise produced modest effects on depression in cancer survivors across cancer types (primarily breast), stages (predominantly early stage) and baseline severity of depressive symptoms (most were not depressed) [7]. The overall effect size, under a random effects model, was −0.22 (CI −0.43, −0.09, $p=0.04$). Significant moderating variables ($p<0.05$) were exercise location, exercise supervision, and exercise duration. The authors concluded that exercise had modest positive effects on depressive symptoms with larger effects for programs that were supervised or partially supervised, not performed at home, and at least 30 min in duration. Limitations included that only one study identified depression as the primary endpoint [7].

## *Cancer-Related Fatigue*

Cancer related fatigue is one of the most commonly reported symptoms by cancer survivors [8]. Fatigue has been reported as a side effect of all types of cancer treatment [9], impacting almost all cancer survivors and sometimes continuing to be problematic for years after completion of treatment ([10, 11], Chapter 20). The suggestion that exercise may have a useful role in reducing fatigue is of great interest considering that cancer survivors have reported fatigue to be a more distressing than other symptoms related to cancer or its treatment including pain, nausea, and vomiting [12–14].

Brown et al. investigated the efficacy of exercise in reducing cancer related fatigue in a meta-analysis of 44 RCTs including 3254 participants. Overall they concluded that exercise reduced fatigue among cancer survivors when compared to controls. Furthermore, fatigue levels improved in direct proportion to the intensity of resistance exercise ($\beta=0.60$, $P=0.01$), and was reduced to a greater extent in older cancer survivors ($\beta=0.24$, $P=0.04$) [15].

## *Quality of Life*

Cancer and its treatment can have a negative impact on quality of life (QOL) [16]. QOL incorporates physical, emotional, and social well-being [17]. One meta-analysis of 78 studies and 3629 participants explored the efficacy of exercise in improving QOL in cancer survivors and found that exercise had a positive and significant effect on the QOL of cancer survivors. The authors also found that interventions were especially successful in women and when the aim was intense aerobic exercise [18].

## *Impact of Exercise on Bone Health*

Bone health is particularly important in breast cancer survivors as treatment may increase the risk of osteoporosis and fractures (Chap. 14). Estrogens play a key role in bone protection and reduced levels (as a result of chemotherapy, endocrine therapy or surgery) may contribute to bone loss. Nutrition, including vitamin D and calcium supplementation (Chap. 9), smoking cessation and medication, including bisphosphonates are important osteoporosis management strategies in the general population as well as breast cancer survivors. However weight-bearing exercises, such as walking, climbing stairs, weight training and dancing, may also help prevent bone loss and may be an additional reason to encourage physical activity in breast cancer survivors [19].

Peppone et al. conducted a pilot study looking at Tai Chi Chuan (TCC), a moderate form of weight-bearing exercise equivalent to walking, which improves aerobic capacity and strength among breast cancer survivors [20]. They randomly assigned 16 breast cancer survivors to TCC (3 times per week, 60 min per session for 12 weeks) or standard support therapy (exercise control). Serum levels of *N*-telopeptides of type I collagen (NTx), a marker of bone resorption, and bone-specific alkaline phosphatise (BSAP), a marker of bone formation, were measured at baseline and after the intervention. Survivors in the TCC group had a greater increase in levels of bone formation and a significant decrease in bone resorption compared with the control group. This pilot study suggested that weight-bearing exercise exerts positive effects on bone loss through increased bone formation and decreased bone resorption in breast cancer survivors [20]. Other small studies have demonstrated the apparent benefits of resistance training on bone densitometry [21]. Winters-Stone et al., conducted a randomized, controlled trial in 106 postmenopausal women with early stage breast cancer who had completed adjuvant chemotherapy and/or radiotherapy [22]. Patients were required to be free from osteoporosis and were randomly assigned to participate in 1 year of three times-weekly progressive, moderate-intensity resistance and impact exercise or in a similar frequency and length control program of progressive, low-intensity stretching. Women who were assigned to the resistance and impact training program preserved bone mineral density at the lumbar spine (0.47 vs. –2.13 %; $P=0.001$) and had lower markers of bone turnover compared with controls. Whilst long-term follow-up studies and documentation of improvements in clinically relevant fracture rates have not been demonstrated in large populations of breast cancer survivors, the benefits of exercise on bone health in the non-cancer population are likely to be replicable in breast cancer survivors.

## *Adherence to Endocrine Therapy*

Up to 50 % of breast cancer survivors who are taking aromatase inhibitors (AI) suffer from arthralgia, which may contribute to non-adherence and discontinuation rates of up to 20 % in the first year of use [23–25]. In the HOPE (Hormones and Physical Exercise) study, breast cancer survivors who had been taking an AI for at least 6 months and reported ≥3 of 10 for worst joint pain on the Brief Pain Inventory (BPI) were randomly assigned to an exercise intervention or usual care for 1 year [26]. The exercise intervention comprised 150 min/week of moderate-intensity aerobic exercise and twice-weekly supervised resistance exercise sessions. One hundred and twenty-one women were randomized and it was found that AI-associated arthralgia symptoms worsened over time in women randomly assigned to usual care (according to BPI and other measures). However in those women assigned to exercise, worst pain scores reduced by approximately 29 % or 1.6 points. On average, pain scores in women randomly assigned to exercise decreased from moderate at baseline to mild at the end of intervention period (BPI worst pain score of approximately 6 to 4 points). Women randomly assigned to exercise also experienced increase in cardiorespiratory fitness, upper and lower body strength and losses in body weight [26]. Given the impact of arthralgia on quality of life, and the long term impact of AI non-adherence on breast cancer outcomes [27], exercise has the potential to provide a substantial health benefit to women with AI-associated arthralgia.

## Levels of Physical Activity in Breast Cancer Survivors

The data discussed in the preceding sections provides some evidence that exercise might be beneficial in breast cancer survivors. However, perhaps one of the biggest challenges is in encouraging and enabling women to take the prescribed levels of physical activity. Zhao et al. examined the prevalence of lifestyle-related risk factors among 7443 women aged ≥18 years and reported a prevalence estimate of 53.8 % for engaging in physical activity ≥150 min/week [28]. Those women answering questionnaires may of course tend to be those who are more aware and engaged with lifestyle factors and therefore this study may over-estimate the levels of physical activity.

The HEAL study demonstrated declines in physical activity, by an estimated 2 h per week and 11 % ($P < 0.05$), following a diagnosis of early breast cancer. A 50 % decrease in physical activity was observed among women who were treated with radiation and chemotherapy and a 23 % ($P < 0.05$) decrease in those who were treated with radiation only [29]. Therefore not only are many women not taking the recommended levels of exercise following a diagnosis of breast cancer, but levels of exercise may actually decline. The reasons for this are likely to be multifactorial and there is clear evidence that an intervention is warranted.

## Interventions to Increase Levels of Physical Activity

Successful interventions to increase levels of activity in breast cancer survivors will need to provide counseling to explain the justification for the recommendations, as well as practical advice and encouragement to enable patients to exercise more in a sustainable manner.

In one randomized controlled trial breast cancer survivors were assigned either to usual care or 12 weeks of a home based walking intervention. The intervention was a single 30 min face-to-face counseling session followed by five 15 min telephone counseling sessions. Patients were instructed to increase walking frequency, duration and intensity. Physical activity was recorded by pedometers. Adherence was 94 % and those undergoing the intervention reported significantly increased levels of physical activity compared with those undergoing usual care [30]. There are a number of other examples of bespoke physical activity interventions for cancer survivors [31, 32] although an important aspect will be whether the lifestyle changes made will be sustainable over time. A number of studies are ongoing to attempt to identify the optimal means by which to increase exercise behavior in breast cancer survivors. However in the meantime, given the recommendations for breast cancer survivors are no different to those of the general population, it may be appropriate to simply signpost patients to existing Department Health/NHS England initiatives to increase physical activity [33] with the emphasis to women that the recommendations have particular relevance given their previous breast cancer.

## Conclusions

There is evidence to suggest that breast cancer survivors who take more physical exercise have lower risks of breast cancer recurrence, and may experience a number of additional health benefits. There is no randomized clinical trial evidence, but such a trial would be methodologically and ethically challenging to conduct. Furthermore these apparent benefits are in addition to the well-established benefits of exercise in terms of cardiovascular and cerebrovascular disease which remain relevant to breast cancer survivors many of whom will die from competing causes of mortality and not breast cancer. Therefore breast cancer survivors should be recommended to take regular exercise along the lines for current guidelines for the general population (Tables 8.1 and 8.2). In the longer term, ongoing studies may identify specific bespoke interventions which are more suited to the needs and abilities of breast cancer survivors, to enhance adherence and sustainability of lifestyle change.

## References

1. Department of Health. Physical activity guidelines for Adults, NHS choices. Available at: http://www.nhs.uk/Livewell/fitness/Pages/physical-activity-guidelines-for-adults.aspx. Access verified 7 Apr 2016.
2. Office for National Statistics. Measuring national well-being: life in the UK, 2015. Available at: http://www.ons.gov.uk/peoplepopulationandcommunity/wellbeing/articles/measuringnationalwellbeing/2016. Access verified 7 Apr 2016.
3. McTiernan A. Mechanisms linking physical activity with cancer. Nat Rev Cancer. 2008; 8:205–11.
4. Neilson HK, Friedenreich CM, Brockton NT, et al. Physical axtivity and postmenopausal breast cancer; proposed biological mechanisms and areas for future research. Cancer Epidemiol Biomarkers Prev. 2009;18:11–27.

5. Schmid D, Leitzmann MF. Association between physical activity and mortality among breast cancer and colorectal cancer survivors: a systematic review and meta-analysis. Ann Oncol. 2014;25:1293–311.
6. Holmes MD, Chen WY, Feskanich D, Kroenke CH, Colditz GA. Physical activity and survival after breast cancer diagnosis. JAMA. 2005;293:2479–86.
7. Craft LL, Vanlterson EH, Helenowski IB, Rademaker AW, Courneya KS. Exercise effects on depressive symptoms in cancer survivors: a systemic review and meta-analysis. Cancer Epidemiol Biomarkers Prev. 2012;21(1):3–19.
8. National Comprehensive Cancer Network Clinical practice guidelines in oncology. Cancer-related fatigue. J Natl Compr Cancer Netw. 2010; 8:904–31.
9. Schmitz KH, Courneya KS, Mathews C, Denmark-Wahnefriend W, Galvao DA, Pinto BM, Irwin ML, Wolin KY, Segal RJ, Lucia A, Schneider CM, von Gruenigen VE, Schwartz AL. American college of sports medicine roundtable on exercise guidelines for cancer survivors. Med Sci Sports Exerc. 2010;42:1409–26.
10. Hofman M, Ryan JL, Figueroa-Moseley CD, Jean-Pierre P, Morrow GR. Cancer – related fatigue: the scale of the problem. Oncologist. 2007;12 Suppl 1:4–10.
11. Servaes P, Verhagen S, Bleijenberg G. Determinants of chronic fatigue in disease – free breast cancer patients: a cross-sectional study. Ann Oncol. 2002;13:589–98.
12. Crom DB, Hinds PS, Gattuso JS, Tyc V, Hudson MM. Creating the basis for a breast health programme for female survivors of Hodgkin disease using a participatory research approach. Oncol Nurs Forum. 2005;32:1131–41.
13. Dow KH, Ferrell BR, Leigh S, Ly J, Gula-sekaram P. An evaluation of the quality of life among long-term survivors of breast cancer. Breast Cancer Res Treat. 1996;39:261–73.
14. Janda M, Gerstner N, Obermair A, Fuerst A, Wachter S, Dieckmann K, Potter R. Quality of life changes during conformal radiation therapy for prostate carcinoma. Cancer. 2000;89:1322–8.
15. Brown JC, Huedo-Medina TB, Pescatello LS, Pescatello SM, Ferrer RA, Johnson BT. Efficacy of exercise interventions in modulating cancer-related fatigue among adult cancer survivors: a meta-analysis. Cancer Epidemiol Biomarkers Prev. 2011;20(1):123–33.
16. Victorson D, Barocas J, Song J, Cella D. Reliability across studies from the functional assessment of cancer therapy-general (FACT-G). Qual Life Res. 2008;17:1137–46.
17. Cella DF, Tulsky DS. Quality of life in cancer: definition, purpose, and method of measurement. Cancer Invest. 2009;11:327–36.
18. Ferrer RA, Huedo-Medina TB, Johnson BT, Ryan S, Pescatello L. Exercise interventions for cancer survivors: a meta-analysis of quality of life outcomes. Ann Behav Med. 2011;41:32–47.
19. National Institute of Health. What breast cancer survivors need to know about osteoperosis. 2015. http://www.niams.nih.gov/Health_Info/Bone/Osteoporosis/Conditions_Behaviors/osteoporosis_breast_cancer.asp. Access verified 7 Apr 2016.
20. Peppone LJ, Mustian KM, Janelsins MC, Palesh OG, Rosier RN, Piazza KM, Purnell JQ, Darling TV, Marrow GR. Effects of a structured weight-bearing exercise program on bone metabolism among breast cancer survivors: a feasibility trial. Clin Breast Cancer. 2010;10(3):224–9.
21. Hojan K, Milecki P, Molinkska-Glura M, et al. Effect of physical activity on bone strength and body composition in breast cancer premenopausal women during endocrine therapy. Eur J Phys Rehabil Med. 2013;49(3):331–9.
22. Winters-Stone KM, Dobek J, Nail L, Bennett JA, Leo MC, Naik A, et al. Strength training stops bone loss and builds muscle in postmenopausal breast cancer survivors: a randomized, controlled trial. Breast Cancer Res Treat. 2011;127:447–56.
23. Murphy CC, Bartholomew LK, Carpentier MY, et al. Adherence to adjuvant hormonal therapy among breast cancer survivors in clinical practice: a systematic review. Breast Cancer Res Treat. 2012;134:459–78.
24. Crew KD, Greenlee H, Capodice J, et al. Prevalence of joint symptoms in postmenopausal women taking aromatase inhibitors for early-stage breast cancer. J Clin Oncol. 2007;25:3877–83.

25. Stestak I, Cuzick J, Sapunar F, et al. Risk factors for joint symptoms in patients enrolled in the ATAC trial: a retrospective, exploratory analysis. Lancet Oncol. 2008;9:866–72.
26. Irwin M, Cartmel B, Gross CP, et al. Randomized exercise trial of aromatase inhibitor–induced arthralgia in breast cancer survivors. J Clin Oncol. 2015;33(10):1104–11.
27. Hershman DL, Shao T, Kushi LH, et al. Early discontinuation and non-adherence to adjuvant hormonal therapy are associated with increased mortality in women with breast cancer. Breast Cancer Res Treat. 2011;126:529–38.
28. Zhao G, Li C, Okoro CA, Li J, Wen XJ, White A, Balluz LS. Trends in modifiable lifestyle-related risk factors following diagnosis in breast cancer survivors. J Cancer Surviv. 2013; 7(4):563–9.
29. Irwin M, Crumley D, McTiernan A, Bernstein L, Baumgartner R, Gilliland FD, Kriska A, Ballard-Barbash R. Physical activity levels before and after a diagnosis of breast carcinoma: the Health, Eating, Activity and Lifestyle (HEAL) study. Cancer. 2003;97(7):1746–57.
30. Matthews CE, Wilcox S, Hanby CL, Der Ananian C, Heiney SP, Gebretsadik T, Shintani A. Evaluation of a 12-week home-based walking intervention for breast cancer survivors. Support Care Cancer. 2007;15(2):203–11.
31. Macmillan cancer support. Available at: http://www.macmillan.org.uk/Documents/AboutUs/Commissioners/Physicalactivityevidencereview.pdf. Access verified 7 Apr 2016.
32. Macmillan cancer support. Available at: http://www.macmillan.org.uk/Documents/AboutUs/Health_professionals/PhysicalActivityEvidenceBasedGuidance.pdf Access verified 7 Apr 2016.
33. Department of health, UK. Available at: https://www.gov.uk/government/publications/let-s-get-moving-revised-commissioning-guidance. Access verified 7 Apr 2016.

# Chapter 9
# Dietary Components and Breast Cancer Survivorship

**Clare Shaw**

**Abstract** The development of breast cancer is multi-factorial and lifestyle factors, including diet, have been implicated in its etiology. The relative influence of different lifestyle factors on breast cancer risk varies between individuals. However the factors for which there is the most evidence of risk modification are maintaining a healthy weight, being physically active and not drinking alcohol. Many other factors have been suggested to be beneficial in terms of cancer prevention and prevention of recurrence: including the optimal balance of the diet, the consumption of fruit and vegetables, use of dairy products, soy foods, vitamin and mineral supplements. This chapter will concentrate on the concerns of women who have undergone treatment, many of whom may change their behavior with the aim of influencing the course of their disease and their overall health. This change in health related behavior may occur at diagnosis, during treatment or at the end of treatment and the time may be different for each individual. The seeking of relevant information and subsequent change in behavior has been identified as the changeable moment and it is important that people have access to balanced, evidenced based information to support their choices.

**Keywords** Diet • Alcohol • Soy • Vitamins • Weight • Weight loss • Body composition and dairy

## Introduction

The development of breast cancer is multi-factorial and lifestyle factors, including diet, have been implicated in its etiology. The relative influence of different lifestyle factors on breast cancer risk varies between individuals. However the factors for which there is the most evidence of risk modification are maintaining a healthy weight, being physically active and not drinking alcohol [1]. Many other factors have been

C. Shaw, BSc (Hons) Nutrition, PhD, RD
Department of Nutrition and Dietetics, The Royal Marsden NHS Foundation Trust, London, UK
e-mail: clare.shaw@rmh.nhs.uk



A. Ring, M. Parton (eds.), *Breast Cancer Survivorship*,
DOI 10.1007/978-3-319-41858-2_9

suggested to be beneficial in terms of cancer prevention and prevention of recurrence: including the optimal balance of the diet, the consumption of fruit and vegetables, use of dairy products, soy foods, vitamin and mineral supplements. This chapter will concentrate on the concerns of women who have undergone treatment, many of whom may change their behavior with the aim of influencing the course of their disease and their overall health. This change in health related behavior may occur at diagnosis, during treatment or at the end of treatment and the time may be different for each individual. The seeking of relevant information and subsequent change in behavior has been identified as the changeable moment and it is important that people have access to balanced, evidenced based information to support their choices.

## Weight Gain and Changes in Body Composition During and After Cancer Treatment

Weight gain is common for women undergoing treatment for early breast cancer and has been identified as occurring in both pre and postmenopausal women. Early studies identified that this weight gain could be as much as up to 11 kg in 25 % of women receiving adjuvant chemotherapy [2]. In this study women who were under observation, but did not receive chemotherapy, also gained a median of 1.8 kg following diagnosis over a 60 week period. In recent years there appears to be a reduction in the magnitude of weight gain with reports of median weight gains of 1.0 kg, 2.0 kg and 1.0 kg documented at 6, 18 and 36 months post-diagnosis respectively [3]. The underlying relative contributions of chemotherapy, endocrine therapy and lifestyle changes associated with a diagnosis of breast cancer to weight gain are not clear. Irrespective, weight gain continues to affect a high proportion of women being treated for breast cancer with 50–96 % of women being affected [4].

Body composition refers to the proportion of fat and fat-free mass (water, muscle and bone) in the body, and is an important prognostic factor in cancer patients. The presence of sarcopenia, the severe depletion of skeletal muscle, can be present in those who are of a normal weight or are overweight. As being overweight or obese is a risk factor for post-menopausal breast cancer, this condition is often left undiagnosed. A cohort of 514 women participants in the Health, Eating, Activity and Lifestyle (HEAL) study underwent measurements in body composition via whole body dual-energy X-ray absorptiometry (DEXA) scanning at baseline and at 2 years post diagnosis [5]. A total of 68 % of women gained weight and 74 % gained body fat. Data were also collected on physical activity and exercise. There was a significant trend of increasing gains in weight for those who had a decrease in sports or recreational physical activity. This was most notable in younger post-menopausal women compared to older post-menopausal women and pre- menopausal women. Weight gained during chemotherapy was associated with an increase in fat mass and a decrease in lean body mass, a pattern known as sarcopenic obesity. This has implications for dietary advice regarding weight management in women following a diagnosis of breast cancer as it is important that advice is directed both at overall weight loss and also preservation of lean body mass.

## Implications of Weight Gain Following Breast Cancer Treatment

Increased body weight is known to be a risk factor for the development of post-menopausal breast cancer. Furthermore a number of studies have identified that being obese *following* a diagnosis of breast cancer confers worse breast cancer and overall survival compared with women of normal weight. A systematic review combining the results from 82 studies, including over 213,000 breast cancer survivors, concluded that being overweight or obese increased the risk of dying in both pre and post-menopausal women [6]. The relative risks (RRs) of total mortality were 1.41 (95 % confidence interval (CI) 1.29–1.53) for obese women (BMI >30 kg/m$^2$) and 1.07 (95 % CI 1.02–1.12) for overweight (BMI >25.0 to <30 kg/m$^2$) women.

Aside from body weight assessed at a single time point, *changes* in body weight may also be important; particularly as these changes may occur during or after treatment for breast cancer. The systematic review by Chan et al examined the risk associated with weight gain before diagnosis, less than 12 months after diagnosis and 12 months or more after diagnosis of breast cancer [6]. Data were analyzed with respect to the increased risk conferred by gain of 5 kg/m$^2$ increments of BMI before, less than 12 months after, and more than 12 months after diagnosis. Increased risks of 17 %, 11 % and 8 % for total mortality and 18 %, 14 % and 29 % for breast cancer mortality were observed, respectively [6]. In addition to its effects on survival outcomes, obesity and/or weight gain may also adversely affect surgical outcomes with higher rates of infection and poor wound healing, fatigue, lymphedema and functional decline [7, 8]. There may also be an impact for some women in terms of body-image and quality of life.

Weight management is therefore a priority for women following treatment for breast cancer, although it should be recognized that there is a paucity of evidence as to the relative impact this has on rates of recurrence and survival.

## Interventions for Weight Management After Breast Cancer Treatment

Intervention studies in women without a diagnosis of breast cancer have focused on both dietary intervention and exercise as means of influencing body composition, aiming to preserve lean body mass and reduce body fat. A study in overweight, physically inactive women used a tailor-made dietary program for all participants. In addition some women were randomized to a program of weight loss induced mainly by an exercise program [9]. The primary the aim was to reduce body weight by 5–6 kg. Participants were monitored with respect to dietary intake and exercise, via an exercise log, and had frequent contact with their dietitian or physiotherapist. A control group aimed to remain weight stable by following a standardized diet and their usual physical activity patterns. Changes in body composition were measured using DEXA scanning. Two hundred and thirty-two (95.5 %) of women completed the 16 week trial. All anthropometric measurements showed a significant decrease in both intervention groups versus the control group [9]. The mainly exercise group showed a greater decrease in waist and hip circumference although the results were not significant. Decreases in body fat were statistically significantly greater in the mainly exercise group versus the diet group. Lean mass was preserved in the mainly exercise group compared with control whereas the diet group lost lean mass [7].

This model of losing weight whilst maintaining fat free mass has been used as an approach in a small study in breast cancer. A study enrolled 28 survivors of triple negative breast cancer who were overweight (BMI >25 kg/m$^2$) in a randomized, controlled trial of moderate intensity aerobic exercise and diet counseling compared to usual care [10]. Twenty-three women completed the study and over the period of the study there was a significant reduction in body weight, BMI and body fat was observed when compared to controls [8].

This and other studies are important as they support successful weight reduction in women who have completed treatment for breast cancer, something that many women do not feel is possible [8, 11]. Of great interest is whether particular dietary approaches support better adherence to dietary change and if they are able to influence metabolic parameters such as insulin sensitivity and lipid profiles. One such dietary approach that has attracted much interest is the use of intermittent energy restriction (IER) compared to the conventional approach of daily energy restriction (DER) [12]. In the popular press this is often referred to as the 2 day diet or intermittent fasting and has been used for overall weight loss, not just in breast cancer. The approach is to restrict dietary intake for two consecutive days a week to 2500–2717 kJ/day and less than 40 g carbohydrate using a relatively high protein intake to maximize satiety. This is compared with dietary advice that is aimed at reducing energy intake by 25 % on a daily basis, following a Mediterranean style diet. This approach was trialed in a group of women at high risk of breast cancer and indicated that, in the short term, the IER was superior to DER with respect to the improvements in insulin sensitivity and the loss of body fat [12]. This approach is currently being trialed in conjunction with 150 min of moderate exercise per week in 170 women who are having chemotherapy after surgery for breast cancer. Outcomes being measured include weight, body fat and muscle mass, blood levels of hormones and inflammation linked to the risk of recurrence, well-being and side effects from chemotherapy [13].

## Diet After Cancer Treatment

Much is written in the research literature and popular mass media about diet and breast cancer. Many beliefs about food and breast cancer persist in the absence of supporting scientific evidence [14]. A comprehensive review of worldwide research on breast cancer survivors was published by the World Cancer Research Fund in October 2014 and provides a thorough systematic review of the literature.

Women often make changes to their diet following a diagnosis of breast cancer, however, their understanding of what constitutes an optimal dietary intake is not always in accordance with dietary current recommendations [15]. Similarly, implementing what women think of as a healthy diet is not always achieved with some not consuming the recommendations for fruit and vegetables and dietary fiber nor the limits for saturated fat and energy intake [15].

## *General Recommendations*

A number of randomized trials have been carried out which have aimed to establish the optimal overall balance of the diet with respect to reducing breast cancer incidence and the risk of recurrence. Interest in the consumption of dietary fat originated from animal experiments in the 1950s which demonstrated the promotion of tumor growth with high fat diets. The Woman's Health Initiative (WHI) dietary modification trial randomized over 48,000 women with no prior history of breast cancer to a reduction in the intake of dietary fat to 20 % of their total energy intake, or to a control group. There was a reduction in the number of cancers in the women who ate a reduced fat intake (HR 0.91, 95 % CI 0.83–1.01) although this was not statistically significant [16].

Later the Women's Intervention Nutrition Study (WINS) randomized 2437 postmenopausal women with early-stage breast cancer to a reduced fat diet of 15 % of energy from fat or a control group. Women in the intervention group successfully reduced their fat intake and lost weight and showed an improved relapse-free survival although statistically this was deemed to be of borderline significance (hazard ratio 0.76, 95 % CI: 0.60–0.98, P=0.03 from Cox Proportional Hazard model). A survival analysis was completed at 108 months follow-up, and there was no statistically significant difference between the groups overall (HR 0.8, 95 % CI: 0.64–1.07, P=0.146). However, in a subgroup analysis, there was an apparent improved survival in women with ER negative, PR negative breast cancers, assigned to the intervention (HR 0.3, 95 % CI: 0.18–0.74, P=0.003). Long term dietary studies of this type are difficult to manage and expensive, particularly with respect to long term dietary compliance. In the WINS study there was a large reduction in the proportion of women who did not complete the dietary assessments with only 40 % responding at 5 years. It is unlikely that those that did not respond had maintained such strict dietary habits for the duration of the study and this would ultimately affect the ability of the study to detect whether adherence to a low fat diet does influence outcome [17, 18].

The Women's Healthy Eating and Living (WHEL) randomized trial used a combined dietary approach and aimed to assess whether a major increase in the consumption of vegetables, fruit and dietary fiber in conjunction with a reduction in dietary fat would influence invasive breast recurrence, the presence of a new primary or death [19]. A total of 3088 women previously treated for early stage breast cancer, aged 18–70 years old at diagnosis were recruited to the study. Those in the intervention group were counseled to consume a daily target of 5 vegetable servings, 16 oz vegetable juice, 3 fruit servings, 30 g of dietary fiber and 15–20 % of energy intake from fat. The control group were provided with printed material on the usual 5-a-day dietary guidelines. The intervention group successfully made dietary changes in accordance with the counseling during the first 4 years. Follow up at 7.3 years did not show any significant difference between the two groups in terms of breast cancer events or mortality. Following a secondary analysis of the WHEL study population, it was identified that the women with the highest reported intakes of total vegetable intake at their baseline measurement had an overall lower hazard for breast cancer recurrence or the development of a new primary [20]. This potentially protective effect was greater in women receiving tamoxifen and was greatest for women who consumed high levels of cruciferous vegetables such as broccoli, cauliflower and cabbage. Whilst this analysis points to a potentially protective effective of vegetables in those receiving tamoxifen the results cannot be generalized to the whole breast cancer population.

A number of lifestyle intervention studies are currently in progress. One of these is the SUCCESS C study [21]. This is a study in 3547 women with early stage HER2 negative breast cancer in the adjuvant setting, where patients undergo two randomizations. The first of these compares anthracycline-taxane adjuvant chemotherapy with a taxane-only regimen. The second randomizes women with a BMI 24–40 kg/m$^2$ to a lifestyle intervention or observation. The lifestyle intervention involves a low fat, low energy diet in combination with physical activity provided by dietitians, a lifestyle coach, trained nurses, physicians and psychologists [21]. More randomized intervention studies of this type are required to ascertain the effect of changes in diet and body composition.

The World Cancer Research Fund International Continuous Update Project has reviewed the evidence for diet, nutrition, physical activity in breast cancer survivors [22]. The report identified limitations in either design or execution of published research meaning that the data is still not strong enough to make specific recommendations for breast cancer survivors. Some evidence suggests that improved survival after breast cancer is linked with a healthy body weight, being physically active, eating foods containing dietary fiber and having a lower intake of total fat, and in particular, saturated fat. However overall, breast cancer survivors are generally advised to follow the general recommendations for a healthy lifestyle to reduce cancer as shown in Table 9.1.

**Table 9.1** General recommendations for a healthy lifestyle to reduce cancer risk [23]

| |
|---|
| Be a healthy weight: Keep weight as low as you can within the healthy range |
| Move more: Be physically active for at least 30 min every day and sit less |
| Avoid high-calorie foods and drinks: Limit high calorie foods and avoid sugary drinks |
| Enjoy more grains, vegetables, fruits and beans |
| Limit red meat and avoid processed meat: Eat no more than 500 g (cooked weight) a week of red meat and eat little, if any processed meat |
| For cancer prevention, don't drink alcohol: If you do, limit alcoholic drinks to two for men and one for women a day |
| Eat less salt: Limit your salt intake to less than 6 g (2.4 g sodium) a day by adding less salt and eating less food processed with salt |
| Don't rely on supplements: Eat a healthy diet rather than relying on supplements to protected against cancer |

## *Specific Considerations*

### Alcohol

The consumption of alcohol has been identified as a risk factor for the development of breast cancer from large prospective cohort studies [24] although the mechanisms are unclear. It is also unclear as to whether alcohol consumption following diagnosis influences survival. Whilst individual studies have indicated that alcohol consumption adversely affects prognosis, a recent meta-analysis of 11 studies concluded that moderate post diagnosis alcohol consumption was not associated with overall survival (HR, 0.95; 95 % CI, 0.85–1.05) [25]. This was also the conclusion of the World Cancer Research Fund review of the evidence in their Continuous Update Programme [22]. Advice on alcohol consumption following treatment for breast cancer should therefore be in keeping with the general recommendations for health (Table 9.1).

### Dairy Foods

Dairy foods such as milk, yogurt, butter and cheese have been the subject of some controversy with respect to breast cancer etiology and following diagnosis. A number of reports in the mass media have encouraged women to reduce their intake of dairy foods and this is a common change that women make following diagnosis [26]. Concern has been expressed over the high dietary fat content of dairy foods, contaminants in milk and hormones in milk such as estrogens and Insulin like growth factor (IGF-1) [14]. However, dairy foods are also a good source of calcium so their overall contribution to dietary intake of minerals is an important consideration, particularly in a population of women who may be at risk of bone mineral density loss as a result of their breast cancer treatment (Chap. 15).

Studies have failed to provide a link between the consumption of dairy foods and recurrence or breast cancer specific survival [27]. One study suggested that high-fat dairy intake, but not a low fat dairy intake, was related to poorer overall survival in long term breast cancer survival [28]. This suggests that it is not dairy foods per se which may influence outcome but may be present in those taking a high fat diet. Current evidence indicates that it is not necessary to reduce or exclude dairy foods from the diet following treatment for breast cancer [22].

### Soy Foods

Soy food consumption varies greatly around the world with higher levels of consumption in Asian populations compared to Western countries. Soy foods have attracted attention with relation to breast cancer due to their isoflavone content. These compounds bind to estrogen receptors and exert estrogen like activity and therefore have been called phyto-estrogens. Their cellular action appears to vary in different tissues and is due to selective binding and activation of ER β receptors in comparison to ER α receptors [29]. Soy beans contain a number of isoflavones including genistein, daidzein and glycitein. The processing of soy beans can alter the amount of isoflavones contained in the food with a much reduced quantity in products such as isolated soy protein. Fermentation of soy beans in foods such as natto and miso does not alter the isoflavone concentration. The availability of phytoestrogenic activity may vary also between individuals as it is partially dependent on the production of more metabolically active compounds through metabolism by gut microbiota. For example the isoflavone daidzein may be metabolized to the more easily absorbed and more metabolically active equal in the gut of some individuals.

There is concern as to how phyto-estrogens may influence cellular activity, particularly growth of breast cancer cells. These concerns arose from in vitro studies, where isoflavones were found to promote mammary tumor growth in animal models, and potentially interfere with the activity of tamoxifen [29, 30]. There have been no intervention studies which have examined the influence of phytoestrogen intake on breast cancer survival. However, some evidence from epidemiological studies indicates that consumption of 10 mg or more of isoflavones confers a benefit in terms of a reduction of total mortality, breast cancer specific mortality and breast cancer recurrence when compared with a consumption of less than 4 mg. These results are from the pooling of 3 large studies with a total of 9514 breast cancer patients who were followed up for a mean of 7.4 years [29, 30]. Some of these studies have focused on populations of Asian women where intake of isoflavones is higher than in Western populations and can range from 10 to 40 mg per day.

The World Cancer Research Fund Continuous update concluded that although the evidence was limited it was generally consistent and suggestive of an inverse relationship between consumption of foods containing soy and all-cause mortality [22]. Nonetheless there remains concern about the use of concentrated isoflavone supplements (such as red clover) in women with breast cancer, and their use is not recommended. These supplements provide a much greater concentration of phytoestrogens and may have adverse interactions with biological mechanisms or prescribed medication [14].

## Vitamins and Mineral Supplementation

There has been much interest in whether vitamins, minerals and bioactive compounds found in food can confer protection against cancer both in terms of prevention and in the reduction of risk after diagnosis. The potential for these compounds to exert their action may be via a direct effect on cellular growth or via other biological systems, for example, influence over the hormonal axis.

The use of vitamin and mineral supplementation is common amongst women diagnosed with breast cancer. Studies report usage among cancer patients and longer-term survivors of 64–81 %, which is higher than the usage of 50 % in the general American population [31]. Usage is especially high in people with breast cancer and in those with a higher level of education. In other cancer diagnoses, such as lung cancer, stomach cancer and colorectal adenomas the use of vitamins and minerals supplements has been demonstrated to have an adverse effect on outcome with higher rates of recurrence in people taking high dose supplementation, particularly for beta-carotene and retinol [32]. There is concern that the use of high dose anti-oxidant vitamins may be protective for cancer cells, reducing the efficacy of chemotherapy or radiotherapy although this has not been substantiated in clinical trials [32].

Data on vitamin supplementation after breast cancer diagnosis was collected in a number of cohort studies both in the United States and China [33]. These pooled data suggest that post treatment supplement use of vitamins A, B, C, D, E and multivitamins, assessed 1–5 years post diagnosis, reduced the risk of death by 16 %. Vitamin E was associated with a decreased risk of recurrence (RR: 0.88; 95 % CI 0.79–99) and vitamin C with a decreased risk of death (RR; 0.81: 95 % CI 0.72–0.92) [33]. Other meta analyses have also concluded that the use of vitamin C post diagnosis of breast cancer may be associated with a reduced risk of mortality [34]. It is not clear, however, to what extent vitamin ingestion is associated with healthier lifestyle and better adherence to endocrine therapy which may also explain this observation.

Vitamin D is a fat soluble vitamin that can be obtained from dietary sources such as liver, oily fish, fish liver oil and egg yolks or from the action of ultra violet light on the skin which facilitates the conversion of pre vitamin D3 to 1,25 dihydroxyvitamin D or calcitriol. Vitamin D is important as it promotes the absorption of calcium in the gut and maintains adequate serum calcium and phosphate levels. These in turn enable normal mineralization of bone. Declining bone density is of concern in women following treatment for breast cancer due to the effect of hormone treatment on calcium bone deposition. The optimal level of supplementation of vitamin D and calcium to improve bone density and reduce the risk of fracture has not been determined. A systematic review of calcium and/or vitamin D supplementation and its effect on bone mineral density (BMD) was published in 2013 [35]. Levels of supplementation were 500–1000 mg for calcium and 200–1000 IU for vitamin D and most of the studies were based on assessment of BMD before and after supplementation. These doses of supplementation were found to be inadequate to prevent BMD loss in both pre and postmenopausal women with breast cancer [35]. Close monitoring of bone health is therefore essential in this population (Chap. 15).

There is much interest in other potential effects of vitamin D as some evidence suggests that higher circulating levels of 25-hydroxyvitamin D levels may confer a better prognosis amongst cancer patients, although this requires further studies before recommendations can be extended to women with early breast cancer [36, 37].

## Summary

Diet and lifestyle changes are an important aspect of living with and beyond breast cancer. Many women are interested in changing their diet following treatment. Increasing evidence indicates that body composition, the balance of dietary intake and some specific food groups may influence outcomes in breast cancer, including breast cancer associated morbidity and overall survival.

It is essential that women have access to evidence based dietary information during and after treatment to enable them to make informed choices regarding lifestyle and health related behaviors, some of which may influence the course of their disease.

## References

1. World Cancer Research Fund International. Link between lifestyle and cancer risk 2015. 15 Oct 2015. Available from: http://www.wcrf.org/int/link-between-lifestyle-cancer-risk.
2. Camoriano JK, Loprinzi CL, Ingle JN, Therneau TM, Krook JE, Veeder MH. Weight change in women treated with adjuvant therapy or observed following mastectomy for node-positive breast cancer. J Clin Oncol Off J Am Soc Clin Oncol. 1990;8(8):1327–34.
3. Gu K, Chen X, Zheng Y, Chen Z, Zheng W, Lu W, et al. Weight change patterns among breast cancer survivors: results from the Shanghai breast cancer survival study. Cancer Causes Control. 2010;21(4):621–9.
4. Vance V, Mourtzakis M, McCargar L, Hanning R. Weight gain in breast cancer survivors: prevalence, pattern and health consequences. Obes Rev. 2011;12(4):282–94.
5. Irwin ML, McTiernan A, Baumgartner RN, Baumgartner KB, Bernstein L, Gilliland FD, et al. Changes in body fat and weight after a breast cancer diagnosis: influence of demographic, prognostic, and lifestyle factors. J Clin Oncol : Off J Am Soc Clin Oncol. 2005;23(4):774–82.
6. Chan DS, Vieira AR, Aune D, Bandera EV, Greenwood DC, McTiernan A, et al. Body mass index and survival in women with breast cancer-systematic literature review and meta-analysis of 82 follow-up studies. Ann Oncol. 2014;25(10):1901–14.
7. Demark-Wahnefried W, Campbell KL, Hayes SC. Weight management and its role in breast cancer rehabilitation. Cancer. 2012;118(8 Suppl):2277–87.
8. Shaw C, Mortimer P, Judd PA. A randomized controlled trial of weight reduction as a treatment for breast cancer-related lymphedema. Cancer. 2007;110(8):1868–74.
9. van Gemert WA, Schuit AJ, Van JP, May AM, Iestra JA, Wittink H, et al. Effect of weight loss, with or without exercise, on body composition and sex hormones in postmenopausal women: the SHAPE-2 trial. Breast Cancer Res. 2015;17(1):120.
10. Swisher AK, Abraham J, Bonner D, Gilleland D, Hobbs G, Kurian S, et al. Exercise and dietary advice intervention for survivors of triple-negative breast cancer: effects on body fat, physical function, quality of life, and adipokine profile. Support Care Cancer. 2015;23(10):2995–3003.
11. Rock CL, Flatt SW, Byers TE, Colditz GA, Demark-Wahnefried W, Ganz PA, et al. Results of the Exercise and Nutrition to Enhance Recovery and Good Health for You (ENERGY) Trial: A Behavioral Weight Loss Intervention in Overweight or Obese Breast Cancer Survivors. J Clin Oncol. 2015;33(28):3169–76.
12. Harvie M, Wright C, Pegington M, McMullan D, Mitchell E, Martin B, et al. The effect of intermittent energy and carbohydrate restriction v. daily energy restriction on weight loss and metabolic disease risk markers in overweight women. Br J Nutr. 2013;110(8):1534–47.
13. Genesis Breast Cancer Prevention B-AHEAD Studies 2015. Available from: https://genesisuk.org/preventative-research/research-projects/diet-lifestyle/b-ahead-studies/.
14. Ferrini K, Ghelfi F, Mannucci R, Titta L. Lifestyle, nutrition and breast cancer: facts and presumptions for consideration. Ecancermedicalscience. 2015;9:557.
15. Klassen AC, Smith KC, Brosbe M, Coa K, Hannum S, Caulfield L. What is a healthful diet? Cancer survivors' interpretations of their own dietary recall data. Cancer Res. 2015;75(9 Suppl 1) P1-09-28.
16. Chlebowski RT. Nutrition and physical activity influence on breast cancer incidence and recurrence. Breast. 2013;22:S30–7.

17. Pierce JP. Diet and breast cancer prognosis: making sense of the Women's Healthy Eating and Living and Women's Intervention Nutrition Study trials. Curr Opin Obstet Gynecol. 2009;21(1):86–91.
18. Chlebowski RT, Blackburn GL, Thomson CA, Nixon DW, Shapiro A, Hoy MK, et al. Dietary fat reduction and breast cancer outcome: interim efficacy results from the Women's Intervention Nutrition Study. J Natl Cancer Inst. 2006;98(24):1767–76.
19. Pierce JP, Natarajan L, Caan BJ, Parker BA, Greenberg ER, Flatt SW, et al. Influence of a diet very high in vegetables, fruit, and fiber and low in fat on prognosis following treatment for breast cancer: the Women's Healthy Eating and Living (WHEL) randomized trial. JAMA. 2007;298(3):289–98.
20. Thomson CA, Rock CL, Thompson PA, Caan BJ, Cussler E, Flatt SW, et al. Vegetable intake is associated with reduced breast cancer recurrence in tamoxifen users: a secondary analysis from the Women's Healthy Eating and Living Study. Breast Cancer Res Treat. 2011;125(2):519–27.
21. Rack B, Andergassen U, Neugebauer J, Salmen J, Hepp P, Sommer H, et al. The German SUCCESS C Study – The First European Lifestyle Study on Breast Cancer. Breast Care (Basel). 2010;5(6):395–400.
22. World Cancer Research Fund International/American Institute for Cancer Research Continuous Update Project Report. Diet, Nutrition, Physical Activity, and Breast Cancer Survivors 2014.
23. World Cancer Research Fund. Ways to reduce cancer risk 2016. 20 Jan 2016. Available from: http://www.wcrf-uk.org/uk/preventing-cancer/ways-reduce-cancer-risk.
24. Ferrari P, Licaj I, Muller DC, Kragh Andersen P, Johansson M, Boeing H, et al. Lifetime alcohol use and overall and cause-specific mortality in the European Prospective Investigation into Cancer and nutrition (EPIC) study. BMJ Open. 2014;4(7):e005245.
25. McLaughlin VH, Trentham-Dietz A, Hampton JM, Newcomb PA, Sprague BL. Lifestyle factors and the risk of a second breast cancer after ductal carcinoma in situ. Cancer Epidemiol Biomarkers Prev. 2014;23(3):450–60.
26. Landers P, Tkacheva-Jameson O, Anderson S, Tolma E, Skaggs V. An update on breast cancer in Oklahoma and the dietary changes women make after diagnosis. J Okla State Med Assoc. 2008;101(1):15–9.
27. Zucchetto A, Franceschi S, Polesel J, Parpinel M, Dal Maso L, Prospective Analysis of Case–control Studies on Environmental F, et al. Re: High- and low-fat dairy intake, recurrence, and mortality after breast cancer diagnosis. J Natl Cancer Inst. 2013;105(22):1759–60.
28. Kroenke CH, Caan BJ. Re: High- and low-fat dairy intake, recurrence, and mortality after breast cancer diagnosis. Response. J Natl Cancer Inst. 2013;105(22):1761–2.
29. Messina M. Soy foods, isoflavones, and the health of postmenopausal women. Am J Clin Nutr. 2014;100:423S–30.
30. Caan BJ, Natarajan L, Parker B, Gold EB, Thomson C, Newman V, et al. Soy food consumption and breast cancer prognosis. Cancer Epidemiol Biomarkers Prev. 2011;20(5):854–8.
31. Velicer CM, Ulrich CM. Vitamin and mineral supplement use among US adults after cancer diagnosis: a systematic review. J Clin Oncol Off J Am Soc Clin Oncol. 2008;26(4):665–73.
32. Harvie M. Nutritional supplements and cancer: potential benefits and proven harms. American Society of Clinical Oncology educational book/ASCO American Society of Clinical Oncology Meeting. 2014:e478–86.
33. Poole EM, Shu X, Caan BJ, Flatt SW, Holmes MD, Lu W, et al. Postdiagnosis supplement use and breast cancer prognosis in the after Breast Cancer Pooling Project. Breast Cancer Res Treat. 2013;139(2):529–37.
34. Harris HR, Orsini N, Wolk A. Vitamin C and survival among women with breast cancer: a meta-analysis. Eur J Cancer. 2014;50(7):1223–31.
35. Datta M, Schwartz GG. Calcium and vitamin D supplementation and loss of bone mineral density in women undergoing breast cancer therapy. Crit Rev Oncol Hematol. 2013;88(3):613–24.
36. Hines SL, Jorn HKS, Thompson KM, Larson JM. Breast cancer survivors and vitamin D: a review. Nutrition. 2010;26(3):255–62.
37. Toriola AT, Nguyen N, Scheitler-Ring K, Colditz GA. Circulating 25-hydroxyvitamin D levels and prognosis among cancer patients: a systematic review. Cancer Epidemiol Biomarkers Prev. 2014;23(6):917–33.

# Part III
# Sequelae of Early Breast Cancer and Its Treatment

# Chapter 10
# Identifying and Managing the Consequences of Treatment for Early Breast Cancer

**Natalie Doyle, Nicola Cunningham, and Richard Henry**

**Abstract** Increasing numbers of women are living for significant periods of time after diagnosis and treatment for early breast cancer. For many of these women the consequences of cancer treatments can be debilitating and distressing yet little is known about their experience of survival. The Recovery Package facilitates the identification and management of the consequences of treatment. This is achieved through the offer of a structured, person centered means of assessing and delivering the appropriate levels of support to these women at a time and in a way that is consistent with their wishes and needs.

**Keywords** Consequences of treatment • Supported Self-Management • Person Centered Care • Recovery Package

## Introduction

The incidence of cancer has risen significantly in recent years. One in three people will develop cancer and half of adults diagnosed with the disease are predicted to survive 10 years or more [1]. Current estimates by the National Cancer Survivorship initiative (NCSI) suggest that almost 1.8 million people in England are living with and beyond cancer and that this number is rising by over 3 % per annum [2].

Eighty percent of women with breast cancer might expect to live 5 years or more after their initial treatment with many going on to live at least a further decade and over 60 % likely to live at least 20 years [3]. This means that, in the

N. Doyle, DNurs, MSc, BSc
The Royal Marsden NHS Foundation Trust, London, UK

N. Cunningham, BSc (Hons) Physiotherapy, PGCert
London Cancer Alliance, London, UK

R. Henry, MSc, BSc, BA (✉)
Medical Biology Centre, School of Nursing and Midwifery, Queens University Belfast, Belfast, UK
e-mail: henry@qub.ac.uk



A. Ring, M. Parton (eds.), *Breast Cancer Survivorship*,
DOI 10.1007/978-3-319-41858-2_10

UK, whilst 48,000 women are at the point of diagnosis or undergoing treatment and another 44,000 at the rehabilitative stage, this is by far outweighed by the 222,000 undergoing early monitoring (2–10 years) and a further 226,000 women in late monitoring [4].

## The Experience of Survival

Whilst the chronology of survival can be readily established much less is known about the experience of survival. Brennan et al. [5] maintain that cancer is an inherently distressing experience and all women with breast cancer will live with the consequences of their disease and its treatment. Although many will learn to self-manage (often with appropriate support) an in depth understanding of their outcomes is limited by the unavailability of comprehensive data which addresses the experience of people living with and beyond cancer. The 2014 National Cancer Experience Survey [6] provides some understanding of the experiences of those who are treated as inpatients, but not their ongoing and longer term experiences. The Quality of Life of Cancer Survivors in England [7] reported on the quality of life of people living with and beyond cancer 1, 2, 3 and 5 years after treatment. Women with breast cancer frequently showed ongoing high levels of pain, worry about the future, concern about weight gain, arm swelling and body image issues.

All people with cancer will undergo a life changing experience that begins at the point of diagnosis and evolves over time. Whilst there is a degree of commonality among those with cancer, the experience for each individual will ultimately be distinctive, personal and unique. This may not necessarily be negative as many women report positive outcomes, however, a constant uncertainty persists, particularly after the completion of hospital-based treatment [8].

## The Consequences of Breast Cancer Treatment

Much of the literature on the consequences of cancer treatments focuses on single specific effects of therapy such cardiotoxicity [9], neurotoxicity [10] or anxiety [11]. Whilst this is useful it is important that it should not obscure the reality that the sequelae of cancer treatments are often characterized by multiple effects that can be highly complex and inter related. Early rehabilitation intervention has been shown to either prevent or minimize many of the consequences of breast cancer and its treatments. Thus physical activity can minimize long term cardiac morbidity and, when linked to dietary interventions, can reduce both cancer specific and all-cause mortality [12]. Performance of gentle upper limb exercises immediately post operatively and continued for life reduce the chances of lymphedema developing. However, many of the effects of cancer and its treatment can be obscured or exaggerated by concurrent diseases. Approximately one third of those living with and beyond cancer have one other long term condition whilst a further third have three or more [13].

Many women with breast cancer have undergone prolonged and aggressive multimodal anticancer therapy which is accompanied by significant toxicities. The nature, length and complexity of cancer treatment means that the consequences often vary significantly in frequency, timing, severity and impact on quality of life. Consequently the level, intensity and type of support that is required will vary. The specific effects of radiotherapy, chemotherapy and other treatment approaches are detailed elsewhere in this volume and consideration is given to their acute or long term nature. Many of the most debilitating and demoralizing are ongoing and persistent effects such as fatigue [14] and pain [15] whilst the mental health and psychological support needs of those living with and beyond cancer are only now starting to gain parity of esteem.

Whilst some consequences of treatment might be predictable the response of those affected by the experience may not be. Similarly, other treatment effects may be more difficult to anticipate and the reaction of those affected consequently more uncertain. Successful support of the individual and management of these consequences may ultimately depend upon an individually tailored approach to care and fundamental to this is empowerment of the individual. This is best realized through person centered approaches to care.

## Person Centered Care

The central tenet behind person-centered care is ensuring that the needs and goals of the individual become central to the process of care [16] with an emphasis on what matters to them rather than what is the matter with them [17]. Price [18] suggests that this requires health professionals to work with each person's definition of their situation and that the practice of person-centered care is predicated on supporting people to participate in decision-making and to self-manage their condition wherever possible. This means that the woman with breast cancer should be regarded as a partner rather than passive recipient of care. In addition, healthcare professionals need to comprehend the psychosocial challenges faced by people living with and beyond breast cancer and by what motivates them [19] whilst Collins [20] stresses the importance of an interplay of philosophy, principles and activities (see Fig. 10.1).

1. Affording people dignity respect and compassion
2. Offering coordinated care, support or treatment
3. Offering personalised care, support or treatment
4. Being enabling

**Fig. 10.1** Principles of person centered care [20]

## Self-Management and Self-Efficacy

Foster and Fenlon [21] maintain that reducing dependence on healthcare professionals and increasing a person's sense of control and wellbeing is desirable. According to McCorkle et al. [22] supported self-management empowers the individual with cancer and their carers by bolstering the confidence of those affected by the disease and its treatment. It also prevents or minimizes the longer term complications associated with the disease and reduces the burden on health services [21]. This is achieved by implementing a range of strategies for supporting self-management. These include focusing on self-efficacy, behavior change, technical skills and information provision [23].

Whilst self-management might be regarded as the ideal for women with early breast cancer, they need to be supported in a way that promotes self-efficacy. Bandura [24] regards this as a belief in one's ability to achieve something, and maintained that a person's sense of self-efficacy is principally influenced by their achievements (giving positive performance feedback), followed by their physiological states (experiencing low levels of stress), vicarious experience (seeing others achieve) and verbal persuasion (strengthening their expectations).

The ability to self-manage can be adversely affected by low self-confidence and a feeling of vulnerability whereas a fund of personal and environmental resources, underpinned by a professional attitude and support in secondary and primary care characterized by early intervention can enhance and support self-management [21].

Behavior change can occur at a population, community or individual level, with significant life events acting as a catalyst for individual reassessment [25]. A cancer diagnosis has been shown to provide an opportunity for promotion of health related behavior change [26]. This has been referred to as the 'teachable moment'. Teachable moments are cueing events which occur when life events, such as the experience of cancer, alter the individual's self-concept or social role in a way that prompts the individual to 'take stock' and re-evaluate life, particularly in relation to lifestyle behaviors [27].

## Stratified Follow Up and Supported Self-Management

Stratified follow up envisages that the Multi Professional Team and the individual living with cancer make a decision about the optimal form of aftercare. This is based on disease progression, response to treatment and the perceived needs and circumstances of the person with cancer.

Maximizing the degree of self-management is regarded as the desirable goal in aftercare. This would mean fewer hospital based appointments and a requirement for primary or local secondary care to respond to more routine issues.

Supported self-management may not always be the optimal method of support for those living with and beyond cancer. However, in breast cancer this is rapidly becoming the norm for a majority of people through initiatives such as open access

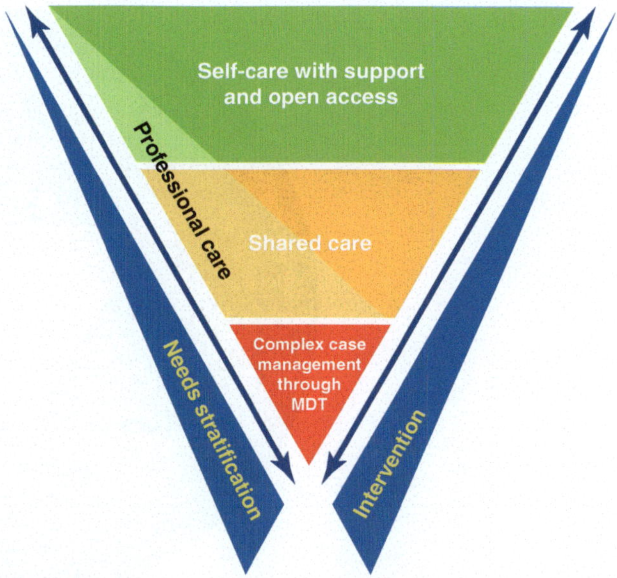


**Fig. 10.2** Stratified pathways of care [2]

follow up. This is enabled by providing those who are deemed eligible for supported self-management with information about signs and symptoms of recurrence, clear pathways to follow if they are concerned and a guarantee of a fast, explicit route to re-access services if necessary [28].

Shared care occurs when those affected by cancer continue to have face-to-face, phone or email contact with professionals as part of continuing follow-up. Thirdly, complex case management occurs when those affected by cancer are given intensive support to manage their cancer and/or other conditions (Fig. 10.2).

## The Recovery Package

The information needed by women living with and beyond breast cancer and their carers can be provided by the Recovery Package [2]. Its overall intention is to support self-management (as outlined previously), the adoption of healthier lifestyles and the reduction of health care service use. The Recovery Package is best delivered in a partnership between a clinical team and a person living with cancer having jointly deciding on the apposite form of stratified aftercare for the individual [29].

The four components of the Recovery Package (Fig. 10.3) contribute to a personalized plan of care for each individual aimed at reducing usage of hospital and primary care services [2]. These components are:

- Holistic Needs Assessment and care planning
- Treatment Summary
- Health and Well Being event
- Cancer Care Review

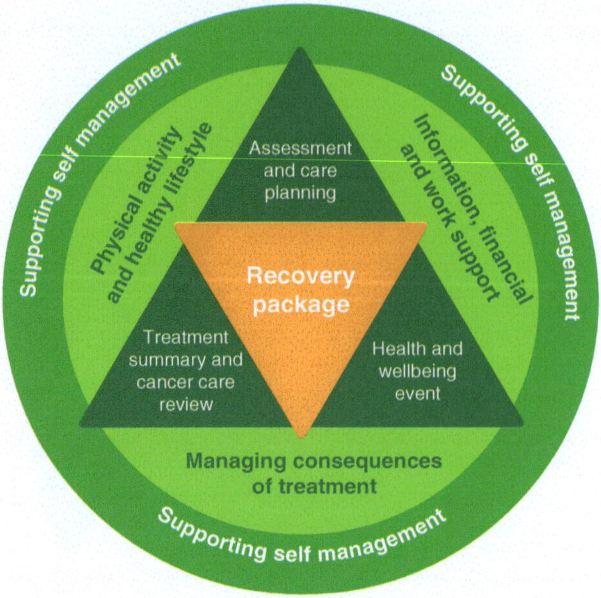


**Fig. 10.3** The recovery package [31]

The Independent Cancer Taskforce [30] advises that everyone with cancer has access to all aspects of the Recovery Package [31] with a recommendation that the necessary services to provide this are commissioned by 2020.

## Treatment Summary

A Treatment Summary should be completed at the end of each treatment phase and given directly to the woman with breast cancer and the Primary Care Team. It provides a summary of the treatments that have been received and outlines their possible consequences such as lymphedema and reduced shoulder range of movement. It includes arrangements for planned follow up including future surveillance (such as mammographic and endocrine monitoring) and it contains alert symptoms that may require re-access to the specialist team. The value of the Treatment Summary is that it supports communication between the cancer center and primary care, empowering the person with cancer and informing the cancer care review.

## Holistic Needs Assessment and Care Planning

The National Cancer Action Team [32] define a Holistic Needs Assessment (HNA) as, “a process of gathering information from the patient and/or carer in order to inform discussion and develop a deeper understanding of what the person understands and needs”. It is concerned with the whole person by incorporating their physical, psychosocial, spiritual and emotional wellbeing into the assessment process.

HNA is undertaken by skilled practitioners who have an intimate knowledge of the practice of caring and working with individuals, an understanding of biological and psychological developments through the lifespan, an appreciation of the needs of this population and the impact of cancer on women with breast cancer

HNA usually comprises a concerns checklist, a distress thermometer and a care plan. The concerns check list allows the woman to specify which issues are of most concern to them. Subsequent discussion with a healthcare professional provides an opportunity to explore the issues raised and to jointly agree how best to address them. Some issues may lend themselves to immediate resolution following discussion and/or imparting of information. Simply allowing the person the opportunity and space to talk may, in itself, be sufficient to ameliorate any concerns. However, other issues may involve prompting or encouraging the individual to take a specific action themselves to address their concern or lead to intervention by a healthcare professional. Finally, there are those issues for which the appropriate response must always be to make onward referral to specialist services. Following the discussion, a care plan is agreed which documents the agreed actions and provides a record of the discussion.

The NCSI [2] suggest a number of key times when a holistic assessment of needs should be conducted. These include when the patient is diagnosed; at the start and end of treatment; when it is determined that the patient cannot be cured; when the patient enters the end-of-life stages; any time that the disease recurs; or whenever a professional caring for the patient feels that it is needed [32]. These deliberately coincide with significant milestones in the pathway where needs might reasonably be expected to change. It may be problematic establishing a categorical link between high levels of distress and specific phases of the patient experience [33] so assessments may also be undertaken at the request of the patient.

The inclusion of HNA onto the National Cancer Outcomes Data Set as a pilot item means that all relevant data will be more readily accessible to inform service improvement initiatives.

## Health and Well Being Events

The NCSI [2] defines health and well-being events as opportunities for those living with and beyond cancer and their carers to get the information they need at the end of treatment to support them to take an active role in their recovery. Whilst they may have value during treatment, for most people they are most usefully offered at the end of treatment. The aim of the health and well-being event is to provide the information to enable those living with and beyond cancer to:

- Promote healthy lifestyle choices
- Make lifestyle changes
- Manage the consequences of cancer and its treatment

Typically, these are group events in which women affected by breast cancer are given the opportunity to engage with others living with and beyond cancer as well as a range of health care professionals e.g. doctors, clinical nurse specialists, allied health professionals, and complementary therapists. They frequently include 'market stalls' of relevant services such as local smoking cessation services, gyms and voluntary agencies. The events also offer expert advice on health promotion in order to minimize risk of recurrence and encourage healthy living. Support is given to underpin the confidence and skills needed to self-manage. Access to financial and benefits advice and vocational rehabilitation as well as specific issues relating to breast cancer such as early detection of recurrence, body image, physical activity, diet, sexual functioning and lymphedema prevention should be addressed

## Cancer Care Review

The Cancer Care Review should be carried out by the women's GP or designated member of the primary care team within 6 months of their cancer diagnosis. It helps people affected by cancer to understand what information and help is available to them in their local community thus underpinning the principles of supported self-management.

## Conclusion

It is essential that pathways and services which can minimize the consequences of breast cancer treatments and address needs are designed and commissioned. The advantages offered by such an approach are that women with early breast cancer will access healthcare services less, that significant economic benefits to the individual and society will be realized and there will be an improved quality of life for all those women who are affected by this disease and its treatment.

Whilst the Recovery Package might be a relatively recent innovation in the management of early breast cancer there are number of ways in which care might be further enhanced. This will involve integrating survivorship care more completely into primary care, embedding the Recovery Package into NHS systems, the development of prehabilitation and better prognostic and predictive factors for the adverse consequences of cancer and its treatment. Improved survivorship intelligence deriving from empowerment of those affected by cancer and healthcare professionals will drive these improvements. This should stem from regular post treatment patient related outcome measures (PROMS) collection together with the development of robust person centered outcome measures (PCOMS) [20].

## References

1. Cancer Research UK (CRUK). Cancer survival statistics. 2014. http://www.cancerresearchuk.org/health-professional/cancer-statistics/survival. Accessed 11 Oct 2015. CRUK 2014.
2. National Cancer Survivorship Initiative. Living with and beyond cancer: taking action to improve outcomes. 2013. Available at: https://www.gov.uk/government/uploads/system/uploads/attachment_data/file/181054/9333-TSO-2900664-NCSI_Report_FINAL.pdf. Accessed 8 Sept 2015.
3. Fenlon D, Frankland J, Foster C, Brooks C, Coleman P, Payne S, Seymour J, Simmonds P, Stephens R, Walsh B, Addington-Hall J. Living into old age with the consequences of breast cancer. Euro J Oncol Nurs. 2013;17(3):311–31.
4. Maher J, McConnell H. New pathways of care for cancer survivors: adding the numbers. Br J Cancer. 2011;105:S5–10.
5. Brennan J, Gingell P, Brant H, Hollingworth W. Refinement of the distress management problem list as the basis for a holistic therapeutic conversation among UK patients with cancer. Psychooncology. 2012;21(12):1346–56.
6. NHS England. Cancer patient experience survey 2014. 2014. https://www.quality-health.co.uk/surveys/national-cancer-patient-experience-survey. Accessed 22 Oct 2015.
7. Department of Health (DH). Quality of life of cancer survivors in England. 2012. https://www.gov.uk/government/uploads/system/uploads/attachment_data/file/267042/9284-TSO-2900701-PROMS-1.pdf. Accessed 22 Oct 2015.
8. Doyle N. Cancer survivorship: evolutionary concept analysis. J Adv Nurs. 2008;62(4):499–509.
9. Schmitz K, Prosnitz R, Schwartz A, Carver R. Prospective surveillance and management of cardiac toxicity and health in breast cancer survivors. Cancer. 2012;118(8):2270–6.
10. Azim H, de Azambuja E, Colozza M, Bines J, Piccart M. Long-term toxic effects of adjuvant chemotherapy in breast cancer. Ann Oncol. 2011;22(9):1939–47.
11. Howard-Anderson J, Ganz P, Bower J, Stanton A. Quality of life, fertility concerns, and behavioral health outcomes in younger breast cancer survivors: a systematic review. J Natl Cancer Inst. 2012;104:386–405.
12. Rock C, Flatt S, Byers T, Colditz G, Demark-Wahnefried W, Ganz P, et al. Results of the Exercise and Nutrition to Enhance Recovery and Good Health for You (ENERGY) Trial: A Behavioral Weight Loss Intervention in Overweight or Obese Breast Cancer Survivors JCO. 2012;33(28):3169–76.
13. Macmillan Cancer Support. 1.8 million people are living with cancer and another long term condition. 2015. http://www.macmillan.org.uk/Aboutus/News/Latest_News/18millionpeoplearelivingwithcancerandanotherlongtermcondition.aspx. Accessed 22 Oct 2015.
14. Mackereth P, Farrell C, Bardy J, Molassiotos A, Finnegan-John J. Legitimising fatigue after breast cancer treatment. Br J Nurs. 2015;24:pS4–S12.
15. Mejdahl M, Andersen K, Gärtner R, Kroman N, Kehlet H. Persistent pain and sensory disturbances after treatment for breast cancer: six year nationwide follow-up study. BMJ. 2013;346:f1865.
16. Draper J, Tetley J. The importance of person-centred approaches to nursing care. 2013. Open Learn, 15 March 2013. [Online]. Available from: The Open University http://www.open.edu/openlearn/body-mind/health/nursing/the-importance-person-centred-approaches-nursing-care. Accessed 4 Oct 2015.
17. The Health Foundation. Person-centred care made simple. What everyone should know about person-centred care. London: The Health Foundation; 2014.
18. Price B. Exploring person-centred care. Nurs Stand. 2006;20(50):49–56.
19. Bibby J. The Health Foundation: Submission of evidence to the Health Select Committees long term conditions inquiry. 2013. [Online]. Available from: http://www.health.org.uk/

areas-of-work/influencing-policy/consultation-responses/the-health-foundation-s-evidence-to-the-health-select-committee-s-inquiry-into-the-management-of-long-term-conditions/. Accessed 22 Oct 2015.
20. Collins A. Measuring what really matters: towards a coherent measurement system to support person-centred care. London: The Health Foundation; 2014.
21. Foster C, Fenlon D. Recovery and self management support following primary cancer treatment. Br J Cancer. 2011;105:S21–8.
22. McCorkle R, Ercolano E, Lazenby M, Schulman-Green D, Schilling L, Lorig K, Wagner E. Self-management: enabling and empowering patients living with cancer as a chronic illness. CA Cancer J Clin. 2011;61(1):50–62.
23. Da Silva D. Helping people help themselves: a review of the evidence considering whether it is worthwhile to support self-management. London: The Heath Foundation; 2011.
24. Bandura A. Self-efficacy: toward a unifying theory of behavioral change. Psychol Rev. 1977;84(2):191–215.
25. NICE. Behaviour changes: general approaches NICE Guidelines. 2007. http://www.nice.org.uk/guidance/ph6/resources/guidance-behaviour-change-the-principles-for-effective-interventions-pdf.
26. Demark-Wahnefried W. Riding the crest of the teachable moment: promoting long-term health after the diagnosis of cancer. J Clin Oncol. 2005;23(24):5814–30.
27. Davies N, Batehup L, Thomas R. The role of diet and physical activity in breast, colorectal and prostate cancer survivorship: a review of the literature. Br J Cancer. 2011;105:52–73.
28. London Cancer Alliance (LCA). Survivorship guidelines. 2015. http://www.londoncanceralliance.nhs.uk/media/112935/lca_survivorshipguidelines2015_web.pdf. Accessed 22 Oct 2015.
29. National Cancer Survival Initiative (NCSI). Innovation to implementation: stratified pathways of care for people living with and beyond cancer. 2011. A how to guide http://www.ncsi.org.uk/wp-content/uploads/howtoguide.pdf. Accessed 5 Oct 2015.
30. Independent Cancer Taskforce. Achieving world class cancer outcomes: a strategy for England. 2015. 2015–2020 http://www.cancerresearchuk.org/sites/default/files/achieving_world-class_cancer_outcomes_-_a_strategy_for_england_2015-2020.pdf. Accessed 22 Oct 2015.
31. Macmillan Cancer Support. The recovery package. 2013. http://www.macmillan.org.uk/Aboutus/Healthandsocialcareprofessionals/Macmillansprogrammesandservices/RecoveryPackage/RecoveryPackage.aspx. Accessed 22 Oct 2015.
32. Team NCA. Holistic common assessment of supportive and palliative care needs for adults with cancer. London: National Cancer Action Team; 2007.
33. Dabrowki M, Boucher K, Ward J, et al. Clinical experience with the NCCN distress thermometer in breast cancer patients. J Natl Compr Canc Netw. 2007;5(1):104–11.

# Chapter 11
# Managing Loco-regional Complications of Breast Cancer Treatment

**Anna M. Kirby**

**Abstract** Most women with breast cancer are treated with surgery and/or radiotherapy during their treatment course. Both of these treatments can be associated with early complications and side-effects which are dealt with by the treating teams in the immediate post-treatment period. However, this chapter discusses the medium- and long-term effects of surgery and radiotherapy, and in particular how these treatments may affect the breast and arm. Three main areas are discussed: post-treatment changes in the breast, lymphedema of the arm, and musculoskeletal effects in the shoulder and arm.

**Keywords** Locoregional complications • Breast surgery • Breast radiotherapy side-effects • Lymphedema • Cording • Shoulder stiffness

## Introduction

Most women with breast cancer are treated with surgery and/or radiotherapy during their treatment course. Both of these treatments can be associated with early complications and side-effects which are dealt with by the treating teams in the immediate post-treatment period. However this chapter discusses the medium- and long-term effects of surgery and radiotherapy, and in particular how these treatments may affect the breast and arm. Three main areas are discussed: post-treatment changes in the breast, lymphedema of the arm, and musculoskeletal effects in the shoulder and arm.

A.M. Kirby, BA, MB, BChir, MA, MRCP, FRCR, MD
Royal Marsden NHS Foundation Trust & Institute of Cancer Research, Surrey, UK
e-mail: anna.kirby@rmh.nhs.uk



A. Ring, M. Parton (eds.), *Breast Cancer Survivorship*,
DOI 10.1007/978-3-319-41858-2_11

## Post-treatment Changes in the Breast

### *Incidence and Risk Factors*

Following surgical wide local excision of breast cancer and/or radiotherapy treatment to the breast and/or regional lymph nodes, medium to long-term complications include breast pain, swelling (Fig. 11.1), firmness, shrinkage and skin changes (Fig. 11.2). Data on the proportion of women affected by these changes, the likely time course, and risk factors comes from long-term follow-up within clinical trials of radiotherapy for breast cancer including the START trials [1] and the Cambridge Intensity-Modulated Radiotherapy (IMRT) Study [2].

Four thousand four hundred and fifty-one women were treated within the START trials between 1999 and 2002. All women had undergone complete surgical excision of breast cancer and were otherwise treated with chemotherapy and/or endocrine therapy according to standard protocols. Women in the START-A trial were then randomized between a radiotherapy treatment regimen of 50Gy delivered in 25 fractions over 5 weeks versus 41.6Gy or 39Gy given in 13 fractions over 5 weeks.

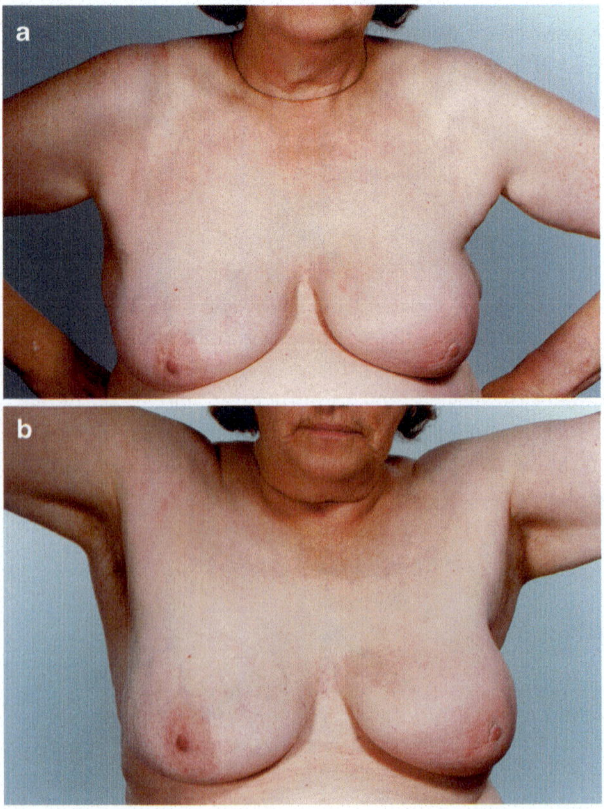


**Fig. 11.1** Change in breast appearance in a woman treated within the START trials from (**a**) before radiotherapy to (**b**) two years after radiotherapy demonstrating mild swelling of the left breast at 2 years

Women in the START-B trial were randomized between 50Gy in 25 fractions over 5 weeks versus 40Gy in 15 fractions over 3 weeks. Of note, most women treated within the START trials received 2-dimensionally (2-D)-planned radiotherapy which was standard at that time. At a median follow-up of almost 10 years, loco-regional relapse rates did not differ significantly between the groups [1]. However, breast firmness, skin changes and breast edema (or swelling) were significantly less common in the 39Gy group of START-A and 40Gy group of START-B as compared to the 50Gy group in each study. In START-A, breast shrinkage and firmness were the most common side-effects at 10 years. Comparing moderate to marked changes in the 50Gy versus 39Gy arms, 27 % versus 23 % experienced breast shrinkage, 23 % versus 18 % breast firmness, 6 % versus 3 % telangiectasia, 13 % versus 7 % breast edema, 12 % versus 9 % shoulder stiffness, and 13 % versus 7 % arm edema. Breast shrinkage and firmness were also the most common side-effects in START-B. Comparing moderate to marked changes at 10 years in the 50Gy versus 40Gy arms, 25 % versus 22 % experienced breast shrinkage, 25 % versus 13 % breast firmness, 5 % versus 3 % telangiectasia, 9 % versus 5 % breast edema, 6 % versus 4 % shoulder stiffness, and 10 % versus 4 % arm edema. Symptomatic rib fractures and lung fibrosis were rare regardless of schedule (around 1 %) and there was only one case of brachial plexopathy out of the 4451 women treated across both START trials. In summary, it is apparent from the START trials that many women experienced noticeable changes in their breast and/or shoulder following the combination of breast surgery and adjuvant radiotherapy.

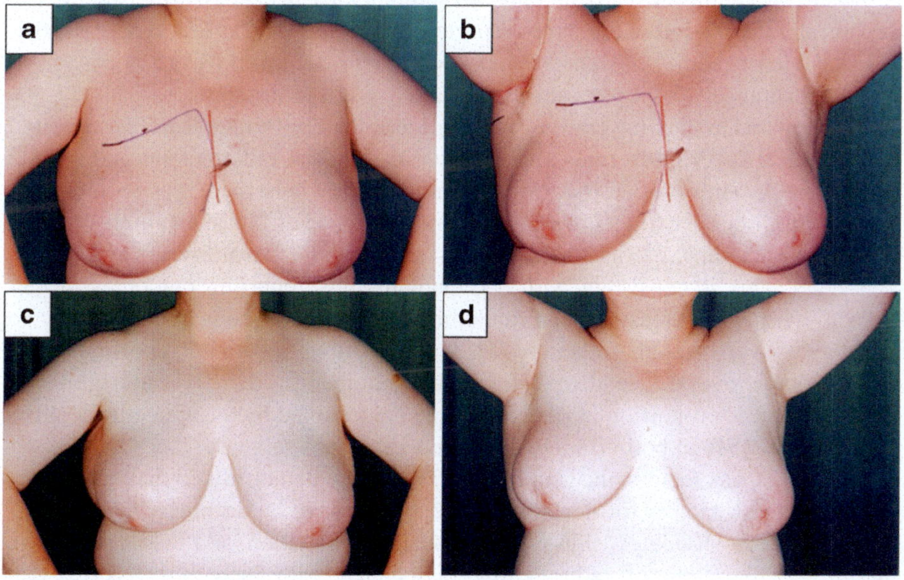


**Fig. 11.2** Change in breast appearance in a woman treated within the START trials from before radiotherapy (**a**, **b**) to 5 years after radiotherapy (**c**, **d**) demonstrating breast shrinkage at 5 years. *Pen markings* illustrate upper inner radiotherapy field edge

Although the START trials provide the longest-term follow-up data, there have been significant improvements in the way we deliver radiotherapy since the women in the START trials were treated. A study comparing 2-D-planned radiotherapy against 3-dimensionally (3-D)-planned or intensity-modulated radiotherapy (IMRT) (in which the radiation dose is delivered more homogeneously across the breast), demonstrated a significant reduction in the proportion of women with any change in breast appearance on clinical photographs taken at 5 years (58 % of 2D-planned patients versus 40 % of 3D-planned patients) [3]. The percentage of women reported to have marked changes in breast appearance was 14 % for the 2-D-planned patients versus 10 % for the 3-D-planned patients, and significantly fewer patients in the 3-D-planned group developed breast firmness as assessed by the clinician in the center of the breast (32 % vs 21 %), upper outer breast (29 % vs 22 %), inframammary fold (24 % versus 17 %) and tumor bed (61 % versus 37 %). However, the differences in breast appearance and palpable breast firmness were not associated with any detectable quality-of-life differences between the two techniques.

Following on from this study, the Cambridge Intensity-Modulated Radiotherapy (IMRT) Study treated 1145 women between 2003 and 2007, randomizing 815 women with inhomogeneous dose on standard wedged tangents to standard radiotherapy versus simple IMRT [2]. Fewer patients in the simple IMRT group (57 %) developed suboptimal overall cosmesis compared to those treated with standard RT (63 %) but there were no differences in breast shrinkage, firmness or swelling between the groups. Once again, patient-reported outcome measures (PROMs) (assessed using global health and breast symptom-specific questionnaires) showed no benefit of simple IMRT over standard radiotherapy [4]. Reassuringly however, the overall rate of adverse outcomes reported using PROMs was low at 5 years (6 % reported breast pain, 4 % skin problems, <0.5 % breast swelling, 15 % change in breast appearance, 13 % breast shrinkage, and 8 % breast firmness).

With regards to the time course of side-effects, the Cambridge IMRT Trial found no difference in PROMs time trends between standard radiotherapy and simple IMRT groups. However, in the trial population as a whole there was an improvement in PROMs over time. For example, the incidence of breast swelling was 5 % prior to radiotherapy, 7 % at 6-months post-radiotherapy, 2 % at 2-years and <0.5 % at 5-years. This is consistent with a Canadian study reporting outcomes in 837 women with early breast cancer randomized after breast-conserving surgery to radiotherapy versus no radiotherapy [5]. The proportion of patients reporting breast pain decreased over time and, at 2 years after radiotherapy, there was no significant difference in the proportion of patients who were troubled by the appearance of the treated breast (5 % in both irradiated and non-irradiated patients).

In terms of risk factors, the Cambridge IMRT Trial demonstrated that, at 2 years, the greatest risk factors for developing late effects were larger breast size (associated with breast shrinkage, skin telangiectasia, pigmentation, and breast swelling), smoking at the time of radiotherapy (associated with increased risk of skin pigmentation), poor baseline post-surgical cosmesis (associated with greatly increased risk of moderate or poor overall cosmesis), and post-operative infection requiring antibiotics (associated with an increased risk of telangiectasia and breast oversensitivity) [6]. At 5 years, patients with moderate to poor baseline post-surgical cosmesis were again more likely to have persisting suboptimal cosmesis, tumor bed firmness, and breast shrinkage [2], whilst post-operative infection and large breast size were the biggest risk factors for patient-reported breast toxicity [4]. In addition, the presence of easily visible seroma on baseline post-operative radiotherapy-planning CT images was associated with an increased risk of post-operative infection and post-operative hematoma, and was also an independent risk factor for whole breast and tumor bed firmness at 2 and 5 years, and for inferior overall cosmesis at 5 years. There was however no significant association between seroma and late breast shrinkage or pain [7].

Other co-morbidities known to increase the risk of late side-effects in irradiated tissues include diabetes [6] and connective tissue disorders [8]. Genetic factors may also influence a patient's risk of developing radiation-induced toxicity [9]. Small studies suggested an association between TGFB1 single nucleotide polymorphisms and the risk of tissue fibrosis [10, 11] but this has not been validated in a larger study of 778 patients treated with breast radiotherapy [12] such that we are some way from being able to identify patients at higher risk of toxicity in whom we can intervene with strategies to protect against radiation toxicity.

### *Treatment*

Patients can be reassured that changes in breast tissue tend to improve with time even in the absence of intervention. In patients with symptomatic changes in breast tissue, massage techniques are of increasing interest but there is little randomized evidence to demonstrate a benefit in patients specifically with breast edema. One study randomized 21 patients with breast edema following breast conservation surgery to manual lymphatic drainage plus or minus low-intensity low-frequency electrostatic fields. Both treatment groups reported a subjective reduction in breast swelling but this was confirmed on 3D measurement only in the electrostatic field group [13]. Data relating to the use of manual lymphatic drainage, acupuncture and exercise therapies in breast-cancer related lymphedema are reviewed below. With regards to oral therapies, a double-blind placebo-controlled trial of pentoxifylline and vitamin E also failed to show a benefit in breast fibrosis [14]. Therefore no routine prophylactic treatment is generally advised to reduce the risk of post-treatment changes in the breast.

## Lymphedema of the Arm

### *Incidence and Risk Factors*

Breast-cancer related lymphedema (BCRL) refers mainly, in the published literature, to swelling of the arm. BCRL can occur as a result of breast cancer surgery, radiation therapy and/or disease and can cause pain, heaviness, and reduced mobility all of which can negatively impact on daily function, psychological well-being, and quality-of-life [15, 16]. The diagnosis of BCRL is based mainly on patient-reported symptoms together with the clinical finding of differences in arm circumference. Investigations such as bioimpedance spectroscopy may be able to detect preclinical changes in extracellular fluid [17] but, since there are few data to support there being a benefit from pre-clinical interventions in BCRL [18], such measurements are not undertaken routinely. Novel imaging modalities include contrast-enhanced magnetic resonance lymphangiography, whereby the anatomy and function of upper limb lymphatics can be evaluated quantitatively [19] underpinning future studies of treatment interventions.

A recent systematic review and meta-analysis of 72 studies assessing the incidence of, and risk factors for, BCRL gave a pooled estimate for lymphedema incidence of 17 % (or 21 % when restricted to data from 30 prospective cohort studies) [18]. The incidence of BCRL increased up to 2 years following surgery for breast cancer and was more than three times higher in women who had undergone axillary node dissection (20 %) than in women who had undergone sentinel lymph node biopsy (6 %). Other risk factors with a strong level of evidence included the number of lymph nodes dissected, mastectomy as compared to breast conservation surgery, and being overweight. Risk factors with a moderate level of evidence included the presence of metastatic lymph nodes, use of chemotherapy or radiotherapy, and lack of regular physical exercise. A more recent analysis of a recent London teaching hospital cohort of women with node-positive disease treated from 2010 to 2012, all of whom underwent axillary node dissection reported a 27 % rate of BCRL (74 of 273 patients). Patients who had received adjuvant taxanes were nearly three times more likely to develop BCRL than patients who had no chemotherapy (HR 2.82). Interestingly, no association was found between use of taxanes in the neoadjuvant setting and risk of lymphedema [20].

## *Pathophysiology*

BCRL is likely to be the result of several pathophysiological processes beyond the simple slowing or cessation of lymphatic flow through a damaged axilla. One hypothesis is that there may be a more global lymphatic dysfunction in women who develop BCRL. One study [21] measured lower-limb scintigraphy in 30 women who had undergone axillary node dissection at least 3 years previously, 15 of whom had BCRL and 15 of whom did not. The control group was 24 women with no history of cancer or lower-limb lymphedema. They reported reduced lower-limb drainage in those with BCRL versus those without BCRL. Interestingly, 17/30 breast cancer patients had reduced lower-limb lymphatic flow compared with 0/24 controls suggesting that there may be a systemic effect of breast cancer or its treatment upon lymphatic function. In another small study from the same group, upper limb lymphatic flow was reported to be higher in women who went onto develop BCRL than in those who did not, suggesting that higher pre-operative flow may predispose to lymphatic overload and failure.

## *Treatment*

The mainstay of treatment of BCRL is the use of decongestive therapies. Complex decongestive therapy (CDT) is a four-fold conservative treatment which includes manual lymphatic drainage (MLD), compression therapy (using bandages and/or sleeves), skin care and lymph-reducing exercises. It is usually undertaken in two phases, a first phase aiming to reduce swelling, and a second maintenance phase. A recent Cochrane Systematic review of manual lymphatic drainage demonstrated that addition of MLD to compression bandaging may particularly benefit those with mild to moderate BCRL in terms of reduced swelling but be of less additional benefit in those with more severe BCRL [22, 23]. There was no conclusive evidence that addition of MLD to compression bandaging improved function or quality of life but, in the studies measuring pain and heaviness, 60–80 % of patients reported an improvement in symptoms regardless of the treatment received. The addition of kinesio-taping to compression bandaging has not been shown to reduce swelling or improve function over compression bandaging [24], whereas the addition of kinesio-taping to CDT has been shown to be beneficial in further reducing swelling at 10-days post-treatment [25].

Other non-surgical treatment approaches include low-level laser therapy (LLLT), hyperbaric oxygen therapy (HBO) and oral therapies. Meta-analysis of nine studies of LLLT suggests clinically relevant reductions in volume and pain immediately after conclusion of treatments [26]. A non-randomized phase II trial of HBO in 21 patients with chronic arm lymphedema (minimum 30 % increase in arm diameter) following axillary and/or supraclavicular radiotherapy (18/21 had undergone axillary surgery) demonstrated a statistically significant but clinically modest reduction in ipsilateral volume compared with baseline [27]. However, a subsequent randomized phase II trial failed to show a benefit of HBO in treating arm lymphedema with almost no reduction in arm volume in both the treatment and control groups [28]. A double-blind placebo-controlled trial of pentoxifylline and vitamin E also failed to show a benefit in arm lymphedema [14].

Surgical approaches to the management of upper limb lymphedema are discussed in Chap. 12.

Exercise programs may be helpful. For example, a recent systematic review showed that progressive resistance training (including resistive exercises using body weight, free/machine weights and/or elastic bands) reduced the risk of breast-cancer related lymphedema in randomized controlled trials [29]. Another systematic review however found no effect of exercise interventions on lymphedema symptoms although it was reassuring that regular exercise did not appear to worsen lymphedema symptoms [30]. Of note, there was insufficient evidence to confirm or refute the current clinical recommendation to wear compression garments during regular exercise.

A pilot study of acupuncture in women with chronic arm lymphedema demonstrated a 33 % reduction in arm circumference [31] in 33 evaluable patients. Importantly, there were no infections or exacerbations of swelling after 255 treatments and 6 months of follow-up suggesting that the use of acupuncture needles in patients with BCRL is safe.

Finally, with regards to lymphedema prevention strategies, a recent Cochrane systematic review found no effect of early post-operative exercise, ongoing progressive resistance exercise therapy, or manual lymphatic drainage on the risk of developing BCRL [32]. Nonetheless patients should be advised to maintain a healthy weight, try and avoid trauma to the arm on the treated side (including use of gloves when gardening and cooking, and avoidance of insect bites and sunburn), to obtain antibiotics promptly where infection develops, and to avoid venepuncture from the affected arm [33, 34].

## Musculoskeletal Late Side-Effects in the Upper Limb

### *Chronic Shoulder Pain and Reduced Shoulder Mobility*

Acute shoulder pain and dysfunction are common following surgery for breast cancer [35]. The likelihood of symptoms increases with the extent of surgery with one study reporting, at 2 weeks post-operatively, restricted shoulder movement in 45 % of patients undergoing sentinel-lymph node biopsy and 86 % of those undergoing axillary dissection [36]. Pain and shoulder dysfunction have been reported to affect psychological well-being in up to one-third of patients who have undergone axillary dissection [35].

Fortunately, for the majority of patients, symptoms settle within a few weeks of surgery [36] but, for a proportion of patients, shoulder pain and dysfunction become chronic (i.e. symptoms persist beyond 3 months post-operatively). The relative contribution of surgery versus radiotherapy to the likelihood of chronic pain is difficult to determine but the level of risk is likely to be determined in part by the extent of the radiotherapy field. In the START-A trial, in which all patients were treated with breast or chest wall radiotherapy, but only 14 % with an additional nodal radiotherapy field (predominantly supraclavicular fossa only), 11–18 % of patients were reported to have shoulder stiffness at 10 years [1]. In the START-B trial, in which only 7 % were treated with an additional nodal field, physician-reported shoulder stiffness at 10 years was 8 % in patients who received 50Gy in 25 fractions and 3 % in those who received 40Gy in 15 fractions [1]. The EORTC IM-MS trial of chest wall radiotherapy plus or minus internal mammary and medial supraclavicular radiotherapy reported arm or shoulder function impairment in <0.5 % of patients at 3 years [37]. In the MA-20 study comparing breast plus or minus locoregional lymph node radiotherapy (including axillary, supraclavicular and internal mammary lymph nodes), the rate of delayed joint stiffness more than 3 months after radiotherapy was 1.5 % in the breast only group and 2.4 % in the breast and locoregional lymph node radiotherapy group [38]. In summary, rates of chronic shoulder pain and dysfunction using modern surgical and radiotherapy techniques are much lower than historically reported.

With regards to treatment, a recent Cochrane systematic review of the effect of exercise interventions following treatment of cancers including breast cancer, suggests that exercise interventions may have beneficial effects on quality-of-life including physical and social functioning. More specifically, early intervention with physiotherapy has been shown to improve shoulder mobility, reduce pain and improve quality of life [39]. Physiotherapy programs vary considerably between studies but common themes are that they begin 1–2 days post-operatively with gentle shoulder abduction, flexion and extension exercises (minimizing stress on the surgical incision by keeping the elbow bent), they progress at around a week post-surgery to shoulder flexion, extension, abduction and adduction with the arm extended, and they continue after 2 weeks (once the suture lines are secure) with exercises that will stretch the soft tissues around the shoulder and chest wall [39, 40]. Specialist referral is recommended where arm and shoulder complications persist despite standard post-operative exercise programs.

## *Cording*

Cording describes the post-operative development of fibrous strands beneath the skin of the armpit and radiating down to the elbow, wrist and occasionally chest wall. Also described as "axillary web syndrome", its cause is unclear. However, the leading hypothesis, supported by biopsy evidence, is that axillary surgery causes lymphovenous outflow obstruction which in turn causes a superficial thrombophlebitis of the superficial veins in the arm [41].

Cording occurs in up to 20 % of patients who have undergone sentinel lymph-node biopsy and up to 72 % of patients who have undergone axillary surgery [36, 41, 42]. Risk factors include younger age [43, 44], extent of axillary surgery [43], and low body-mass index [42]. It rarely occurs in the absence of axillary surgery [41]. Where cording does develop, it usually arises 1–8 weeks post-operatively [41]. In some series, the majority of cases of cording resolve spontaneously within 3 months of surgery [41]. In other series, symptoms persist in up to a third of patients at 12 weeks [42].

For some patients, cording is asymptomatic but, for others, it can feel tight and sometimes painful. In up to 74 % of patients, cording can limit movement of the upper limb on the affected side [36]. Symptomatic cording can be treated using physiotherapy exercises along the lines described above and has been specifically described by Kepics [45] and Wyrick et al. [46]. Soft tissue mobilization techniques including modified massage described by Fourie and Robb [47] may also accelerate recovery but have not been tested in randomized controlled trials.

## Summary

As surgical and radiotherapeutic techniques have improved, the incidence of locoregional complications has fallen but nonetheless remains a significant issue for a proportion of patients. Where complications impact on daily function and quality of life, specialist advice in managing complications should be sought as, although complications may not be curable, a broad range of treatments is available to reduce symptoms. Further well-designed randomized trials in the treatment of locoregional complications will be helpful in refining treatment recommendations and identifying preventative strategies.

## References

1. Haviland JS, et al. The UK Standardisation of Breast Radiotherapy (START) trials of radiotherapy hypofractionation for treatment of early breast cancer: 10-year follow-up results of two randomised controlled trials. Lancet Oncol. 2013;14(11):1086–94.
2. Mukesh MB, et al. Randomized controlled trial of intensity-modulated radiotherapy for early breast cancer: 5-year results confirm superior overall cosmesis. J Clin Oncol. 2013; 31(36):4488–95.
3. Donovan E, et al. Randomised trial of standard 2D radiotherapy (RT) versus intensity modulated radiotherapy (IMRT) in patients prescribed breast radiotherapy. Radiother Oncol. 2007;82(3):254–64.
4. Mukesh MB, et al. Patient reported outcome measures (PROMs) following forward planned field-in field IMRT: results from the Cambridge Breast IMRT trial. Radiother Oncol. 2014; 111(2):270–5.
5. Whelan TJ, et al. The effects of radiation therapy on quality of life of women with breast carcinoma: results of a randomized trial. Ontario Clinical Oncology Group. Cancer. 2000;88(10): 2260–6.
6. Barnett GC, et al. The Cambridge Breast Intensity-modulated Radiotherapy Trial: patient- and treatment-related factors that influence late toxicity. Clin Oncol (R Coll Radiol). 2011;23(10):662–73.
7. Mukesh MB, et al. Association of breast tumour bed seroma with post-operative complications and late normal tissue toxicity: results from the Cambridge Breast IMRT trial. Eur J Surg Oncol. 2012;38(10):918–24.
8. Holscher T, Bentzen SM, Baumann M. Influence of connective tissue diseases on the expression of radiation side effects: a systematic review. Radiother Oncol. 2006;78(2):123–30.
9. Barnett GC, et al. A genome wide association study (GWAS) providing evidence of an association between common genetic variants and late radiotherapy toxicity. Radiother Oncol. 2014;111(2):178–85.
10. Andreassen CN, et al. Prediction of normal tissue radiosensitivity from polymorphisms in candidate genes. Radiother Oncol. 2003;69(2):127–35.
11. Giotopoulos G, et al. The late radiotherapy normal tissue injury phenotypes of telangiectasia, fibrosis and atrophy in breast cancer patients have distinct genotype-dependent causes. Br J Cancer. 2007;96(6):1001–7.
12. Barnett GC, et al. No association between SNPs regulating TGF-beta1 secretion and late radiotherapy toxicity to the breast: results from the RAPPER study. Radiother Oncol. 2010;97(1):9–14.
13. Jahr S, Schoppe B, Reisshauer A. Effect of treatment with low-intensity and extremely low-frequency electrostatic fields (Deep Oscillation) on breast tissue and pain in patients with secondary breast lymphoedema. J Rehabil Med. 2008;40(8):645–50.
14. Gothard L, et al. Double-blind placebo-controlled randomised trial of vitamin E and pentoxifylline in patients with chronic arm lymphoedema and fibrosis after surgery and radiotherapy for breast cancer. Radiother Oncol. 2004;73(2):133–9.
15. Hayes SC, et al. Upper-body morbidity after breast cancer: incidence and evidence for evaluation, prevention, and management within a prospective surveillance model of care. Cancer. 2012;118(8 Suppl):2237–49.

16. Maunsell E, Brisson J, Deschenes L. Arm problems and psychological distress after surgery for breast cancer. Can J Surg. 1993;36(4):315–20.
17. Cornish BH, et al. Early diagnosis of lymphedema using multiple frequency bioimpedance. Lymphology. 2001;34(1):2–11.
18. DiSipio T, et al. Incidence of unilateral arm lymphoedema after breast cancer: a systematic review and meta-analysis. Lancet Oncol. 2013;14(6):500–15.
19. Borri M, et al. Quantitative contrast-enhanced magnetic resonance lymphangiography of the upper limbs in breast cancer related lymphedema: an exploratory study. Lymphat Res Biol. 2015;13(2):100–6.
20. Cariati M, et al. Adjuvant taxanes and the development of breast cancer-related arm lymphoedema. Br J Surg. 2015;102(9):1071–8.
21. Bains SK, et al. Global abnormalities in lymphatic function following systemic therapy in patients with breast cancer. Br J Surg. 2015;102(5):534–40.
22. Ezzo J, et al. 'Manual lymphatic drainage for lymphedema following breast cancer treatment', Cochrane Database Syst Rev. 2015; 5: CD003475.
23. Gradalski T, Ochalek K, Kurpiewska J. Complex decongestive lymphatic therapy with or without vodder II manual lymph drainage in more severe chronic postmastectomy upper limb lymphedema: a randomized non-inferiority prospective study. J Pain Symptom Manage. 2015;50(6):750–7.
24. Taradaj J, et al. The influence of Kinesiology Taping on the volume of lymphoedema and manual dexterity of the upper limb in women after breast cancer treatment. Eur J Cancer Care (Engl). 2016;25(4):647–60.
25. Pekyavas NO, et al. Complex decongestive therapy and taping for patients with postmastectomy lymphedema: a randomized controlled study. Eur J Oncol Nurs. 2014;18(6):585–90.
26. Smoot B, et al. Effect of low-level laser therapy on pain and swelling in women with breast cancer-related lymphedema: a systematic review and meta-analysis. J Cancer Surviv. 2015;9(2):287–304.
27. Gothard L, et al. Non-randomised phase II trial of hyperbaric oxygen therapy in patients with chronic arm lymphoedema and tissue fibrosis after radiotherapy for early breast cancer. Radiother Oncol. 2004;70(3):217–24.
28. Gothard L, et al. Randomised phase II trial of hyperbaric oxygen therapy in patients with chronic arm lymphoedema after radiotherapy for cancer. Radiother Oncol. 2010;97(1): 101–7.
29. Cheema BS, et al. Safety and efficacy of progressive resistance training in breast cancer: a systematic review and meta-analysis. Breast Cancer Res Treat. 2014;148(2):249–68.
30. Singh B, et al. Systematic review and meta-analysis of the effects of exercise for those with cancer-related lymphedema. Arch Phys Med Rehabil. 2016;97(2):302–315.e13.
31. Cassileth BR, et al. Acupuncture in the treatment of upper-limb lymphedema: results of a pilot study. Cancer. 2013;119(13):2455–61.
32. Stuiver MM, et al. Conservative interventions for preventing clinically detectable upper-limb lymphoedema in patients who are at risk of developing lymphoedema after breast cancer therapy, Cochrane Database Syst Rev. 2015;(2):CD009765.
33. Harris SR, et al. Clinical practice guidelines for breast cancer rehabilitation: syntheses of guideline recommendations and qualitative appraisals. Cancer. 2012;118(8 Suppl): 2312–24.
34. Poage E, et al. Demystifying lymphedema: development of the lymphedema putting evidence into practice card. Clin J Oncol Nurs. 2008;12(6):951–64.
35. Caffo O, et al. Pain and quality of life after surgery for breast cancer. Breast Cancer Res Treat. 2003;80(1):39–48.
36. Leidenius M, et al. Motion restriction and axillary web syndrome after sentinel node biopsy and axillary clearance in breast cancer. Am J Surg. 2003;185(2):127–30.
37. Poortmans PM, et al. Internal mammary and medial supraclavicular irradiation in breast cancer. N Engl J Med. 2015;373(4):317–27.
38. Whelan TJ, et al. Regional nodal irradiation in early-stage breast cancer. N Engl J Med. 2015;373(4):307–16.

39. Testa A, Iannace C, Di Libero L. Strengths of early physical rehabilitation programs in surgical breast cancer patients: results of a randomized controlled study. Eur J Phys Rehabil Med. 2014;50(3):275–84.
40. Harmer V. Breast cancer nursing care and management. 2nd ed. Chichester: Wiley; 2011.
41. Moskovitz AH, et al. Axillary web syndrome after axillary dissection. Am J Surg. 2001;181(5): 434–9.
42. Koehler LA, et al. Movement, function, pain, and postoperative edema in axillary web syndrome. Phys Ther. 2015;95(10):1345–53.
43. Fukushima KF, et al. Frequency and associated factors of axillary web syndrome in women who had undergone breast cancer surgery: a transversal and retrospective study. Springerplus. 2015;4:112.
44. O'Toole J, et al. Cording following treatment for breast cancer. Breast Cancer Res Treat. 2013;140(1):105–11.
45. Kepics J. Physical therapy treatment of axillary web syndrome. Rehabil Oncol. 2004;22:21–2.
46. Wyrick SL, Waltke LJ, Ng AV. Physical therapy may promote resolution of lymphatic cording in breast cancer survivors. Rehabil Oncol. 2006;24(1):29–34.
47. Fourie WJ, Robb KA. Physiotherapy management of axillary web syndrome following breast cancer treatment: discussing the use of soft tissue techniques. Physiotherapy. 2009;95(4): 314–20.

# Chapter 12
# The Role of Surgery in Breast Cancer Survivors

**Rachel L. O'Connell and Jennifer E. Rusby**

**Abstract** The vast majority of women diagnosed with breast cancer undergo some form of surgery to the breast, with or without surgery to the axilla. Approximately half undergo breast-conserving therapy (wide local excision/lumpectomy with or without radiotherapy) and the remainder undergo a mastectomy (removal of all of the breast tissue), with or without immediate reconstruction.

However, even after primary treatment (which may include surgery, chemotherapy and radiotherapy), the patient may require further surgical procedures by choice or necessity during the course of their survivorship. These can range from small procedures performed as a day case under local anesthetic to a long and complex conversion from an implant-based to autologous reconstruction.

Reasons for surgery can be classified into:

- Delayed breast reconstruction
- Surgery for late complications
- Other aesthetic adjustment (to improve appearance, usually after the primary reconstruction)
- Contralateral symmetrization surgery
- Contralateral risk-reducing mastectomy
- Surgery for lymphedema

In this chapter, we will discuss the indications, outcome and possible complications of these procedures.

## Introduction

The vast majority of women diagnosed with breast cancer undergo some form of surgery to the breast, with or without surgery to the axilla. Approximately half undergo breast-conserving therapy (wide local excision/lumpectomy with or

R.L. O'Connell, MBBS, BSc, MRCS • J.E. Rusby, BM, BCh, DM, FRCS (✉)
The Breast Unit, The Royal Marsden NHS Foundation Trust, Surrey, UK
e-mail: jennifer.rusby@rmh.nhs.uk



A. Ring, M. Parton (eds.), *Breast Cancer Survivorship*,
DOI 10.1007/978-3-319-41858-2_12

without radiotherapy) and the remainder undergo a mastectomy (removal of all of the breast tissue), with or without immediate reconstruction [1].

However, even after primary treatment (which may include surgery, chemotherapy and radiotherapy), the patient may require further surgical procedures by choice or necessity during the course of their survivorship. These can range from small procedures performed as a day case under local anesthetic to a long and complex conversion from an implant-based to autologous reconstruction.

Reasons for surgery can be classified into:

- Delayed breast reconstruction
- Surgery for late complications
- Other aesthetic adjustment (to improve appearance, usually after the primary reconstruction)
- Contralateral symmetrization surgery
- Contralateral risk-reducing mastectomy
- Surgery for lymphedema

In this chapter, we will discuss the indications, outcome and possible complications of these procedures. We will not discuss surgery for recurrence as management of recurrent disease is not within the scope of this book.

## Delayed Breast Reconstruction

Immediate breast reconstruction is performed at the same time as the mastectomy. Delayed breast reconstruction is performed months, or years after the mastectomy. NICE guidelines [2] on the treatment of early and locally advanced breast cancer state that immediate breast reconstruction should be discussed with all patients who are considering mastectomy, and offered except where significant comorbidity or the need for adjuvant therapy preclude this option. The caveat regarding adjuvant therapy usually relates to post mastectomy radiotherapy (PMRT). Radiotherapy causes fibrosis of the reconstructed breast. It increases the risk of fat necrosis in an autologous reconstruction (see section "Fat Necrosis After Free Flap Transfer") and capsular contracture in an implant based reconstruction (see section "Capsular Contracture"). At worst it may result in failure of the reconstruction so that the implant or autologous reconstruction must be removed prematurely. Therefore if the patient is known to require PMRT, many surgeons recommend avoidance of free flaps in the immediate setting. While the dogma that autologous flaps, especially abdominal-based flaps, should not be irradiated is now being tested [3, 4], this would not be regarded as a standard approach. The options remaining include a simple mastectomy (i.e. no reconstruction) or immediate, implant-based reconstruction in which the intention may be that the definitive reconstruction is implant-based, or that the implant will be replaced by a definitive autologous reconstruction after radiotherapy.

Other women may feel at the time of diagnosis that they wish to focus on the oncological treatment and cannot cope with the complex decision making required for reconstruction or need more time to consider the reconstructive options. Therefore they may choose a therapeutic mastectomy without reconstruction, and some will request a delayed reconstruction, months or years after the original surgery.

There are various surgical techniques available for delayed reconstruction. The choice will depend on patient preferences, surgeon expertise and patient factors such as whether the patient had PMRT, body mass index (BMI), smoking status and medical co-morbidities.

## *Autologous Reconstruction*

This type of reconstruction uses the patient's own tissue from elsewhere in the body which is moved to the breast either keeping the blood supply intact (pedicled flap) or by dividing the blood vessels supplying the flap of tissue and then re-joining them using microsurgery to vessels near the breast. Flaps may be taken from the abdomen (DIEP, deep inferior epigastric perforator flap, SIEA, superficial inferior epigastric artery flap or TRAM, transverse rectus abdominis myocutaneous flap), upper back (LD, latissimus dorsi flap), thigh (TUG, transverse upper gracilis) or buttock (IGAP, inferior gluteal artery perforator flap or SGAP, superior gluteal artery perforator flap). One final consideration is that a DIEP flap is a "once in a lifetime opportunity", so if a woman is considering delayed DIEP flap reconstruction and contralateral risk-reducing surgery (see section "Contralateral Mastectomy for Risk Reduction"), these should be planned as a simultaneous procedure so that (if of sufficient volume) the DIEP flap can be used to reconstruct both breasts to maximize symmetry.

## *Implant Based Reconstruction*

This accounts for approximately 16 % of delayed reconstructions in the UK and may be done in one or two stages. An inflatable implant or tissue expander (TE) may be inserted into a pocket created by the surgeon under the pectoral muscle and fascia to the infra-mammary fold. Over several weeks the TE is filled with saline to stretch the pocket so eventually it can be removed and replaced by the definitive implant (usually made of silicone) of the correct volume. Direct to fixed volume implant (one stage) reconstruction may be undertaken if the surgeon is confident that enough space can be created in the pocket though this is unusual in the delayed setting even for small breasts. Achieving coverage of the inferior pole of the implant may be achieved by recruiting a portion of the serratus muscle laterally. More recently acellular dermal matrixes (ADM) which are collagen sheets derived from porcine, bovine or human tissue and synthetic mesh have been developed to provide lower pole coverage, though these are rarely used in delayed breast reconstruction as an ellipse of skin is removed at mastectomy and needs to be replaced by tissue expansion or autologous tissue transfer.

**Table 12.1** Advantages and disadvantages of reconstructive options in the delayed setting

| Type of reconstruction | Advantages | Disadvantages |
|---|---|---|
| Implant | No donor site scar | Difficult to expand in irradiated tissue<br>Artificial shape<br>Risk of capsular contracture |
| Latissimus dorsi (LD) flap | Autologous flap brings skin as well as volume<br>Widely available | Donor site scar on back<br>Risk of shoulder weakness<br>May not carry sufficient volume |
| Combined LD and implant | Addresses volume issues of LD alone | Disadvantages as for implant and LD |
| DIEP flap | Autologous flap bringing skin as well as volume<br>Natural breast-like texture<br>Abdominal wall musculature preserved<br>"Tummy tuck" due to the removal of the abdominal skin and fat from the lower abdomen | Complex microsurgery<br>Long operation and recovery time<br>Long donor site scar |
| Thigh flap | May be suitable for women who do not have an adequate abdominal pannus | Initial wound-related complications owing to inner thigh location |
| Buttock flap | May be suitable for women who do not have adequate abdominal pannus | Buttock asymmetry<br>Donor site scar<br>Fat of buttock is firmer so reconstruction less natural in texture than DIEP |

Table 12.1 **summarizes some of the advantages and disadvantages of reconstructive options in the delayed setting. A review by Thiruchelvam et al**. [5] **and the MacMillan Understanding Breast Reconstruction patient information booklet** [6] **provide further information about post-mastectomy breast reconstruction.**

Figure 12.1 shows a patient before and after delayed DIEP reconstruction, illustrating the need for contralateral symmetrization reduction, dog-ear removal and the appearance without nipple reconstruction.

## *Delayed Partial Breast Reconstruction for Focal Deficit After Breast Conserving Surgery*

The intention of modern oncoplastic breast conserving surgery is to repair the defect in the breast during the primary procedure either by tissue displacement (ranging from simple parenchymal advancement to complex mammoplasty techniques) or volume replacement techniques. Occasionally, however, patients are seen with a very poor aesthetic outcome after primary breast conserving therapy and it is necessary to replace lost volume. This could be using lipomodelling (outlined below), or using a partial breast reconstruction with volume replacement (such as LD miniflap, or now muscle-sparing local perforator flaps such as LICAP, lateral intercostal

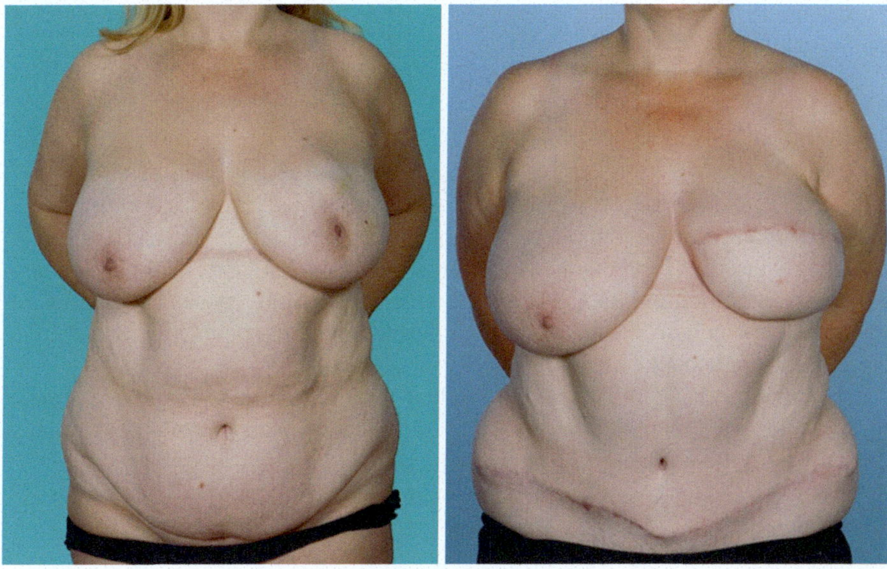

**Fig. 12.1** A patient before and after delayed DIEP reconstruction, illustrating the need for contralateral symmetrization reduction, dog-ear removal and the appearance without nipple reconstruction

artery perforator flaps or TDAP, thoracodorsal artery perforator flaps). Sometimes the deficit is felt to be so extensive that a completion mastectomy and whole breast reconstruction is recommended.

## Surgery for Late Complications

### *Infection*

Implant removal because of infection or skin necrosis is most common in the early post-operative period, but infection can occur many years later, presumably via hematogenous spread. If planning allows, an immediate autologous salvage reconstruction can be performed. Generally, however, the implant is removed, the cavity washed out thoroughly and left free of foreign material for several months. At a later stage a salvage reconstruction may be performed.

### *Capsular Contracture*

It is normal for a capsule to form around an implant as the host response to foreign material is to wall it off. However, that capsule may thicken and contract making the reconstruction firmer. In more severe cases, capsular contracture may lead to a change in shape and thus symmetry of the reconstruction, and even pain or displacement.

## *Implant Rupture*

This is fortunately rare with modern implants, the exception being the series of Poly Implant Prosthèse (PIP) implants which came to light in 2012 [7]. These used unapproved silicone filler and were associated with higher rupture rates. Symptoms of implant rupture include change in shape or development of palpable regional lymph nodes which contain silicone.

For both capsular contracture and implant rupture, the options include simple removal and adjustment of the pocket to a flat chest wall, or more commonly replacement of the implant (with excision (capsulectomy) or release (capsulotomy) of the tight capsule in cases of contracture) or conversion to an autologous reconstruction.

## *Latissimus Dorsi Muscle Twitching*

When used in a reconstruction, the LD muscle is moved from the patient's back to an anterior position over the chest wall. The muscle may remain active, causing movement of the reconstruction, known as animation, and a sense of tightness, in the absence of clinically obvious capsular contracture. Division of the thoracodorsal nerve is not often done during initial operation because it is thought that denervation will lead to muscle volume loss, and for fear of damaging the vascular pedicle. When the muscle remains active, delayed division of the thoracodorsal nerve via an axillary incision will stop the twitching, decrease the resting tone of the muscle and, in most patients, offers significant relief from symptoms of tightness and movement [8]. More recently the use of Botulinum toxin A (botox injection) to cause functional denervation of the muscle fibers at the neuromuscular junction by inhibiting the release of acetylcholine from the thoracodorsal nerve terminals has been reported [9].

## *Fat Necrosis After Free Flap Transfer*

Occasionally women develop small areas of fat necrosis within a free flap and may present, concerned because they have found a lump in their reconstruction. Usual diagnostic protocols should be followed and most women can be reassured. Rarely, the process is painful, particularly if it occurs over a wider area and consideration should then be given to removal by excision, liposuction or image-guided vacuum excision.

## Surgery to Donor Sites

As described above, in autologous reconstruction tissue is 'donated' to the breast from another site. There may be morbidity associated with the donor site. There are some specific complications that may require further surgery in the longer term.

### *Abdominal Hernias*

The important difference between TRAM and DIEP flaps is that the former sacrifices part of the rectus abdominis muscle of the abdominal wall to carry the blood supply to the reconstruction and is, therefore, associated with double the rate of abdominal hernia compared with DIEP reconstructions [10]. Patients may present with a palpable abdominal swelling, which may cause an aching or dragging sensation. The defect in the rectus muscles may be repaired by a surgical procedure and usually requires the insertion of a mesh which can be synthetic or made of an ADM. This may be performed by the same plastic surgeon that performed the original DIEP or a general surgeon. Some plastic surgeons routinely insert mesh at the primary operation to prevent this complication.

### *Chronic Seromas*

Most women develop a seroma after simple mastectomy, axillary dissection and at donor sites (back and abdomen), but it is unusual for this to remain in the long term. Those that do may be uncomfortable, or form an awkward lump. They can be managed by opening the cavity and quilting (suturing the anterior wall to the posterior wall), and insertion of suction drains which should be left for up to 2 weeks. Although this is without much scientific evidence, anecdotally, they seem rarely to recur.

## Symmetrizing Reduction/Augmentation

The ultimate aim of oncoplastic breast surgery is to remove the tumor safely whilst maintaining symmetry with the contralateral breast. If the patient has large or ptotic breasts, maintaining symmetry may not be possible, and this may also be the case if the breasts are small. Symmetrizing surgery refers to the adjustment of the contralateral, healthy breast to match the index, treated breast.

Surgical options for the opposite breast include:

- Reduction (reduction mammoplasty)
- Enlargement (augmentation)

- Breast uplift (mastopexy)
- Enlargement and uplift (augmentation mastopexy)

If a patient wishes to undergo symmetrizing surgery, a careful discussion between the patient and surgeon must take place towards understanding the patient's goals and aligning expectations to the likely possible outcome. Timing of the surgery is controversial. It may be possible to carry out a symmetrizing procedure at the same time as the index breast surgery, however, the effect of radiotherapy and "settling" of a reconstruction lead to unpredictability of the target shape and size. In addition, simultaneous symmetrization increases the operation length and carries the risk of complications which might delay adjuvant treatment. Conversely, planning a two-stage procedure incurs logistical considerations, such as finding space on operating lists and the prioritization of oncological procedures ahead of aesthetic procedures. Thus the patient often has to endure a prolonged period of marked asymmetry, throughout their adjuvant treatment, and when on the waiting list for an elective non-cancer procedure.

Figure 12.2 shows a patient before and at increasing time intervals after bilateral therapeutic mammoplasty. It demonstrates the impact of post-radiotherapy shrinkage of the index right breast over time, leading to asymmetry. It also illustrates a patient before and after nipple reconstruction and areola tattooing.

The patient should be warned that after symmetrizing surgery, the breasts may undergo further changes due to gravity or fluctations in body weight so that asymmetry may recur. A review by Rizki et al. [11] describes surgical management of the contralateral breast in post-mastectomy breast reconstruction in more detail.

## Contralateral Mastectomy for Risk Reduction

At the time of diagnosis, particularly if undergoing mastectomy, many women enquire about their contralateral risk and whether a contralateral risk-reducing mastectomy is warranted. Most accept the explanation of low risk of contralateral relative to distant disease, and the need to focus treatment on the index cancer and their anxiety wanes over time. A few women will return to clinic during their survivorship requesting contralateral risk-reducing mastectomy. Occasionally this is because new diagnoses within the family or lower thresholds for genetic testing have led to the patient being tested and found to carry a pathogenic mutation in, for example, one of the BRCA genes (Chap. 5). More often, however, a woman finds herself psychologically unable to move on for fear of a contralateral cancer. The issues may include unwillingness to go through treatment again (particularly chemotherapy) and a lack of faith in surveillance imaging (especially if the index tumor was imaging-occult). While the surgery itself is similar to therapeutic mastectomy and immediate reconstruction, the pre-operative discussions are often complex. Many women over-estimate their risk of contralateral breast cancer [12] and underestimate their risk of distant disease, leading them to believe that contralateral risk-reducing mastectomy

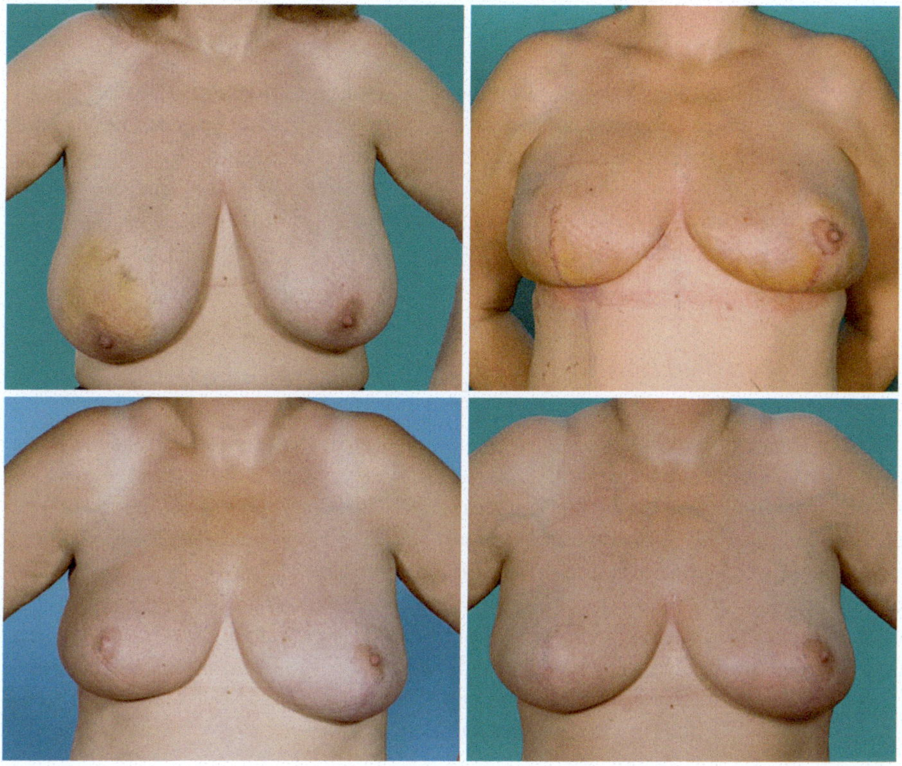

**Fig. 12.2** Clockwise from *top left*: a patient before and at increasing time intervals after bilateral therapeutic mammoplasty. This figure demonstrates the impact of post-radiotherapy shrinkage of the index right breast over time, leading to asymmetry. It also illustrates a patient before and after nipple reconstruction and areola tattooing

may improve their overall survival. In fact, this has only been suggested in BRCA carriers [13] but a Cochrane review concluded that there is insufficient evidence to support this in the general breast cancer population [14], and this should be emphasized. Furthermore, contralateral surgery adds morbidity, carrying a similar complication profile to therapeutic surgery, but with higher expectations. It remains to be seen whether "optional" surgery with no clear oncological benefit will continue to be funded by tax-funded national health services or indeed private insurers.

## Adjustment Surgery

Most indications for adjustment surgery are relative, and depend upon the patient's desire to undergo repeated operations. Patients' expectations of the likely benefit of aesthetic adjustments must be managed.

## *Removal of Dog Ears*

"Dog ears" describe the folds of excess skin and fat that may remain at either end of a scar. They may occur after a simple mastectomy, or at the LD or abdominal donor sites, especially if the closure was tight. These may be unsightly or rub against clothes, though can be excised or reduced using liposuction as a day case procedure. There may also be an overhang of tissue above an abdominal scar, which may be amenable to liposuction.

## *Nipple Reconstruction*

The nipple is usually preserved in breast conserving surgery unless there is evidence of involvement by the malignant process. Similarly, there is now a move towards nipple-sparing mastectomy when immediate breast reconstruction is planned. There are challenges with this approach, including identifying malignant involvement which would make preservation unwise, maintaining blood supply to the nipple and controlling position of the nipple on the reconstructed breast. If the nipple-areola complex is sacrificed then it can be reconstructed at a later date. This is usually several months after the surgery has taken place to allow the reconstruction to 'settle'. There are several techniques described and a decision is made between the surgeon and patient as to which method is best. Options include:

- Raising a local flap. This is the most common method, but such flaps may be subject to loss of projection over time due to retraction forces from the surrounding skin and tenuous blood supply. Figure 12.3 shows a nipple reconstruction 2 weeks post-operation.
- Flap with autologous graft. This technique has developed to try and overcome the problem of projection loss. Auricular or costal cartilage or fat grafting may be used to act as a scaffold to maintain flap projection.

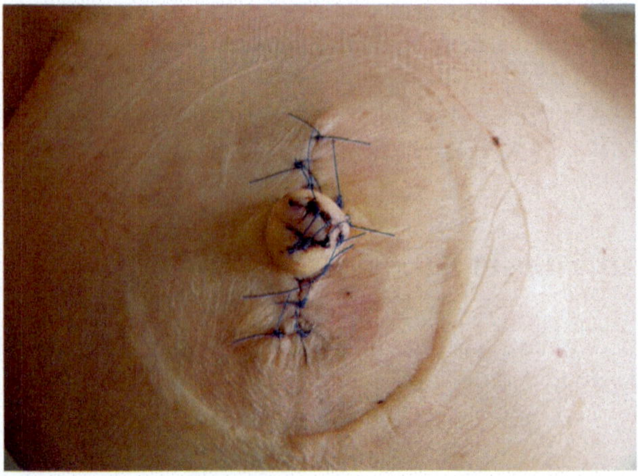

**Fig. 12.3** A nipple reconstruction 2 weeks post-operation

- Flap with alloplastic augmentation. Materials such as hyaluronic acid and calcium hydroxyapatite may be used as a scaffold. This avoids donor site morbidity, however there is a risk of infection and extrusion of the foreign material. The use of acellular dermal matrix has also been reported.
- Taking a graft from the contralateral nipple, termed nipple sharing. A good technique if the patient has a very projected nipple on the contralateral side, however some women will prefer not to have surgery on the unaffected breast.

## *Areola Reconstruction*

This requires recreation of the pigmentation and texture of the native areola. This may be achieved by skin grafting or tattooing. The skin graft may be taken from the contralateral areola, inner thigh or an area where there is excess skin and is usually done at the same time as the nipple reconstruction. A tattoo may be used to define the areola. This allows excellent color match, however a 'touch up' may be required after a few years. This may be performed by a hospital tattoo artist who solely does medical related tattoos, or a commercial tattoo artist. Some tattoo artists are skilled in shading and shadowing so that the illusion of a nipple can be created without the use of a nipple reconstruction as above. Nimboriboonporn et al. [15] have reviewed techniques for NAC reconstruction.

## *Lipomodelling*

Liposuction may be performed on an autologous reconstruction to shape it or reduce its volume. Generally, however, lipomodelling (also known as fat transfer or fat grafting) uses fat harvested from patient's thighs, flank or abdomen, injected into the reconstructed or conserved breast to replace volume loss or fill focal deficits. The fat is harvested from the donor sites by aspiration, then may be washed and/or centrifuged and injected into the area required. There is always a degree of fat resorption and several sessions may be required to fill a larger deficit. NICE guidelines [16] on lipomodelling were published in 2012 and state that there is no evidence that the procedure has any influence on recurrence of breast cancer. The guidelines state that in large case series of lipomodelling after breast reconstruction the majority of patients had significant improvement in the breast shape/size. In a series of patients undergoing lipomodelling after breast conservation, 90 % were judged to have a 'very good' or 'good' result. There were initial concerns that architectural changes as a result of lipomodelling may interfere with surveillance imaging. NICE guidelines advised that this 'ought not to be an issue with current techniques for lipomodelling and with expert interpretation of subsequent images'. The risks of lipomodelling are local infection (1 %), fat necrosis (3 %), and there was one report of a pneumothorax.

## Surgical Management of Lymphedema of the Arm

Breast cancer related lymphedema (BCRL) is the accumulation of protein-rich fluid in the subcutaneous tissues and skin secondary to dysfunction of the lymphatic system. This may be due to surgery and radiotherapy to the axilla as well as chemotherapy. BRCL affects around one third of women who have undergone axillary lymph node dissection and a between 5 and 17 % of patients who undergo sentinel lymph node biopsy. The rates of lymphedema in the medical literature vary according to the diagnostic threshold and length of follow up, though it is clear that it is associated with significant physical and psychological morbidity in many sufferers. BCRL is principally managed by conservative therapies (Chap. 11) however in some refractory cases surgery may be indicated. Surgery may be reductive (such as excision or liposuction) or physiological. Recently, physiological approaches have undergone a revival of interest and these options will be described. This highly specialized area of reconstructive surgery requires careful patient selection and work up.

### *Lymph Node Transfer*

This is the transfer of a healthy vascularized lymph node within a block or flap of tissue from the groin to the affected limb. The mechanism of action is unknown. It is thought that it may encourage new lymphatic vessels to develop in the region or by draining excess lymph fluid via intra-flap lymphatico-venous connections.

### *Lymphatico-Lymphatic Bypass*

Grafts of healthy lymphatic vessels or veins may be harvested from the thigh and anastomosed between the lymphatics of the affected arm to central lymphatics in the neck to bypass the area of obstruction in the axilla. This method has the disadvantage of a long scar in the leg and risk of lymphedema at the donor site.

### *Lymphaticovenous Anastomosis*

Lymphatic fluid may be diverted into the venous system before it reaches areas of obstruction by anastomosing the lymphatics to veins to bypass the obstruction. Indocyanine green (ICG) fluorescence lymphography is used preoperatively and intraoperatively to map the lymphatic channels. Figure 12.4 shows a patient before and after lymphatico-venous anastomosis, and an intraoperative image showing dye crossing an anastomosis from a lymphatic into a venule.

A recent review by Leung et al. [17] describes the modern techniques for the surgical treatment of lymphedema.

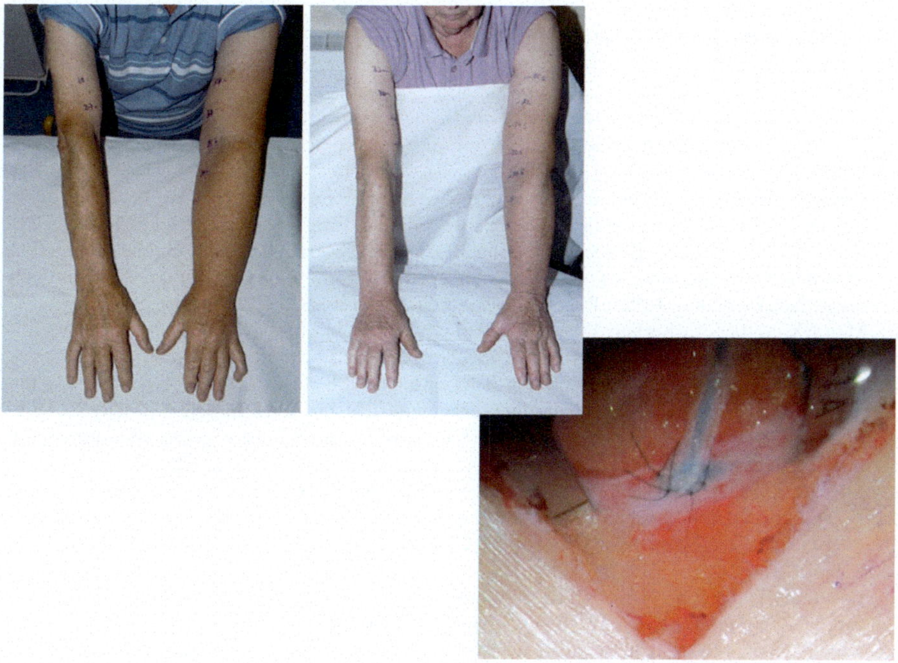

**Fig. 12.4** A patient before and after lymphatico-venous anastomosis, and an intraoperative image showing dye crossing an anastomosis from a lymphatic into a venule

## Conclusion

As discussed, many women reach a point of considering surgery to improve their survivorship. Some of the indications are clear, some are more subjective. When deciding to take a healthy survivor back to the operating theater for a cosmetic procedure, the benefit of a team approach cannot be over-emphasized. Discussion with colleagues, ideally in an oncoplastic multidisciplinary meeting [18] helps ensure the correct balance between pragmatism and the pursuit of aesthetic perfection.

## References

1. Jeevan RCD, Browne J, van der Meulen J, Caddy CM, Pereira J, et al. Second annual report of the National Mastectomy and Breast Reconstruction Audit 2009. Centre NI, editor. 2009.
2. NICE guidelines [CG80]. Early and locally advanced breast cancer: diagnosis and treatment. 2009.
3. Chatterjee JS, Lee A, Anderson W, Baker L, Stevenson JH, Dewar JA, Thompson AM. Effect of postoperative radiotherapy on autologous deep inferior epigastric perforator flap volume after immediate breast reconstruction. Br J Surg. 2009;96(10):1135–40.
4. Taghizadeh R, Moustaki M, Harris S, Roblin P, Farhadi J. Does post-mastectomy radiotherapy affect the outcome and prevalence of complications in immediate DIEP breast reconstruction? A prospective cohort study. J Plast Reconstr Aesthet Surg. 2015;68(10):1379–85.

5. Thiruchelvam PT, McNeill F, Jallali N, Harris P, Hogben K. Post-mastectomy breast reconstruction. BMJ. 2013;347:f5903.
6. Understanding Breast Reconstruction, Macmillan Cancer Support, January 2014. 11th ed. MAC 11660.
7. https://www.gov.uk/government/publications/poly-implant-prosthese-pip-implants--toxicology-testing/poly-implant-prosthese-pip-implants-toxicology-testing. Accessed 17 Nov 2015.
8. Halperin TJ, Fox SE, Caterson SA, Slavin SA, Morris DJ. Delayed division of the thoracodorsal nerve: a useful adjunct in breast reconstruction. Ann Plast Surg. 2007;59(1):23–5.
9. Figus A, Mazzocchi M, Dessy LA, Curinga G, Scuderi N. Treatment of muscular contraction deformities with botulinum toxin type A after latissimus dorsi flap and sub-pectoral implant breast reconstruction. J Plast Reconstr Aesthet Surg. 2009;62(7):869–75.
10. Man LX, Selber JC, Serletti JM. Abdominal wall following free TRAM or DIEP flap reconstruction: a meta-analysis and critical review. Plast Reconstr Surg. 2009;124(3):752–64.
11. Rizki H, Nkonde C, Ching RC, Kumiponjera D, Malata CM. Plastic surgical management of the contralateral breast in post-mastectomy breast reconstruction. Int J Surg. 2013;11(9):767–72.
12. Abbott A, Rueth N, Pappas-Varco S, Kuntz K, Kerr E, Tuttle T. Perceptions of contralateral breast cancer: an overestimation of risk. Ann Surg Oncol. 2011;18(11):3129–36.
13. Metcalfe K, Gershman S, Ghadirian P, Lynch HT, Snyder C, Tung N, Kim-Sing C, Eisen A, Foulkes WD, Rosen B, Sun P, Narod SA. Contralateral mastectomy and survival after breast cancer in carriers of BRCA1 and BRCA2 mutations: retrospective analysis. BMJ. 2014; 348:g226.
14. Lostumbo L, Carbine NE, Wallace J. Prophylactic mastectomy for the prevention of breast cancer. Cochrane Database Syst Rev. 2010;(11): CD002748.
15. Nimboriboonporn A, Chuthapisith S. Nipple-areola complex reconstruction. Gland Surg. 2014;3(1):35–42.
16. NICE interventional procedure guidance [IPG417]. Breast reconstruction using lipomodelling after breast cancer treatment. 2012.
17. Leung N, Furniss D, Giele H. Modern surgical management of breast cancer therapy related upper limb and breast lymphoedema. Maturitas. 2015;80(4):384–90.
18. Rusby JE, Gough J, Harris PA, MacNeill FA. Oncoplastic multidisciplinary meetings: a necessity or luxury? Ann R Coll Surg Engl. 2011;93(4):273–4.

# Chapter 13
# Management of Menopausal Symptoms in Breast Cancer Survivors

**Helen Mitchell and Anne C. Armstrong**

**Abstract** Menopausal symptoms are a common consequence of systemic therapy for breast cancer and can significantly impact on quality of life as well as affect treatment compliance. The most effective treatments available using exogenous hormones are generally cautioned against in women with a history of breast cancer and management of such symptoms can therefore pose a challenge to the health care professional. This chapter focuses on the current options for the treatment of vasomotor and urogenital symptoms in women who have had treatment for breast cancer.

**Keywords** Vasomotor symptom • HRT • Menopausal symptoms • Urogenital symptoms • Atrophic vaginitis

## Introduction

Breast cancer survival in England and Wales is highest for women diagnosed aged 40–69, traditionally the peri/post menopausal years, with 65 % of all women diagnosed surviving their disease in excess of 20 years [1]. Breast cancer treatments are known to both induce and exacerbate menopausal symptoms [2], resulting in significant related morbidities for many patients regardless of age. Reasons for this include iatrogenic ablation of ovarian function with either chemotherapy or with the use of Luteinizing Hormone Releasing Hormone (LHRH) agonists, oophorectomy as a prophylactic treatment option for women with BRCA mutations, as a side-effect of endocrine therapy or as a consequence of stopping HRT abruptly when diagnosed with breast cancer [3]. Women already postmenopausal at diagnosis are also more likely to develop further menopausal symptoms as a result of treatment and symptoms are more likely to be intense [4] and experienced for prolonged periods [5].

H. Mitchell, BSc (Hons), MA, MSc, DMedEth
Department of Clinical Oncology, The Christie NHS Foundation Trust, Withington, Manchester, UK

A.C. Armstrong, MB, ChB, PhD (✉)
The Christie NHS Foundation Trust, Wilmslow, Manchester, UK
e-mail: anne.armstrong@christie.nhs.uk



A. Ring, M. Parton (eds.), *Breast Cancer Survivorship*,
DOI 10.1007/978-3-319-41858-2_13

## Vasomotor Symptoms

Vasomotor symptoms are common and experienced by about 75 % of postmenopausal women. The prevalence and severity of hot flushes is higher in women with breast cancer than in women who undergo a natural menopause, particularly as cessation of menses often occurs at an early age [4]. Hot flushes and night sweats are the most commonly reported vasomotor symptoms [6], and are often associated with palpitations, anxiety and irritability [7]. Such symptoms can be debilitating for breast cancer patients [8] and can exert a profound impact on quality of life particularly as sequelae such as insomnia can further impact on quality of life contributing to overall fatigue [9].

### *Pathophysiology*

Changes in levels of estrogens are thought to affect the functioning of the thermoregulatory center in the hypothalamus [10] possibly via changes in neurotransmitter levels [11] such as norepinephrine and serotonin (5-HT). Changes in these neurotransmitter levels in response to reduced estrogens are thought responsible for reducing the thermoregulatory set point, inducing heat loss strategies such as sweating [11]. These observations have led to investigation of drugs known to interfere with the adrenergic and neurosynaptic pathways such as Clonidine, Venlafaxine and Paroxetine.

### *Management Options*

The European Menopause and Andropause Society (EMAS) advocates a personalized approach according to individual needs [12]. The advice that healthcare professionals offer their patients can range from simple practical solutions (Tables 13.1 and 13.2) to complete lifestyle management strategies [13]. Sometimes, just taking the woman's concerns seriously can have a positive impact on symptom management [14]. Positive reinforcement of advice given in a face to face meeting by appropriately qualified staff has been found to result in the most effective and enduring lifestyle changes [13] and referral to specialist menopausal clinics may also be helpful.

#### Complementary Medicine and Alternative Therapies

Blaes et al. [3] report that cancer survivors are 36 % more likely than the general population to use complementary and alternative therapies. Women with breast cancer form one of the highest user groups [15] with approximately 50–75 % of postmenopausal women utilizing alternative therapies to manage symptoms. Whilst

**Table 13.1** Practical advice for breast cancer patients with menopausal hot flushes

| |
|---|
| Identify and avoid triggers such as caffeine/alcohol/spicy foods/nicotine |
| Use fans to cool room/hand held fan for facial cooling |
| Use a cooling facial mist spray |
| Wear light layers of loose clothing |
| Have layers of bedclothes that can be removed |
| Wear cotton or linen fabrics, avoid man made materials |
| Have cool water available to sip regularly |
| Consider the use of a cooling pillow pad for night time sweats |
| Discuss diet/exercise/weight control/stress management and relaxation strategies (Cognitive Behavioral Therapy) with your healthcare professional team |
| Discuss the use of recommended prescribed medication such as venlafaxine/paroxetine/gabapentin/clonidine |

**Table 13.2** Guidance for healthcare professionals to manage menopausal hot flushes in breast cancer patients

| |
|---|
| Establish frequency/intensity/impact of symptoms on quality of life. |
| Take a full medical/medicine history, particularly the use of over the counter medication and dietary supplements and ongoing breast cancer treatments such as tamoxifen |
| Discuss potential triggers and offer lifestyle advice regarding exercise/diet/stress management |
| Consider Cognitive Behavioral Therapy (CBT) if available |
| Consider using a menopausal symptom rating scale to assess pre and post intervention |
| Consider use of recommended prescribed medication and tailor to the patient's individual needs: |
| SSRIs/SNRIs (venlafaxine (37.5–75 mg/day) or citalopram (10–20 mg/day) favored over paroxetine or fluoxetine for patients taking tamoxifen) |
| Gabapentin (start at 300 mg nocte then titrate to 300 mg three times per day over 9 days) |
| Clonidine (0.1 mg/day) |
| Access specialist services which may be offered by local breast care nursing team such as CBT |
| Consider referral to specialist menopause clinics if available and/or referral back to oncologist for discussion of changing endocrine therapy |
| **It is important to reassess and evaluate any interventions regularly** |

women may favor the use of non-prescribed interventions such as vitamin E and Evening Primrose Oil, research evidence does not demonstrate a consistent benefit with their use in comparison to placebo. (For a comprehensive review see Borrelli and Ernst [16]). Other interventions such as "Ladycare" magnets, worn inside women's underwear, are claimed by the company website to 'rebalance part of the autonomic nervous system' and reduce hot flushes [17] although the Royal College of Gynecologists [18] found no evidence to support their use. Similarly, 'chillow pillows' which provide a cooling cushion for patients to use at night, aimed at reducing night sweats, have been extremely popular but lack an evidence base [19].

Women also seek relief from their hot flushes using acupuncture and whilst some studies have shown a benefit to acupuncture over control procedures a recent systematic review of acupuncture failed to find sufficient evidence to either support or refute the benefits of this therapy [20]. Small studies have shown a benefit for cognitive behavioral therapy (CBT) with some data to suggest the symptomatic improvement is due to changing beliefs and improving mood and sleep [21].

## Lifestyle Advice

Women with a history of breast cancer are likely to benefit from maintaining a healthy weight, being physically active, limiting alcohol consumption and stopping smoking. Some of these lifestyle interventions may also impact on vasomotor symptoms. Smokers are more likely than non-smokers to experience hot flushes, the mechanism of which is unclear but decreased levels of bioavailable estrogen and interference with thermoregulatory pathways may be implicated [21]. These authors performed a longitudinal study of 761 peri-menopausal women and found that women who stopped smoking were not only less likely to experience hot flushes but were less likely to experience severe hot flushes or have frequent hot flushes compared to those women who smoked, (OR = 0.55, 0.80, 0.76). Similarly, some women find that alcohol, hot drinks and spicy foods may exacerbate hot flushes.

## Hormonal Agents

The most effective therapeutic option for the management of hot flushes is estrogen replacement therapy and this is often used in women without a history of breast cancer. Hormone replacement therapy (HRT) would render aromatase inhibitors ineffective and current guidelines discourage the use of topical or systemic estrogens in all women with a history of breast cancer. The results of the Women's Health Initiative (WHI) in the USA [22] and the Million Women Study in the UK [23] demonstrated an increased incidence of breast cancer in postmenopausal women treated with the use of estrogen and progestins as HRT [22]. Two randomized trials have looked at the use of HRT in breast cancer survivors. The HABITS (Hormonal Replacement Therapy after Breast Cancer - Is it safe?) trial was stopped early after a median follow-up of 2 years when a statistically significant increase in breast cancer recurrence was seen with therapy [24]. In a second study, the Stockholm trial, use of HRT was not associated with more recurrences [25]. The reasons behind these conflicting results are not clear.

A more recent study, LIBERATE (Livial Intervention Following Breast Cancer, Efficacy, Recurrence and Tolerability) aimed to demonstrate that tibolone, a synthetic steroid with a pharmacological profile different to that of conventional sex steroids, known to be a useful treatment for hot flushes and poor bone health, was non-inferior to placebo regarding risk of recurrence in breast cancer patients. Unfortunately the trial was terminated early due to an increased risk of recurrence in women taking tibolone. After a median follow up of 3.1 years 237 of 1556 (15.2 %) women on tibolone experienced a recurrence compared to 165 (10.7 %) on placebo. Whilst the hazard ratio for recurrence was lower in ER- (HR 1.15) than ER+ women (HR 1.56) the authors conclude that it is not possible to identify a subgroup for whom tibolone can be safely used [26].

The most effective non-estrogenic agents for the treatment of hot flushes are progesterone analogs with reductions in hot flushes similar to reductions seen with estrogen therapy. In one study intramuscular medroxyprogesterone acetate (MPA, 500 mg on days 1,14,28) was compared to a 6 week course of oral megestrol acetate (40 mg) [27]. Whilst both treatments had a similar reduction in hot flushes at week 6 (~85 %) i.m MPA provided better long term relief (89 % at week 24 compared to 45 % in the megestrol group ($p=0.03$)). In a separate study a single dose of MPA was more effective at reducing hot flushes than venlafaxine [28].

The safety of progesterones after a diagnosis of breast cancer remains uncertain though the role of the progesterone receptor in breast cancer is complex and incompletely understood. Whilst synthetic progestins used in HRT increase the risk of breast cancer, in cell lines that express both estrogen and progesterone receptors progesterone inhibits proliferation [29]. There remains a reluctance to prescribe systemic estrogens or progesterones after a diagnosis of breast cancer and non-hormonal options should be exhausted before they are considered.

## Non-hormonal Agents

Prescribed medications including clonidine, gabapentin, paroxetine and venlaflaxine are endorsed and recommended by EMAS and North American Menopause Society. Clonidine, a centrally acting alpha2-adrenergic agonist, has been found in a systematic review and meta-analysis to show a significant benefit over placebo [30], However, this drug can enhance the effects of antihypertensives, anxiolytics and alcohol and have prohibitive adverse effects including dry mouth, dizziness, postural hypotension and constipation.

In the 1980s selective serotonin reuptake inhibitors (SSRIs) and serotonin/norepinephrine reuptake inhibitors (SNRIs) were anecdotally noted to reduce hot flushes. Placebo-controlled, double-blinded randomized control trials followed, with a subsequent meta-analysis demonstrating decreased hot flash scores for paroxetine, venlafaxine, fluoxetine and sertraline of 41 %, 33 %, 13 % and 3–18 % respectively compared to placebo [31]. Since this meta-analysis trials using other antidepressants, desvenlafaxine (for a meta-analysis see Berhan and Berhan [32]) and citalopram [33] have been published. Both drugs significantly reduce hot flushes compared to placebo, though in the single published trial citalopram appears to be better tolerated with no statistically different adverse events compared to placebo whereas discontinuation rates of desvenlafaxine are high. Efficacy of SSRIs/SNRIs does not appear to be dose dependent for either paroxetine [34] or citalopram [33] and adverse events are lower with lower doses.

Much of the anti-estrogenic activity of tamoxifen resides in its active metabolite, endoxifen. The rate-limiting step in converting tamoxifen to endoxifen is the highly polymorphic cytochrome P450 CYP2D6 enzyme with considerable variation between individuals in the amount of CYP2D6 enzyme produced. Drugs such as tamoxifen that are metabolized by CYP2D6 may be eliminated quickly (by extensive metabolizers) or slowly (by poor metabolizers). Some, but by no means all, studies have suggested inferior clinical outcomes for patients who metabolize tamoxifen poorly due to a loss of function genetic polymorphism (see Johnson et al. [35] for further information) or due to co-administration with drugs that inhibit CYP2D6 [36]. The SSRIs paroxetine and fluoxetine are both potent inhibitors of CYP2D6 and reduce endoxifen levels to those seen in poor metabolizers. Sertraline and citalopram are weaker inhibitors of CYP2D6 and cannot convert extensive metabolizers into poor metabolizers. Venlafaxine has no effect on CYP2D6. For tamoxifen users at least, it seems preferable to avoid paroxetine and fluoxetine when an SSRI/SNRI is prescribed for the management of vasomotor symptoms.

Gabapentin is a gamma-aminobutyric acid analog, conventionally used to treat epilepsy and migraine but more recently has shown activity as a treatment for hot flushes. Its mechanism of action is uncertain but it may reduce noradrenergic activity. Interest in the use of the drug as a treatment for hot flushes arose after a case series report. Placebo controlled trials followed, with a subsequent meta-analysis confirming that, compared to placebo, this drug reduced the frequency and severity of hot flushes by 20–30 % [37]. This is comparable to improvements seen with SSRIs/SNRIs. Again, adverse events, which include somnolence and dizziness, preclude its use for some women. Four weeks of therapy of gabapentin and venlafaxine were directly compared in an open-labeled, randomized cross over trial [38]. Whilst both drugs were similarly effective at reducing the hot flash score (66 % reduction), 38 of 56 patients who expressed a preference preferred taking venlafaxine to gabapentin. Pregabalin, although less well studied, has been found to be similarly effective at reducing hot flushes [39].

#### Stellate Ganglion Block

The use of Stellate Ganglion Block (SGB), in which local anesthetic is injected into the sympathetic nerves of the stellate ganglion under fluoroscopic guidance, has been investigated as a treatment option for vasomotor symptoms. The largest and only randomized sham-controlled trial was performed by Walaga et al. [40]. Forty women with moderate to severe hot flushes were randomized to the use of SGB or sham injection and followed for a 6 month period with an improvement in hot flushes seen. No study related adverse effects were reported. Further investigation of this technique is warranted but the costs involved in this procedure may be prohibitive.

### *Urogenital Symptoms*

Urogenital symptoms due to estrogen deprivation are a common consequence of adjuvant systemic therapy for breast cancer. The prevalence of such symptoms after a diagnosis of breast cancer is somewhat challenging to quantify due the variety of quality of life scoring systems used in the literature but it is clear that urogenital symptoms are common, with an increased incidence of such symptoms following the use of chemotherapy and/or endocrine therapy. Crandall et al. [41], using data from a tumor based registry of breast cancer survivors, reported vaginal dryness in over 60 % of postmenopausal survivors compared to 23 % of premenopausal women.

Quality of life outcomes from the ATAC (Arimidex, Tamoxifen Alone or in Combination) trial, where postmenopausal women were randomized to tamoxifen or anastrazole for 5 years, reported more frequent dyspareunia with anastrazole compared to tamoxifen (17 % vs 8 %) as well as vaginal dryness (18 % vs 9 %) and reduced libido (34 % vs 26 %) [42]. Recent data suggest that the addition of ovarian function suppression to either tamoxifen or exemestane as adjuvant endocrine therapy in premenopausal women is associated with an improvement in relapse free survival and its use is likely to become more widespread in future years [43, 44]. Such women, but particularly those treated with exemestane and ovarian suppression, are at high risk of urogenital side effects with women reporting more vaginal dryness and sexual symptoms compared to those taking tamoxifen and ovarian suppression [45].

Unlike vasomotor symptoms, which generally improve over time, urogenital symptoms persist throughout postmenopausal life and may therefore have a prolonged effect on quality of life [46].

## *Pathophysiology*

The female reproductive tract, including the vulva, vagina, pelvic floor musculature, bladder and urethra is rich in estrogen receptors [47, 48] and is therefore highly sensitive to estrogen deprivation. Falling estrogen levels result in thinning of the epithelial cells of the vulvovaginal area, the vaginal walls become thinner and loose elasticity. The uterus, ovaries, vagina, and vulva all shrink in size. With a reduction in the vaginal epithelia fewer cells are shed into the vagina. As epithelial cells die they release glycogen which is hydrolyzed to glucose, which in turn is broken into lactic acid by lactobacillus species [49]. The consequence of reduced shedding of the epithelial cells is increased vaginal alkalinity and an overgrowth of other bacteria which can further increase the risk of urinary infections.

## *Management Options*

### Non Hormonal Treatments

Lifestyle modifications may be helpful at ameliorating the symptoms of urogenital atrophy (UA) in women with a history of breast cancer. Cigarette smoking may accelerate UA and smoking cessation should be advised. Scented hygiene products should be avoided. There is also evidence that regular sexual intercourse may be helpful as sexually active women have fewer symptoms and less physical evidence of vaginal atrophy [50]. Vaginal lubricants (such as K-Y Jelly®) may be useful to reduce discomfort during intercourse but have a short duration of action and are not considered to be vaginal moisturizers.

A wide range of vaginal moisturizers (e.g. Replens®) are available and have been investigated in women with and without a history of breast cancer. Two small studies have compared the use of Replens with topical estrogen preparations suggesting equivalent benefit with both preparations [51, 52]. However when Replens was tested against placebo in breast cancer survivors superior efficacy was not seen [53]. One study with the specific aim of improving the symptoms of dyspareunia in breast cancer survivors compared saline with the use of 4 % aqueous lidocaine used just before intercourse. In the blinded phase, patients on lidocaine reported less dyspareunia (median score 1/10) compared with saline (5.3/10, $p=0.015$) [54]. In subsequent open-label use of lidocaine seventeen of twenty previous abstainers (85 %) resumed intercourse.

## Hormonal Agents

In women without a history of breast cancer symptoms, of UA can be alleviated by systemic or topical estrogen therapy. Where systemic treatment is not needed for other reasons local estrogen therapy is preferable to avoid systemic adverse events. In comparison to placebo or non-hormonal gels the Cochrane Overview in 2003 found vaginal estrogen (VE) preparations were superior as a treatment for the management of UA in post-menopausal women (without a history of breast cancer) [55]. Estrogen is absorbed through the vaginal epithelium and as such there maybe systemic effects of local estrogen therapy. This is relevant to women with a history of hormone receptor positive breast cancer, and particularly important for women taking aromatase inhibitors compared with those on tamoxifen. The risk of systemic absorption of VE is greater at the beginning of treatment when the vaginal epithelium is still atrophic; as it matures in response to therapy less estrogen is absorbed with lower doses required to prevent recurring symptoms [56]. Low dose VE preparations (Vagifem 10 μg) are now available which appear to have minimal systemic absorption [57].

Few studies have investigated the safety or otherwise of topical estrogens as treatment for UA in women with a history of breast cancer. Wills et al. [58], investigated the effects of VE on serum estradiol levels in postmenopausal women at risk of breast cancer and taking an aromatase inhibitor or selective estrogen receptor modulator as breast cancer prevention. In this group of women use of VE rings and VE tablets resulted in increased estradiol levels even though the women were eligible only if they had been on the estrogenic preparations for 3 months prior to study entry and would therefore be expected to have a mature vaginal epithelium. The authors concluded VE regardless of type should be used in caution in women treated with aromatase inhibitors. Two studies have reported the use of VE in women with a history of breast cancer. Simmons et al., in an open label randomized comparison of Vagifem ® or Estring® for 12 weeks found an improvement in quality of life scores (FACT-ES, sexual health) vaginal maturation index and pH. Serum estradiol rose in all patients by week 2 but fell to undetectable levels by week 12 [59]. The study closed early due to poor accrual. The second study investigated the use of an ultra-low dose vaginal estriol and Lactobacillus combination vaginal tablet. Estriol preparations, which cannot be metabolized into more potent estrogens such as estradiol or estrone may have advantages in women with a history of breast cancer. In this phase 1 study in 8 of 16 women small increases in serum estriol but not estradiol or estrone were seen and UA improved [60].

Large, prospective randomized trials to determine the safety of VE in breast cancer patients are lacking. However a large population-based cohort study from the Danish Breast Cancer Group provides interesting data. The database was used to identify 2 cohorts of women, a cohort of 5900 who had not received systemic therapy of which 996 had filled a prescription for VE and a cohort of 6529 postmenopausal women who had been treated with an AI or Tamoxifen of whom 1096 had been prescribed VE therapy. With a median FU of 8.5 years the use of VE did not impact on prognosis with an adjusted relative risk for recurrence and death among users were 0.93 ($p=0.51$) and 0.79 ($p=0.001$) respectively [61]. The effect was independent of whether patients received adjuvant endocrine therapy.

## Summary

Menopausal symptoms are a common consequence of treatment for breast cancer. Appropriate management of symptoms is crucial not only to maintain quality of life but also to enable as many women as possible to complete their planned endocrine therapy with data clearly demonstrating that poor compliance results in increased recurrence rates and poorer survival [62].

## References

1. Cancer Research UK (CRUK, 2011). www.cancerresearchuk.org/cancerstats/types/breast/incidence. Accessed 1 Oct 2015.
2. Anderson DJ, Yates P, McCarthy N, Porter-Steele J. Younger and older womens concerns about menopause after breast cancer. Eur J Cancer Care. 2011;2:285–94.
3. Blaes AH, Kreitzer MJ, Torkelson C, Haddad T. Nonpharmacologic complementary therapies in symptom management for breast cancer survivors. Semin Oncol. 2011;38:394–402.
4. Carpenter JS, Andrykowski MA, Cordova M, et al. Hot Flashes in postmenopausal women treated for breast carcinoma. Prevelence, severity, correlates, management, and relation to quality of Life. Cancer. 1998;82:1682–91.
5. Harris PF, Remington PL, Trentham-Dietz A, et al. Prevalence and treatment of menopausal symptoms among breast cancer survivors. J Pain Symptom Manage. 2002;23:501–9.
6. Dennerstein L, Dudley EC, Hooper JL, et al. A prospective population based study of menopausal symptoms. Obstet Gynecol. 2000;96:351–8.
7. Kronenberg F. Hot Flashes: epidemiology and physiology. Ann N Y Acad Sci. 1990;592:52–86.

8. Mom CH, Buijs C, Willemse PHB, et al. Hot flushes in breast cancer patients. Critical Reviews Oncology/Haematology. 2006;57:63–77.
9. Savard J, Simard S, Blanchet J, et al. Prevalence, clinical characteristics and risk factors for insomnia in the context of breast cancer. Sleep. 2001;24:583–90.
10. Stearns V, Ullmer L, Lopez L, et al. Hot flushes. Lancet. 2002;360:1851–61.
11. Rosenberg J, Holst-Larsen S. Hypothesis: pathogenesis of postmenopausal hot flushes. Med Hypotheses. 1991;35:349–50.
12. Neves-e-Castro M, Birkhauser M, Samsioe G G, et al. EMAS position statement: the ten point guide to the integral management of menopausal health. Maturitas. 2015;81:88–92.
13. Anderson D, Seib C, McGuire A, Porter-Steele J. Decreasing menopausal symptoms in women undertaking a web-based multimodal lifestyle intervention: The Women's Wellness Program. Maturitas. 2015;81:69–75.
14. Schover LR, Jenkins R, Sui D, et al. Randomised trial of peer counselling on reproductive health in African American breast cancer survivors. J Clin Oncol. 2006;24:1620–6.
15. Greenlee H, Balneaves LG, Carlson LE, et al. Clinical practice guidelines on the use of integrative therapies as supportive care in patients treated for breast cancer. J Natl Cancer Inst Monogr. 2014;50:346–58.
16. Borrelli F, Ernst E. Alternative and complementary therapies for the menopause. Maturitas. 2010;66:333–43.
17. Ladycare USA. 2015. http://www.ladycareusa.com/faqs. Accessed 27 Oct 2015.
18. Royal College of Obstetricians and Gynaecologists. Alternatives to hormone replacement therapy for the management of symptoms of the menopause. 2010. 2010 Scientific Impact Paper No 6 September RCOG.
19. Royal College of Nursing (RCN). Menopause: lifestyle and therapeutic approaches. RCN guide for nurses, midwives and health visitors. London: RCN; 2014.
20. Garcia MK, Graham-Getty L, Haddad R, et al. Systematic review of acupuncture to control hot flashes in cancer patients. Cancer. 2015;121:3948–58.
21. Smith RL, Flaws JA, Gallicchio L. Does quitting smoking decrease the risk of hot flashes? A longitudinal analysis. Maturitas. 2015;82:123–7.
22. Rossouw JE, Anderson GL, Prentice RL, et al. Risks and benefits of estrogen plus progestin in healthy postmenopausal women: principal results from the Women's Health Initiative randomized controlled trial. JAMA. 2002;288:321–33.
23. Beral V, Million Women Study Collaborators. Breast cancer and hormone-replacement therapy in the Million Women Study. Lancet. 2003;362:419–27.
24. Holmberg L, Iversen OE, Rudenstem CM. Increased risk of recurrence after hormone replacement therapy in breast cancer survivors. J Natl Cancer Inst. 2008;100:475–82.
25. Von Schoultz E, Rutqvist LE, Stockholm Breast Cancer Study Group. Menopausal hormone replacement therapy in breast cancer survivors. J Natl Cancer Inst. 2008;100:475–8.
26. Kenemans P, Bundred NJ, Foldart J, et al. Safety and efficacy of tibolone in breast-cancer patients with vasomotor symptom: a double-blind, randomized, non-inferiority trial. Lancet Oncol. 2009;10:135–46.
27. Bertelli G, Venturini N, Del Mastro L, et al. Intramuscular depot medroxyprogesterone versus oral megestrol for the control of postmenopausal hot flashes in breast cancer patients: a randomized study. Ann Oncol. 2002;13:883–8.
28. Loprinzi CL, Levitt R, Barton D, et al. Phase III comparison of depomedroxyprogesterone acetate to venlafaxine for managing hot flashes: North Central Cancer Treatment Group Trial N99C7. J Clin Oncol. 2006;24:1409–14.
29. Mohammed H, Russell JA, Stark R, et al. Progesterone receptor modulates ERα action in breast cancer. Nature. 2015;523:313–7.
30. Nelson HD, Vesco KK, Haney E, et al. Nonhormonal therapies for menopausal hot flashes: systematic review and meta-analysis. J Am Med Asso. 2006;295:2057–71.
31. Loprinzi CL, Sloan J, Stearns V, et al. Newer antidepressants and gabapentin for hot flashes: an individual patient pooled analysis. J Clin Oncol. 2009;27:2831–7.

32. Berhan Y, Berhan A. Is desvenlafaxine effective and safe in the treatment of menopausal vasomotor symptom? A meta-analysis and meta-regression of randomized double-blind controlled studies. Ethiop J Health Sci. 2014;24:209–18.
33. Barton DL, LaVasseur BI, Sloan JA, et al. Phase III placebo-controlled trial of three doses of citalopram for the treatment of hot flashes: NCCTG Trial N05C9. J Clin Oncol. 2010;28:3278–83.
34. Stearns V, Beebe KL, Ivengar M, Dube E. Paroxetine controlled release in the treatment of menopausal hot flashes: a randomized controlled trial. JAMA. 2003;289:2827–34.
35. Johnson JA, Hamadeh IS, Langaee TY. Loss of heterozygosity at the CYP2D6 locus in breast cancer: implications for tamoxifen pharmacogenetic studies. J Natl Cancer Inst. 2015;107:dju437.
36. Jin Y, Desta Z, Stearns V, et al. CYP2D6 genotype, antidepressant use, and tamoxifen metabolism during adjuvant breast cancer treatment. J Natl Cancer Inst. 2005;97:30–9.
37. Toulis KA, Tzellos T, Kouvelas D, Goulis DG. Gabapentin for the treatment of hot flashes in women with natural or tamoxifen-induced menopause: a systematic review and meta-analysis. Clin Ther. 2009;31:221–35.
38. Bordeleau L, Pritchard KI, Loprinzi CL, et al. Multicenter, randomized, cross-over clinical trial of venlafaxine versus gabapentin for the management of hot flashes in breast cancer survivors. J Clin Oncol. 2010;28:5147–52.
39. Loprinzi CL, Qin R, Balcueva EP, et al. Phase III randomized, double-blind, placebo-controlled evaluation of pregabalin for alleviating hot flashes, N07C1. J Clin Oncol. 2010;28:641–7.
40. Walaga DR, Rubin LH, Banuvar S, et al. Effects of stellate ganglion block on vasomotor symptoms: findings from a randomised clinical trial in postmenopausal women. Menopause. 2014;21:807–14.
41. Crandall C, Petersen MS, Ganz PA, Greendale GA. Association of breast cancer and its therapy with menopause-related symptoms. Menopause. 2004;11:519–30.
42. Cella D, Fallowfield L, Barker P, et al. Quality of life of postmenopausal women in ATAC ("Arimidex", tamoxifen, alone or in combinations) trial after completion of 5 years adjuvant treatment for early breast cancer. Breast Cancer Res Treat. 2006;100:273–84.
43. Pagani O, Regan MM, Francis PA, et al. International Breast Cancer Study Group. Exemestane with ovarian suppression in premenopausal breast cancer. N Engl J Med. 2014;371:1358–9.
44. Francis PA, Regan MM, Fleming GF, et al. Adjuvant ovarian suppression in premenopausal breast cancer. N Engl J Med. 2015;372:436–46.
45. Bernhard J, Luo W, Ribi K, et al. Patient-reported outcomes with adjuvant exemestane versus tamoxifen in premenopausal women with early breast cancer undergoing ovarian suppression (TEXT and SOFT): a combined analysis of two randomised phase 3 trials. Lancet Oncol. 2015;16:848–58.
46. Nappi RE, Palacios S. Impact of vulvovaginal atrophy on sexual health and quality of life at postmenopause. Climacteric. 2014;17:3–9.
47. Weigerink MA, Poortman J, Agema AR, Thijssen JH. Estrogen receptors in human vaginal tissue. Maturitas. 1980;2:59–67.
48. Iosif CS, Batra S, Ek A, Astedt B. Estrogen receptors in the human female lower urinary tract. Am J Obstet Gynecol. 1981;141:817–20.
49. Roy S, Caillouette JC, Roy T, et al. Am J Obstet Gynecol. 2004;190:1272–7.
50. Leiblum S, Bachmann G, Kemmann E, et al. Vaginal atrophy in postmenopausal women. The importance of sexual activity and hormones. JAMA. 1983;249:2195–8.
51. Bygdeman M, Swahn ML. Replens versus dienoestrol cream in the symptomatic treatment of vaginal atrophy in postmenopausal women. Maturitas. 1996;23:259–63.
52. Nachtigall LE. Comparative study: replens versus local estrogen in menopausal women. Fertil Steril. 1994;61:178–80.
53. Loprinzi CL, Abu-Ghazaleh S, Sloan JA, et al. Phase III randomized double-blind study to evaluate the efficacy of a polycarbophil-based vaginal moisturizer in women with breast cancer. J Clin Oncol. 1997;15:969–73.

54. Goetsch MF, Lim JY, AB C. A practical solution for dyspareunia in breast cancer survivors: a randomized controlled trial. J Clin Oncol. 2015;33:3394–400.
55. Suckling J, Lethaby A, Kennedy R. Local oestrogen for vaginal atrophy in postmenopausal women. Cochrane Database Syst Rev. 2003;(4):CD001500.
56. Nilsson K, Helmer G. Low-dose oestradiol in the treatment of urogenital oestrogen deficiency-a pharmacokinetic and pharmacodynamics study. Maturitas. 1992;15:121–7.
57. Notelovitz M, Funk S, Nanavati N, Mazzeo M. Estradiol absorption from vaginal tablets in postmenopausal women. Obstet Gynecol. 2002;99:555–62.
58. Will S, Ravipati A, Venuturumilli P, et al. Effects of vaginal estrogens on serum estradiol levels in postmenopausal breast cancer survivors and women at risk of breast cancer taking an aromatase inhibitor or a selective estrogen receptpr modulator. J Oncol Pract. 2012;8:144–8.
59. Simmons CE, Kuchuk I, Freedman OC, et al. Are Estring® and Vagifem® equally effective and safe for the treatment of urogenital atrophy in breast cancer patients on aromatase inhibitor therapy? Clin Oncol (R Coll Radiol). 2012;24:e128–9.
60. Donders G, Bellen G, Neven P, et al. Effects of ultra-low-dose estriol and lactobacilli vaginal tablets (Gynoflor®) on inflammatory and infectious markers of the vaginal ecosystem in post-menopausal women with breast cancer on aromatase inhibitors. Eur J Clin Microbiol Infect Dis. 2015;34:2023–8.
61. Cold S, Cold F, Jensen MB, et al. Vaginal estrogens and risk of recurrence or death in women treated for estrogen receptor positive breast cancer. 2015. European Cancer Congress Vienna 25–29 Sept 2015.
62. Makubate B, Donnan PT, Dewar JA, et al. Cohort study of adherence to adjuvant endocrine therapy, breast cancer recurrence and mortality. Br J Cancer. 2013;108:1515–24.

# Chapter 14
# Bone Health

**Amy Kwan, Omar S. Din, and Matthew C. Winter**

**Abstract** Bone health is an important, though sometimes neglected, part of the treatment of early breast cancer patients. The use of chemotherapy, ovarian suppression and aromatase inhibitors has the potential to induce significant bone loss and increase skeletal morbidity including osteoporosis and fracture. As most women are likely to be long-term survivors after a diagnosis of early breast cancer, recognition of patients at risk and introduction of bone-targeted therapy forms a crucial part of early breast cancer management. A large number of studies have demonstrated the efficacy of bisphosphonates in the prevention of cancer treatment-induced bone loss and risk-adapted treatment guidelines have been published for both pre- and post-menopausal women. The use of denosumab, an anti-RANK ligand antibody, in reducing fracture risk associated with aromatase-inhibitor therapy has also been reported. In addition, exciting new data suggest that bisphosphonates may also modify the metastatic disease process with recently published meta-analyses data demonstrating a reduction in bone recurrence and an improvement in breast cancer survival in post-menopausal women.

**Keywords** Adjuvant therapy • Bisphosphonate • Bone health • Bone mineral density • Denosumab • Early breast cancer • Fracture risk • Osteoporosis

## Introduction

The management of early breast cancer has become increasing successful with a number of effective chemotherapeutic agents and the addition of endocrine therapy for patients with estrogen receptor (ER) positive disease. The 5-year relative survival is 99.1 % for patients diagnosed with stage 1 disease and 87.6 % for patients with stage 2 disease [1]. However, randomized clinical trials have shown that these

A. Kwan, MBBS, BSc • O. S. Din • M.C. Winter, MB, ChB, MSc, MD, FRCP (✉)
Specialised Cancer Services, Weston Park Hospital, Sheffield Teaching Hospitals NHS Foundation Trust, Sheffield, South Yorkshire, UK
e-mail: matthew.winter@sth.nhs.uk



A. Ring, M. Parton (eds.), *Breast Cancer Survivorship*,
DOI 10.1007/978-3-319-41858-2_14

therapies are associated with bone mineral density loss in both the pre-menopausal and post-menopausal setting. This occurs either through a direct cytotoxic effect on bone cells, inhibition of production of gonadal steroid hormones, or inhibiting aromatase activity leading to the inhibition of conversion of androgens to estrogens in peripheral tissue. As estrogen plays a key role in the negative regulation of osteolysis, low physiological levels of estrogen significantly increase the risk of osteoporosis, fractures and longer-term morbidity [2], in addition to increased health-care costs. As long term survivors are increasingly common in the early breast cancer setting and bone loss occurs naturally with age, it is imperative that bone health features in survivorship plans.

Osteoporosis is a skeletal disorder, characterized by reduced bone mass and micro-architectural deterioration of bone tissue predisposing individuals to a high risk of fracture [3]. The World Health Organization (WHO) defined osteoporosis as a bone mineral density of 2.5 or less standard deviations from that expected of a normal individual [4]. This is assessed by a dual energy x-ray absorptiometry (DEXA) scan. Bone loss is common with increasing age, with 1 in 3 women over the age of 50 sustaining an osteoporotic fracture of the wrist, hip or vertebrae [5, 6]. Bone loss in itself is asymptomatic with morbidity occurring only after fracture has been sustained. After development of an osteoporotic hip fracture there is significant mortality and morbidity, with a 20 % increased risk of dying within 12 months [7].

BMD is not the only important factor determining fracture risk, as a significant proportion of women with fractures do not have osteoporosis as defined above, likely due to the fact that other factors that influence bone strength such as bone size, geometry and microarchitectural change are not captured by BMD assessment [8, 9]. Measurement of BMD should therefore be combined with other recognized risk factors to determine an overall fracture risk assessment, leading to lifestyle modification recommendations and a risk-stratified approach to prophylactic bone-directed therapy. To guide the decision to use a prophylactic anti-osteoporotic treatment, an important advance was the development of the online FRAX algorithm [10, 11]. This uses the recognized clinical risk factors of age, sex, body mass index, previous history of fracture, family history of fracture, use of corticosteroids, lifestyle factors including smoking and alcohol >3 units/day and co-morbidities such as rheumatoid arthritis and secondary osteoporosis with or without femoral neck BMD T-score to calculate a 10-year fracture risk adapted for different countries. However the FRAX score was not designed to evaluate fracture risk in women with breast cancer, as it does not take into account the effect of anti-cancer treatments. More specific guidelines related to the prevention and treatment of breast cancer treatment-induced bone loss have been developed over the last 7 years, and are covered at a later stage.

## Pharmacology of Bone-Directed Therapy

Bisphosphonates are the mainstay for the treatment of established osteoporosis. Bisphosphonates are stable synthetic analogs of pyrophosphate and have a P-C-P backbone that acts as a bone hook (see Fig. 14.1). There are two covalently bound

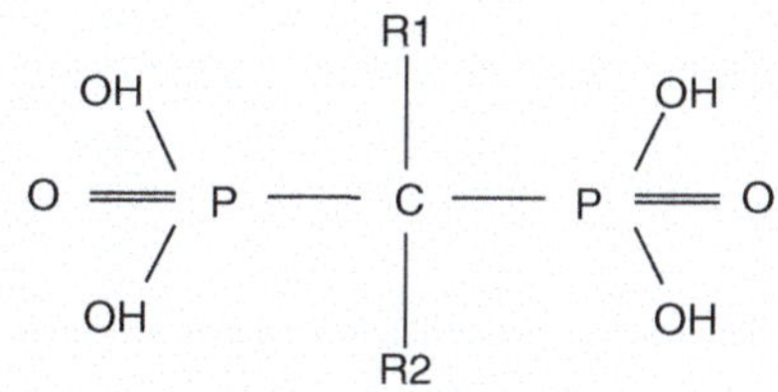


**Fig. 14.1** The chemical structure of bisphosphonates (Reproduced from Winter et al. [48], with permission from Elsevier)

side chains to the carbon atom, R1 and R2, that determine biological activity, with the presence of a nitrogen atom in the R2 side chain increasing potency and divides bisphosphonates into nitrogen containing and non-nitrogen containing bisphosphonates [12, 13]. Following either oral or intravenous administration they accumulate in bone and are selectively internalized by osteoclasts during bone reabsorption. The metabolism of non-nitrogen containing bisphosphonates to ATP-analogs results in osteoclast apoptosis [12]. Nitrogen containing bisphosphonates inhibit farnesyl diphosphate synthase in the mevalonate pathway, disrupting the prenylation of important signaling GTPases, ultimately inducing osteoclast apoptosis (see Fig. 14.2) [14].

Bisphosphonates are generally well tolerated and toxicity is related to mode of administration. Oral bisphosphonates can cause gastrointestinal complications including gastrointestinal bleeding. Intravenous bisphosphonates are associated with infusion reactions, metabolic effects (hypocalcaemia) and renal toxicity. A rare, but serious side effect is the development of osteonecrosis of the jaw [15]. The risk of developing this with zoledronic acid is 0.12–0.7 % if used biannually [16]. The pathogenesis of this is unclear and may be largely avoided with patient education and pre-treatment dental evaluation.

## Cancer Treatment-Induced Bone Loss

Pre-menopausal women are at significant risk of accelerated bone loss from adjuvant treatments including chemotherapy, tamoxifen and ovarian suppression, resulting from suppression of estrogen levels and premature ovarian failure [17]. Furthermore, cytotoxic chemotherapy may also directly negatively affect bone health.

### *Tamoxifen and Bone Mineral Density Loss*

Tamoxifen is a selective estrogen receptor modulator, and has mixed pro- and anti-estrogenic activities. It is one of the most commonly used treatments in patients with estrogen receptor (ER) positive breast cancer, with the effect on the bone being dependent on menopausal status. In the post-menopausal setting, tamoxifen has been shown to increase bone mineral density of the spine and hip. In the premenopausal setting it has a predominantly anti-estrogen effect resulting in a small (1–2 %)

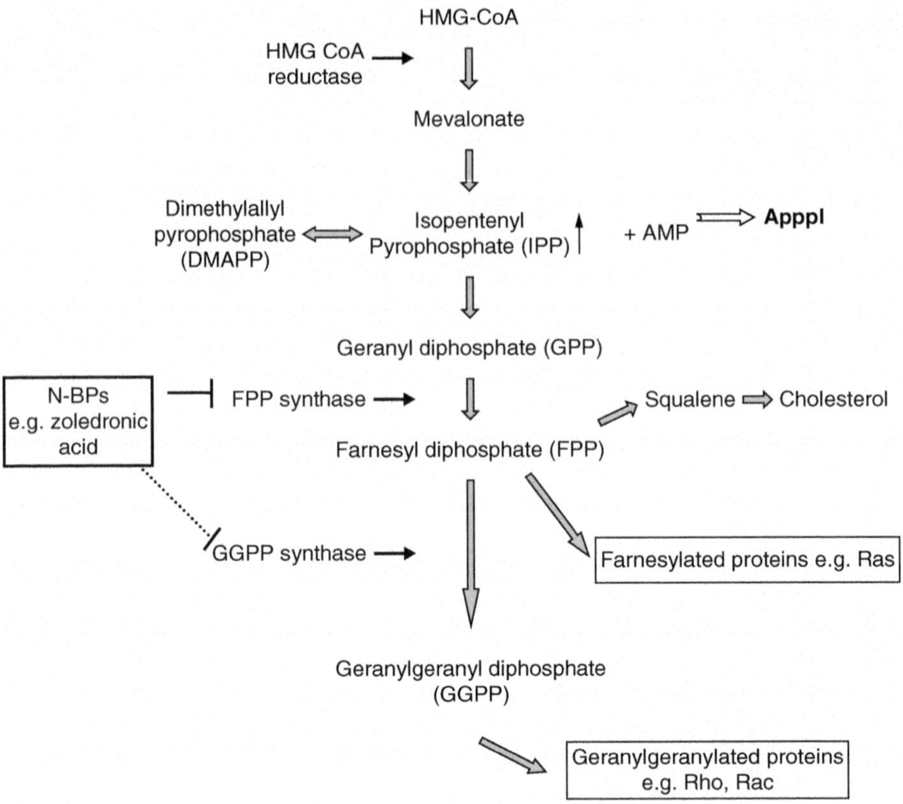


**Fig. 14.2** Schematic diagram of the mevalonate pathway demonstrating the inhibition of FPP synthase, and the proposed inhibition of GGPP synthase, by N-BPs. This results in the inhibition of formation of FPP and GGPP which are required for the post-translational prenylation of important small signaling GTPases, ultimately leading to apoptosis. Inhibition of FPP synthase by N-BPs also results in accumulation of IPP and the biosynthesis of ApppI, an ATP analog capable of inducing apoptosis in osteoclasts (Reproduced from Winter et al. [48], with permission from Elsevier)

increased loss of bone mineral density. This is not clinically significant and no bone protection in recommended in this setting.

## *Chemotherapy and Bone Mineral Density Loss*

Combination cytotoxic chemotherapy is used in the treatment of early breast cancer to prevent disease recurrence and improve breast cancer related mortality. In premenopausal patients, the use of such treatments can result in either temporary or permanent ovarian failure. Approximately 68 % of patients, ranging from 20 to 100 % depending on age >40 years, cytotoxic agent and cumulative dose, will experience chemotherapy-induced primary ovarian failure [17–19]. This results in the potential for rapid decrease in BMD of up to 7 % within 1 year [20].

There are a small group of studies investigating whether early intervention with bisphosphonates can counteract the loss of BMD following adjuvant chemotherapy alone. Risedronate, clondronate and zolendronic acid have been investigated in this setting, with more intensive treatment doses than conventionally used for osteoporosis. Saarto et al. [21] randomized 148 patients to receive clodronate at a dose of 1600 mg daily or control in addition to receiving six cycles of CMF chemotherapy. BMD of lumbar spine and femoral neck was measured at 1 and 2 years. Patients who did not become amenorrheic during chemotherapy only experienced marginal BMD changes, but in patients developing amenorrhea, both treatment groups developed bone density loss. The use of clodronate significantly reduced bone loss in comparison to controls (lumbar spine (−5.9 % vs. 9.5 %) and femoral neck (−0.4 % vs. −4.6 %).

In a small study by Delmas et al. [22], breast cancer patients with artificially induced menopause following chemotherapy were treated with risedronate (30 mg/day or placebo for 2 weeks, followed by 10 weeks of no treatment, repeated over 2 years) or placebo. In the risedronate group, there was an increase in BMD at 24 months, compared to a significant decrease in BMD at the lumbar spine and hip in placebo (mean difference: 2.5 ± 1.2 %, [95 % confidence interval [CI], 0.2–4.9] at the lumbar spine, $p=0.041$; and 2.6 ± 1.1 %, [95 % CI, 0.3–4.8] at the femoral neck, $p=0.029$). Of interest, on treatment withdrawal, patients experienced bone loss suggesting maintenance of treatment, or a more potent bisphosphonate, is required for ongoing beneficial effect. Dosing regimen is clearly important as risedronate, in a conventional osteoporosis schedule of 35 mg weekly did not prevent bone loss caused by chemotherapy induced ovarian suppression in a study by Hines et al. [23].

These data suggest an intravenous schedule in this setting may therefore be required. In the largest study of zoledronic acid (CALGB 79809) [24], at a dose of 4 mg every 3 months for 2 years, was given to 439 women either starting immediately or 1 year after completion of chemotherapy. The primary endpoint, percentage change in BMD in lumbar spine (LS) from baseline to 12 months in the zoledronic acid and control groups, was evaluated in those women developing chemotherapy-induced ovarian failure. Median percent change at 1 year was +1.2 % and −6.7 %, ($p<0.001$), in the immediate versus delayed groups. Final results at 3 years reported +1.0 % and −0.5 %, $p=0.019$, in immediate versus delayed groups respectively. These results show that immediate zoledronic acid was able to prevent bone loss compared to the control group where there was a significant difference in bone loss from baseline to 1 year. However, there are questions that remain unanswered. Firstly there is no long-term follow-up from these trials and consequently the clinical relevance of cancer treatment induced bone loss with respect to longer-term fracture risk is unknown [25]. Additionally, efforts need to focus on trying to identify those women who are likely to develop chemotherapy-induced ovarian failure or those at highest risk of cancer treatment-induced bone loss to enable the selective introduction of earlier therapy, although the optimal schedule of bisphosphonate treatment is not well defined.

## *Ovarian Suppression and Bone Mineral Density Loss*

Studies have also evaluated the prevention of endocrine treatment-induced bone loss in pre-menopausal patients. Recent data has suggested a benefit of the addition of adjuvant ovarian suppression to either tamoxifen or exemestane in higher risk women in women who remain pre-menopausal after chemotherapy [26]. In view of this, the use of ovarian suppression and exemestane may play an important role in high-risk patients under the age of 35 who have premenopausal levels of oestradiol levels following chemotherapy. Ovarian suppression can be obtained medically or surgically, with medical ovarian suppression utilizing GnRH analogs (including goserelin, triptorelin, leuprolide) to suppress the release of gonadotrophins (FSH/LH) and thus reversibly inhibit gonadal activity and estrogen production. Studies from their use in benign conditions have demonstrated a bone mineral density loss of 4–5 % in the lumbar spine over the first 6 months of therapy [27]. In pre-menopausal breast cancer patients, ABCSG-12 randomized 1803 patients with hormone-receptor positive breast cancer to receive endocrine treatment (goserelin and tamoxifen or anastrozole, each with or without zoledronic acid every 6 months for 3 years [28, 29]. Data from the bone sub-study (n=404) showed that in patients who did not receive bone protective therapy with zoledronic acid, there was a significant reduction in BMD at 3 years (trochanter −7.3 %, lumbar spine −11.3 %), with a larger detrimental effect in those patients receiving anastrazole. At 5 years, there was only partial recovery with BMD levels remaining less than baseline (trochanter −4.1 %, lumbar spine −6.3 %). In contrast, the addition of zoledronic acid to endocrine therapy alone was associated with stable BMD during the 3 years of treatment with an increase seen at 5 years compared to baseline (trochanter +3.9 %, lumbar spine +4.0 %). Recently published data also show that the addition of zoledronic acid to adjuvant therapies in pre-menopausal women significantly reduce bone turnover markers compared to significant increases in these markers in placebo-treated patients [30]. Longer-term follow-up, from ABCSG-12 particularly, will be crucial to understand whether the treatment-induced rapid bone loss observed in the study in patients without bone protection, with some evidence of partial recovery after treatment stopped, translates into longer-term fracture risk.

## *Aromatase Inhibitor Associated Bone Loss*

In the post-menopausal setting the standard of care for ER positive patients with early breast cancer has shifted from tamoxifen to the use of adjuvant aromatase inhibitors (AI), with data from the most recent meta-analysis showing that 5 years of treatment with AI reduces 10-year breast cancer mortality rates by about 15 % compared with 5 years of tamoxifen [31]. In the post-menopausal setting, circulating estrogen results from the conversion of androgens to estrogen in the peripheral tissue by the enzyme aromatase. Inhibition by either the reversible non-steroidal inhibitors (anastrazole/letrozole) or the irreversible steroidal inhibitor (exemestane) results in almost undetectable levels of circulating estrogen. Aromatase-inhibitor induced bone loss (AIBL) occurs at over double the rate of physiological post-menopausal bone mineral density loss [32] leading to an increased fracture risk.

A bone sub-study as part of the 'Arimidex, Tamoxifen alone, or in combination' (ATAC) trial [33] reported the longer-term effects of BMD following treatment with hormone treatment for 5 years in patients with early breast cancer. A total of 308 women had baseline lumbar and hip BMD assessed by DEXA and then on treatment at 1, 2, and 5 years. Following treatment, 50 patients treated with anastrozole alone had further assessment at years 6–7. Patients treated with anastrozole alone showed a median decrease in BMD of 6.1 % and 7.2 % in the lumbar spine and hip respectively, compared to an increase of 2.77 % and 0.74 % in the lumbar spine and hip respectively in patients receiving tamoxifen. Of note, women who had normal BMD at baseline did not develop osteoporosis.

Following completion of anastrozole treatment, DEXA measurements at 6 and 7 years showed an increased in BMD by 2.35 and 4.02 % at the lumbar spine and 0.71 and 0.5 % at the hip suggesting that treatment related bone loss does not continue beyond treatment [34]. Similar results were seen in the Intergroup Exemestane study [35].

Longer-term follow-up from large phase 3 adjuvant studies directly comparing tamoxifen and aromatase inhibitors have demonstrated that AIs are associated with an increased risk of fractures, maintained for the duration of treatment. At a median follow-up of 100 months in the ATAC study, during active treatment the incidence of fracture in the anastrozole arm was 12 % compared to 7.5 % in patients receiving tamoxifen with an annual rate of 2.93 % and 1.9 % respectively [36]. Similarly, in the BIG 1–98 study, 4895 patients were randomized to receive 5 years of letrozole or tamoxifen, and at a median follow-up of 5 years, the fracture incidence was 9.3 % and 6.5 % in patients receiving letrozole and tamoxifen respectively [37]. Importantly, the fracture rates in ATAC were no different between treatments after treatment was completed, potentially explained in part by the increase in BMD observed off anastrozole treatment [36]. Recognition and treatment of patients at particular risk of fracture will therefore help to select a patient group who would benefit from bone-directed therapy.

## Bisphosphonates in the Treatment of Aromatase Inhibitor Induced Bone Loss

A number of bisphosphonates have undergone clinical trials of efficacy in the prevention of AIBL, and data from over 4000 patients (Table 14.1) have demonstrated that both oral and intravenous bisphosphonates effectively prevent AIBL [2]. Zolendronic acid had been particularly widely studied. In three parallel-designed international trials (Z-FAST [38, 39], ZO-FAST [40] and E-ZO-FAST [41]), and a

4th trial N03CC [42] approximately 2750 post-menopausal women with hormone receptor positive breast cancer receiving 5 years of adjuvant letrozole were randomized to receive zoledronic acid (4 mg q6monthly) either immediately or delayed, if required due to accelerated bone loss (T score $<-2.0$) or fracture. At 12 months, it was demonstrated in all these trials that upfront zoledronic acid effectively prevented letrozole induced bone loss. Ongoing follow-up from these trials, including 5 year final follow-up from both ZO-FAST and Z-FAST, have all reported continued efficacy with the upfront zoledronic acid.

A handful of studies have investigated the efficacy of oral bisphosphonates including the SABRE and ARIBON studies (Table 14.1). These trials, although inclusive of a smaller number of patients and follow-up is shorter, suggest that oral bisphosphonates given in osteoporotic dosing regimens demonstrate efficacy in AIBL, although there are ongoing concerns about compliance with oral bisphosphonates.

## Guidelines for the Monitoring and Treatment of Cancer Treatment-Induced Bone Loss

Over the last few years, recommendations for the management of CTIBL have been published including expert guidelines from the UK and Europe [2, 3, 17, 27, 43].

All patients receiving systemic treatments that have a potential detrimental effect on bone should be recommended to have a calcium-rich diet, regular weight bearing and resistance exercise and take 1000–2000 IU vitamin D daily [3]. Current assessments of fracture risk are based on data from healthy post-menopausal women and therefore are not able to sufficiently evaluate the associated risks of treatment in pre-menopausal women [44]. It is therefore recommended in pre-menopausal women with breast cancer that the potential risk of bone loss should be discussed prior to initiating anti-cancer treatment and that anti-resorptives are commenced when the BMD T-score is below −2 (Fig. 14.3) [3, 17, 27].

In post-menopausal women receiving an AI, with a T-score ≥2 and no other risk factors for fracture, re-assessment of BMD and risk factors is recommended after 1–2 years. If the patient experiences an annual BMD decrease of ≥10, or 4–5 % annual decrease if osteopenic at baseline, then investigations for secondary causes of osteoporosis such as vitamin D deficiency, hyperparathyroidism and hyperthyroidism, together with initiation of bisphosphonate therapy is recommended [2]. Expert panel consensus recommends treatment with an anti-resorptive if the T-score is below −2, or have 2 or more risk factors for fracture (Fig. 14.3) [3]. Once treatment is started, this should be continued for as long as the patient is receiving an AI. Over 5 years, the current data is strongest for zoledronic acid, 4 mg 6-monthly, but other acceptable options are oral alendronate 70 mg weekly, risedronate 35 mg weekly or oral ibandronate 150 mg monthly. Compliance to oral bisphosphonates is a common problem and these patients should receive intravenous zoledronic acid. Recent data also suggest the efficacy of denosumab 60 mg 6-monthly in this setting [45].

**Table 14.1** Randomized controlled trials of bisphosphonates in the prevention of AI associated bone loss in post-menopausal women with invasive breast cancer

| Trial | No. | BP, Dose<br>Duration<br>Comparison<br>Concomitant therapy | L Spine BMD<br>Mean % change from baseline<br>p value | Total Hip BMD<br>Mean % change from baseline<br>p value |
|---|---|---|---|---|
| E-ZO-FAST | 527 | Zol, 4 mg q6m<br>5 years<br>immediate vs. delayed with letrozole | **At 36 month FU**<br>*Immediate vs. delayed*<br>+5.98 % vs.–3.74 %<br>p<0.001 | **At 36 month FU**<br>*Immediate vs. delayed*<br>NR |
| Z-FAST | 602 | Zol, 4 mg q6m<br>5 years<br>immediate vs. delayed with letrozole | **At 61 month FU**<br>*Immediate vs. delayed*<br>+6.19 % vs.–2.42 %<br>p<0.0001 | **At 61 month FU**<br>*Immediate vs. delayed*<br>2.57 % vs.–4.12 %<br>p<0.001 |
| ZO-FAST | 1065 | Zol, 4 mg q6m<br>5 years<br>immediate vs. delayed with letrozole | **At 60 month FU**<br>*Immediate vs. delayed*<br>+4.3 % vs.–5.4 %<br>p<0.0001 | **At 60 month FU**<br>*Immediate vs. delayed*<br>+1.6 % vs.–4.1 %<br>p<0.0001 |
| N03CC | 558 | Zol, 4 mg q6m<br>5 years<br>immediate vs. delayed with letrozole following completion of ≤6 years tamoxifen | **At 24 month FU**<br>*Immediate vs. delayed*<br>+4.94 % vs.–2.28 %<br>p<0.001 | **At 24 month FU**<br>*Immediate vs. delayed*<br>+1.22 % vs.–3.34 %<br>p<0.001 |
| SABRE | 154 | Risedronate/Placebo 35 mg/ week in addition to anastrozole in pts with moderate risk of fracture<br>(T<–1 to≥2) | **At 24 month FU**<br>*Risedronate vs placebo*<br>+2.2 % vs.–1.8 %<br>p<0.001 | **At 24 month FU**<br>*Risedronate vs placebo*<br>+1.8 % vs.–1.1 %<br>p<0.001 |
| ARBI | 70 | Risedronate, 35 mg/week in addition or not to anastrozole in pts with moderate risk of fracture<br>(T<–1 to≥2) | **At 24 month FU**<br>*Risedronate vs not*<br>+5.7 % vs.–1.5 %<br>p<0.006 | **At 24 month FU**<br>*Risedronate vs not*<br>+1.6 % vs.–3.9 %<br>p=0.037 |
| ARIBON | 50 | Ibandronate/Placebo 150 mg q28days in addition to anastrozole in pts with osteopenia<br>(T<–1 to≥2.5) | **At 24 month FU**<br>*Ibandronate vs. placebo*<br>+2.98 % vs.–3.22 %<br>p<0.01 | **At 24 month FU**<br>*Ibandronate vs. placebo*<br>+0.6 % vs.–3.9 %<br>p<0.01 |

Reproduced from Winter et al. [25] with permission from Elsevier

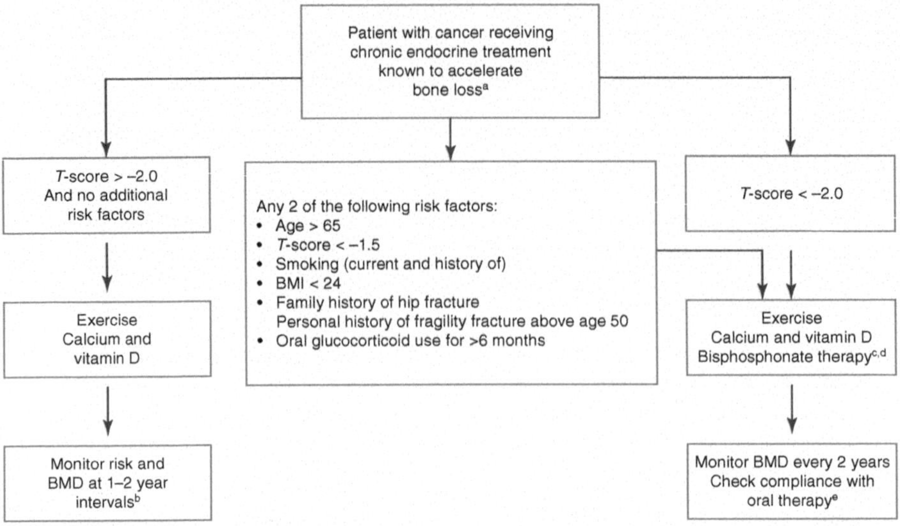


**Fig. 14.3** Recommended algorithm for managing bone health during cancer treatment (Reproduced from Coleman et al. [3], with permission from Oxford University Press). [a]Includes aromatase inhibitors and ovarian suppression therapy/oophorectomy for breast cancer and androgen deprivation therapy for prostate cancer. [b]If patients experience an annual decrease in BMD of ≥10 % (or ≥4–5 % in patients who were osteopaenic at baseline) using the same DXA machine, secondary causes of bone loss such as vitamin D deficiency should be evaluated and antiresorptive therapy initiated. Use lowest *T*-score from spine and hip. [c]Six monthly i.v. zoledronic acid, weekly oral alendronate or risedronate or monthly oral ibandronate acceptable. [d]Denosumab may be a potential treatment option in some patients. [e]Although osteonecrosis of the jaw is a very rare event with bone protection doses of antiresorptives, regular dental care and attention to oral health is advisable. BMD, bone mineral density; BMI, body mass index

## Recent Developments

### *Assessment of Response to Treatment*

Conventionally, response to bisphosphonate treatment has been monitored through serial DEXA scans. These are relatively expensive, need to be performed after a long duration in time to allow for assessment of response and are not best at predicting future fracture risk. Bone turnover markers (BTM) may potentially provide a more dynamic, non-invasive and cheaper assessment of skeletal metabolism [46, 47].

BTM can be divided into two groups; formation and resorption markers. Formation markers reflect the activity of osteoblasts and include bone-specific alkaline phosphatase (BALP) and pro-collagen type 1 amino-terminal propeptide (P1NP). Resorption markers reflect the activity of osteoclast and include cross-linked type 1 collagen (CTX) and type 1 collagen amino-terminal telopeptide (NTX). BTM monitoring may allow for earlier identification of patients with bone mineral density loss. In an exploratory subset analysis of the Z-FAST trial, patients who had BTM assessment suggested that early increase in NTX and BALP were predictive of clinically relevant long-term bone loss [39]. However, further studies are needed to support the use of BTM to tailor anti-resorptive therapies to prevent fractures.

## *Denosumab in the Use of Aromatase Inhibitor Induced Bone Loss*

Denosumab is a fully humanized monoclonal antibody administered subcutaneously that binds to RANK ligand and prevents activation of the RANK receptor on osteoclasts and ultimately inhibits osteoclast activity.

In the recently published ABCSG-18 trial [45], 3420 post-menopausal patients receiving aromatase inhibitors were randomized to denosumab 60 mg ($n=1711$) or placebo ($n=1709$) subcutaneously every 6 months. Primary end-point was time to first fracture. The trial demonstrated patients in the denosumab group had a significantly delayed time to first clinical fracture (hazard ratio [HR] 0.50 [95 % CI 0.39–0.65], $p<0.0001$) and there was a reduction in the overall number of fractures in the denosumab group (92 vs 176 in the placebo group). Treatment was well tolerated. These data suggest that denosumab is an effective alternative therapeutic option to bisphosphonates in this setting.

## *Adjuvant Use of Bisphosphonates in Breast Cancer*

The bone marrow is understood to act as a reservoir for dormant tumor cells. These cells preferentially home to the hematopoietic stem cell niche, where they can reside for years and escape the effects of systemic anti-cancer therapy. For reasons that are not clearly understood, years later, they exit the dormant state and proliferate and metastasize causing an array of clinical problems. The use of adjuvant bisphosphonates to modify disease course and disrupt the metastatic process represents an exciting clinical strategy. Pre-clinical studies have suggested a potential anti-cancer effect of bisphosphonates, but whether this is a direct or indirect effect has long been debated [48].

Several large clinical studies have investigated this effect and have recently been analyzed together in an individual patient data meta-analysis by the EBCTCG [49]. This is discussed in Chap. 7 in greater detail. As a result of these data, practice is now changing. Adjuvant bisphosphonates are considered part of the standard of care for post-menopausal women and are now appearing in adjuvant treatment protocols. In the meantime, trials are already well underway investigating the role of denosumab in reducing the risk of bone recurrence (D-CARE).

## Summary and Key Points

Bone health is an important component of survivorship. A number of early breast cancer treatments can lead to significant BMD loss resulting in increased fracture risk. The groups at most risk are those pre-menopausal women undergoing ovarian suppression and post-menopausal women on aromatase inhibitors. The current standard is to use DEXA scans to monitor BMD, although bone turnover markers may provide a useful adjunct to assessments. Therapeutic strategies to prevent and treat CTIBL have been an important development in breast cancer management and the role of bisphosphonates in this setting is well defined. International expert guidelines for the prevention and treatment of CTIBL have been published, utilizing risk-adapted strategies that define thresholds for introduction of bisphosphonates. Denosumab has also been shown to be efficacious and its mode of delivery may be preferable to some patients. Bisphosphonates have also been used as part of the adjuvant therapy for patients with early breast cancer to prevent cancer recurrence in bone and improve breast cancer survival in post-menopausal patients.

## References

1. CRUK. Cancer Research UK Breast cancer statistics. [Website] 2015. Available from: http://www.cancerresearchuk.org.
2. Hadji P, et al. Management of aromatase inhibitor-associated bone loss in postmenopausal women with breast cancer: practical guidance for prevention and treatment. Ann Oncol. 2011;22(12):2546–55.
3. Coleman R, et al. Bone health in cancer patients: ESMO Clinical Practice Guidelines. Ann Oncol. 2014;Suppl 3:iii124–37.
4. Kanis JA. Assessment of fracture risk and its application to screening for postmenopausal osteoporosis: synopsis of a WHO report. WHO Study Group. Osteoporosis Int J established as result of cooperation between the European Foundation for Osteoporosis and the National Osteoporosis Foundation of the USA. 1994;4(6):368–81.
5. Kanis JA, et al. Long-term risk of osteoporotic fracture in Malmo. Osteoporosis Int J established as result of cooperation between the European Foundation for Osteoporosis and the National Osteoporosis Foundation of the USA. 2000;11(8):669–74.
6. Melton 3rd LJ, et al. Perspective. How many women have osteoporosis? J Bone Miner Res. 1992;7(9):1005–10.
7. Cummings SR, Melton LJ. Epidemiology and outcomes of osteoporotic fractures. Lancet. 2002;359(9319):1761–7.
8. Seeman E, Delmas PD. Bone quality–the material and structural basis of bone strength and fragility. N Engl J Med. 2006;354(21):2250–61.
9. Body JJ. Increased fracture rate in women with breast cancer: a review of the hidden risk. BMC Cancer. 2011;11:384.
10. Kanis JA, et al. FRAX and the assessment of fracture probability in men and women from the UK. Osteoporosis Int J established as result of cooperation between the European Foundation for Osteoporosis and the National Osteoporosis Foundation of the USA. 2008;19(4):385–97.
11. Diseases, W.H.O.C.C.f.M.B. FRAX® WHO fracture risk assessment tool. [Website]. Available from: http://sheffield.ac.uk/FRAX/index.jsp.

12. Rogers MJ, et al. Cellular and molecular mechanisms of action of bisphosphonates. Cancer. 2000;88(12 Suppl):2961–78.
13. Russell RG, Rogers MJ. Bisphosphonates: from the laboratory to the clinic and back again. Bone. 1999;25(1):97–106.
14. Luckman SP, et al. Nitrogen-containing bisphosphonates inhibit the mevalonate pathway and prevent post-translational prenylation of GTP-binding proteins, including Ras. J Bone Miner Res. 1998;13(4):581–9.
15. Coleman R, et al. Safety of zoledronic acid and incidence of osteonecrosis of the jaw (ONJ) during adjuvant therapy in a randomised phase III trial (AZURE: BIG 01–04) for women with stage II/III breast cancer. Breast Cancer Res Treat. 2011;127(2):429–38.
16. Kourie HR, et al. Osteonecrosis of the jaw during biyearly treatment with zoledronic acid for aromatase inhibitor associated bone loss in early breast cancer: a literature review. J Bone Oncol. 2015;4(3):77–9.
17. Hadji P, et al. Cancer treatment-induced bone loss in premenopausal women: a need for therapeutic intervention? Cancer Treat Rev. 2012;38(6):798–806.
18. Bines J, Oleske DM, Cobleigh MA. Ovarian function in premenopausal women treated with adjuvant chemotherapy for breast cancer. J Clin Oncol. 1996;14(5):1718–29.
19. Pfeilschifter J, Diel IJ. Osteoporosis due to cancer treatment: pathogenesis and management. J Clin Oncol. 2000;18(7):1570–93.
20. Lester J, et al. The causes and treatment of bone loss associated with carcinoma of the breast. Cancer Treat Rev. 2005;31(2):115–42.
21. Saarto T, et al. Clodronate improves bone mineral density in post-menopausal breast cancer patients treated with adjuvant antioestrogens. Br J Cancer. 1997;75(4):602–5.
22. Delmas PD, et al. Bisphosphonate risedronate prevents bone loss in women with artificial menopause due to chemotherapy of breast cancer: a double-blind, placebo-controlled study. J Clin Oncol. 1997;15(3):955–62.
23. Hines SL, et al. Phase III randomized, placebo-controlled, double-blind trial of risedronate for the prevention of bone loss in premenopausal women undergoing chemotherapy for primary breast cancer. J Clin Oncol. 2009;27(7):1047–53.
24. Shapiro CL, et al. Zoledronic acid preserves bone mineral density in premenopausal women who develop ovarian failure due to adjuvant chemotherapy: final results from CALGB trial 79809. Eur J Cancer. 2011;47(5):683–9.
25. Winter MC, Coleman RE. Bisphosphonates in the adjuvant treatment of breast cancer. Clin Oncol. 2013;25(2):135–45.
26. Francis PA, Regan MM, Fleming GF. Adjuvant ovarian suppression in premenopausal breast cancer. N Engl J Med. 2015;372(17):1673.
27. Reid DM, et al. Guidance for the management of breast cancer treatment-induced bone loss: a consensus position statement from a UK Expert Group. Cancer Treat Rev. 2008;34 Suppl 1:S3–18.
28. Gnant MF, et al. Zoledronic acid prevents cancer treatment-induced bone loss in premenopausal women receiving adjuvant endocrine therapy for hormone-responsive breast cancer: a report from the Austrian Breast and Colorectal Cancer Study Group. J Clin Oncol. 2007;25(7):820–8.
29. Gnant M, et al. Adjuvant endocrine therapy plus zoledronic acid in premenopausal women with early-stage breast cancer: 5-year follow-up of the ABCSG-12 bone-mineral density substudy. Lancet Oncol. 2008;9(9):840–9.
30. Hadji P, et al. Effects of zoledronic acid on bone mineral density in premenopausal women receiving neoadjuvant or adjuvant therapies for HR+ breast cancer: the ProBONE II study. Osteoporosis Int J established as result of cooperation between the European Foundation for Osteoporosis and the National Osteoporosis Foundation of the USA. 2014;25(4):1369–78.
31. Dowsett M, et al. Aromatase inhibitors versus tamoxifen in early breast cancer: patient-level meta-analysis of the randomised trials. Lancet. 2015;386(10001):1341–52.
32. Hadji P. Aromatase inhibitor-associated bone loss in breast cancer patients is distinct from postmenopausal osteoporosis. Crit Rev Oncol Hematol. 2009;69(1):73–82.

33. Eastell R, et al. Effect of anastrozole on bone mineral density: 5-year results from the anastrozole, tamoxifen, alone or in combination trial 18233230. J Clin Oncol. 2008;26(7):1051–7.
34. Eastell R, et al. Long-term effects of anastrozole on bone mineral density: 7-year results from the ATAC trial. Ann Oncol. 2011;22(4):857–62.
35. Coleman RE, et al. Reversal of skeletal effects of endocrine treatments in the Intergroup Exemestane Study. Breast Cancer Res Treat. 2010;124(1):153–61.
36. Forbes JF, et al. Effect of anastrozole and tamoxifen as adjuvant treatment for early-stage breast cancer: 100-month analysis of the ATAC trial. Lancet Oncol. 2008;9(1):45–53.
37. Rabaglio M, et al. Bone fractures among postmenopausal patients with endocrine-responsive early breast cancer treated with 5 years of letrozole or tamoxifen in the BIG 1–98 trial. Ann Oncol. 2009;20(9):1489–98.
38. Brufsky A, et al. Zoledronic acid inhibits adjuvant letrozole-induced bone loss in postmenopausal women with early breast cancer. J Clin Oncol. 2007;25(7):829–36.
39. Brufsky AM, et al. Final 5-year results of Z-FAST trial: adjuvant zoledronic acid maintains bone mass in postmenopausal breast cancer patients receiving letrozole. Cancer. 2012;118(5):1192–201.
40. Bundred NJ, et al. Effective inhibition of aromatase inhibitor-associated bone loss by zoledronic acid in postmenopausal women with early breast cancer receiving adjuvant letrozole: ZO-FAST Study results. Cancer. 2008;112(5):1001–10.
41. Llombart A, et al. Immediate administration of zoledronic acid reduces aromatase inhibitor-associated bone loss in postmenopausal women with early breast cancer: 12-month analysis of the E-ZO-FAST trial. Clin Breast Cancer. 2012;12(1):40–8.
42. Hines SL, et al. Immediate versus delayed zoledronic acid for prevention of bone loss in postmenopausal women with breast cancer starting letrozole after tamoxifen-N03CC. Breast Cancer Res Treat. 2009;117(3):603–9.
43. Hadji P, et al. Practical guidance for the management of aromatase inhibitor-associated bone loss. Ann Oncol. 2008;19(8):1407–16.
44. Hadji P. Cancer Treatment-Induced Bone Loss in women with breast cancer. BoneKey Rep. 2015;4:692.
45. Gnant M, et al. Adjuvant denosumab in breast cancer (ABCSG-18): a multicentre, randomised, double-blind, placebo-controlled trial. Lancet. 2015;386(9992):433–43.
46. Burch J, et al. Systematic review of the use of bone turnover markers for monitoring the response to osteoporosis treatment: the secondary prevention of fractures, and primary prevention of fractures in high-risk groups. Health Technol Assess. 2014;18(11):1–180.
47. Lipton A, Costa L, Coleman RE. Bone turnover markers: tools for prognosis and monitoring response to bisphosphonates? Breast Dis. 2011;33(2):59–69.
48. Winter M, et al. Exploring the anti-tumour activity of bisphosphonates in early breast cancer. Cancer Treat Rev. 2008;34:453–75.
49. Coleman R, et al. Adjuvant bisphosphonate treatment in early breast cancer: meta-analyses of individual patient data from randomised trials. Lancet. 2015;386(10001):1353–61.

# Chapter 15
# Fertility

**Stuart Lavery and Georgios Christopoulos**

**Abstract** Treatment of early breast cancer effects ovarian function and fertility in pre-menopausal women. Some women now choose to delay conception to a later age, when potentially a diagnosis of breast cancer may occur. Although many women are cured of their breast cancer long term, the opportunity to have children has to be explored at the time of diagnosis to allow the use of potential measures to preserve fertility options in the future. This chapter explores the systemic effects of chemotherapy on ovarian function, and fertility sparing measures available to women. Overall, the evidence in the literature suggests that subsequent pregnancy does not appear to adversely effect long-term breast cancer outcomes.

**Keywords** Fertility • Premature ovarian insufficiency (POI) • AMH • GnRH agonists • IVF • Cryopreservation • Pregnancy

## Introduction

It is estimated that 5–7 % of breast cancers occur in women under the age of 40. As one quarter of first live births occurs between the ages of 30 and 40, many women will be nulliparous at the time of diagnosis [1]. However less than 10 % of women diagnosed with invasive breast cancer less than the age of 40 will subsequently have children after treatment [1]. In a large survey of women with breast cancer, 29 % reported that fertility concerns influenced their treatment decisions and only 51 % felt that these concerns were adequately addressed by their doctors [2].

The potential effect of cancer treatment on fertility and ovarian function should be discussed with all breast cancer patients of reproductive age. An early discussion will allow patients and doctors to consider and plan appropriate fertility preservation

S. Lavery, MBBCh, MSc, MRCOG (✉) • G. Christopoulos, MD, MRCOG
Department of Reproductive Medicine Hammersmith and Queen Charlotte's Hospitals, Imperial College Healthcare NHS Trust, London, UK
e-mail: stuart.lavery@imperial.ac.uk



A. Ring, M. Parton (eds.), *Breast Cancer Survivorship*,
DOI 10.1007/978-3-319-41858-2_15

treatment. Routine fertility preservation strategies, such as oocyte or embryo cryopreservation, usually require at least 2 weeks from the onset of treatment. Consequently any cancer treatment such as chemotherapy may be delayed, sometimes for more than 1 month.

A new diagnosis of breast cancer carries a significant psychological burden. When women with breast cancer are asked to make important decisions regarding their long-term fertility at the same time, they should be offered multidisciplinary support, expert advice and adequate time to reach a decision. Conversely for patients that will not require chemotherapy, an immediate referral to fertility experts for counseling may overestimate the need of fertility preservation strategies, which highlights the complex nature of the timing and content of fertility counseling for these women.

The number of oocytes present in the ovaries progressively declines until the menopause. The maximum number of oocytes is 6–7 million at 20 weeks of gestation in the female fetus. Oocytes will then decrease to approximately 1–2 million at birth. The number of oocytes declines further to 300,000–500,000 at puberty, 25,000 at age 37 years and approximately 1000 at the age of 51. The fecundity of women decreases gradually but significantly, beginning approximately at age 32 years and decreases more rapidly after age 37 years. This primarily reflects a decrease in egg quality and quantity and is associated with a gradual increase in circulating levels of follicle-stimulating hormone. Consequently the long-term postponement of pregnancy through the use of adjuvant tamoxifen for 10 years after the diagnosis of estrogen receptor – positive breast cancer will be associated with a significant decline in natural fertility without accounting for the deleterious effect of chemotherapy, which is discussed below.

## Ovarian Insufficiency Induced by Chemotherapy

Chemotherapy agents used in breast cancer patients can cause premature ovarian insufficiency (POI). The toxic effect to the ovaries can manifest through the impairment of follicular maturation, the depletion of primordial follicles, or both [3, 4]. Chemotherapy-induced gonadotoxicity resembles accelerated ovarian aging [3, 5, 6] with depletion of ovarian follicles through follicular apoptosis and premature atresia and fibrosis of the ovarian cortex, which result in ovarian atrophy [6, 7]. When chemotherapy is administered in the follicular phase of the cycle, the risk of gonadotoxicity increases further [3, 8, 9]. Age is an important prognostic factor of chemotherapy-induced POI [8]. A small number of studies have reported that chemotherapy-induced POI occurred in 22–61 % of women aged less than 40 years old and 61–97 % of women over 40 years old [3, 10, 11].

Alkylating agents are most commonly associated with permanent ovarian failure, partly because their action is not cell cycle-specific (Table 15.1). Consequently both resting and growing primordial follicles can be affected [4, 12]. On the other hand chemotherpautic agents, such as methotrexate, 5-fluorouracil and bleomycin are cell-cycle-specific and demonstrate only mild or no gonadotoxicity. Adriamycin and cisplatin can modestly affect gonadal function. The impact of taxanes on

**Table 15.1** Estimated risk of premature ovarian insufficiency resulting from adjuvant chemotherapy treatment for early breast cancer

| | Single drug | Adjuvant regimens |
|---|---|---|
| Higher risk (>80 %) | Cyclophosphamide<br>Ifosfamide<br>Chlorambucil | |
| | Melphalan, busulfan | CMF, FEC, FAC × 6 cycles in women aged ≥40 years |
| | Nitrogen mustard<br>Procarbazine thiotepa | |
| Intermediate risk | Cisplatin | CMF, FEC, FAC × 6 cycles in women aged 30–39 years |
| | Carboplatin<br>Adriamycin | AC, EC × 4 in women aged ≥40 years |
| | Taxanes | Taxane-containing combinations |
| Lower risk (<20 %) | Bleomycin<br>Dactinomycin | |
| | Vincristine | CMF, FEC, FAC × 6 cycles in women aged <30 years |
| | Vinblastine<br>Methotrexate | |
| | Mercaptopurine | AC, EC × 4 in women aged <40 years |
| | 5-Fluorouracil | |
| To be determined | Trastuzumab, bevacizumab | |
| | Lapatinib | |

chemotherapy-induced POI remains controversial. When taxanes are added to standard chemotherapy, the risk of POI appears to increase [13–18]. This additional risk of POI associated with taxanes is transient, being limited to 12 months following the end of chemotherapy, although the data suggest polychemotherapy schedules increase amenorrhea. Most oncologists select schedules according to breast cancer risk and no particular schedule is deemed low risk for fertility purposes alone.

## The Use of GnRH Agonists During Chemotherapy to Reduce POI

The protective role of GnRH agonists against the gonadotoxic effect of chemotherapy until recently remained controversial. In a randomized trial by Del Mastro et al. [19], premenopausal women with stage I through III breast cancer, who were candidates for adjuvant or neoadjuvant chemotherapy, were randomized to receive chemotherapy alone or combined with triptorelin. Triptorelin was administered intramuscularly at a dose of 3.75 mg at least 1 week before the start of chemotherapy and then every 4 weeks for the duration of chemotherapy. Twelve months after the last cycle of chemotherapy the rate of early menopause was 25.9 % in the chemotherapy-alone group and 8.9 % in the chemotherapy plus triptorelin group (P<.001). Moore et al. [20] randomized 257 premenopausal women with operable hormone-receptor–negative breast cancer to receive standard chemotherapy with the GnRH agonist goserelin or standard chemotherapy without goserelin. The primary end point was the rate of ovarian failure at 2 years. For 135 women with complete primary end-point data, the ovarian failure rate was 8 % in the goserelin group and 22 % in the chemotherapy-alone group. In a meta-analysis of 12 randomized studies including 1231 patients, Lambertini et al. [21] reported that GnRH agonist co-treatment was associated with a significant reduced risk of premature ovarian failure (OR 0.36, 95 % CI 0.23–0.57; P<0.001) and seemed to increase pregnancy rates, without an apparent negative consequence on prognosis.

## Assessment of Ovarian Reserve

Fertility preservation strategies should be patient-tailored, since the effect of chemotherapy and the response of fertility treatment depend on the age and ovarian reserve of each patient. Ovarian reserve is a term used to describe the ovarian reproductive potential based on the number and the quality of the available oocytes. Previous ovarian surgery, smoking and a family history of premature menopause are factors, which may further affect the ovarian reserve of breast cancer patients. The use of ovarian reserve markers such as serum AMH is also useful in the evaluation of chemotherapy-induced gonadotoxicity and can be used as a tool for the comparison of gonadotoxicity of various chemotherapy protocols.

Ovarian reserve can be assessed by serum hormonal markers and ultrasound evaluation of the antral follicle count (AFC). Serum anti-mullerian hormone (AMH) constitutes the most accurate serum marker of ovarian reserve [22–24]. AMH is a dimeric glycoprotein, which is produced by granulosa cells from preantral and antral follicles. Unlike follicle-stimulating hormone (FSH) and 17-beta estradiol levels, serum AMH levels remain stable throughout the menstrual cycle, which allows clinicians to assess the ovarian reserve of patients at the time of presentation. AMH levels decline with age and become undetectable in postmenopausal women.

Antral follicles are ovarian follicles during a certain stage of folliculogenesis, during which a fluid-filled antrum forms adjacent to the oocyte. The assessment of the AFC is based on the number of follicles measuring 2–10 mm in diameter identified by transvaginal ultrasound examination. AFC is strongly related to serum AMH levels because the hormone is actually produced by antral follicles. A major improvement in ultrasound technology has been the use of three-dimensional, automated follicular assessment, which can decrease the intra- and inter-observer variability in the assessment of the size and number of ovarian follicles.

Cut-off levels of serum AMH levels for poor ovarian response vary significantly in the published literature to date. Nelson et al. [22] found a cut-off level of 5 pmol/l (0.7 ng/ml) (DSL assay) to be associated with a sensitivity of 75 % and specificity of 91 %. Al-Azemi et al. [23] found an AMH value of 9.7 pmol/l (1.36 ng/ml) (IBC assay) to be associated with 75.5 % sensitivity and 74.8 % specificity.

Similarly there is considerable variability in AFC cut-off levels for the prediction of poor ovarian response. AFC cut-off values vary between an AFC < 3 [24] and <12 [25]. In clinical practice the most commonly used cut-off values of AFC for prediction of poor response range between <5 and <7 [26, 27].

# Reproductive Procedures to Preserve Fertility

## *In Vitro Fertilization*

IVF treatment consists of sequential steps, which occur continuously during a single menstrual cycle:

*Controlled ovarian stimulation*. Exogenous hormones are administered to the patients to stimulate the ovaries such that multiple follicles containing oocytes develop simultaneously. Conversely during a physiological menstrual cycle, the ovaries typically produce only one follicle containing one oocyte.

- *Preventing a premature LH surge*. A premature surge of luteinizing hormone (LH) could lead to premature ovulation and to a decrease in the number of eggs, which could then be retrieved. The use of GnRH analogs during the phase of stimulation of the ovaries can prevent the LH surge through reversible blockade of the pituitary GnRH receptors.
- *Triggering oocyte maturation*. In order for oocytes to become mature and gain the competence for fertilization by sperm, LH exposure is required. This can be achieved through the bolus administration of pharmacological agents such as hCG, which simulates the effects of the natural mid-cycle LH surge.
- *Oocyte retrieval*. The oocytes are usually retrieved from the ovaries in an outpatient setting 36–38 h after the administration of the oocyte maturation trigger. The operating doctor passes a needle through the vaginal wall under ultrasound guidance and aspirates the fluid from the follicles to retrieve the egg.
- *In vitro fertilization*. The collected oocytes are then placed adjacent to sperm in laboratory petri dish for in vitro fertilization (IVF). Alternatively the embryologist may perform a procedure called intracytoplasmic sperm injection (ICSI), during which a single spermatozoon is injected directly into the oocyte for fertilization.

### Controlled Ovarian Stimulation Protocols

The aim of the initial phase of IVF treatment is to promote multi-follicular growth through pharmacological ovarian stimulation. To achieve this, human menopausal gonadotrophins (hMGs) or recombinant FSH (rFSH) are used. GnRH antagonists are also administered during the phase of ovarian stimulation for the prevention of a premature LH surge during IVF treatment. The main advantage of using GnRH antagonists to prevent premature LH surge is the rapidity of onset of action and the rapidity of offset, due to the fact that they are competitive antagonists and can therefore be displaced from the receptor by a GnRH agonist. The use of GnRH antagonists thus allows for the use of a GnRH agonist to trigger oocyte maturation. The GnRH antagonist (ganirelix or cetrorelix) is administered in daily 0.25 mg doses, from the 6th day of controlled ovarian stimulation onwards [28]. A further variation was introduced to reduce the required number of GnRH antagonist doses by the use of flexible protocols. In a flexible protocol, the GnRH antagonist is commenced when the largest ovarian follicles reach a size >14–16 mm in mean diameter.

A prerequisite for the GnRH antagonist protocol to commence is the occurrence of spontaneous menses, as the phase of controlled ovarian stimulation generally commences on day 2 of the menstrual cycle. This may not always be advisable, however, as the urgency to commence chemotherapy may not allow for further delay in the treatment. For this reason random-start ovarian stimulation protocols have been introduced. With random-start protocols, ovarian stimulation can start in the late follicular phase or the luteal phase following the physiological LH surge or after the induction of ovulation with hCG or a GnRH agonist. Random-start ovarian stimulation protocols appear to be effective as conventional-start protocols in the early follicular phase. Random-start protocols can therefore decrease the duration of the IVF cycle, without compromising the number of oocytes collected before cancer treatment can commence [29].

## Oocyte Maturation Triggers

During a natural cycle, the mid-cycle surge of pituitary LH secretion induces ovulation. Exogenous hCG (at doses of 5000–10,000 IU) has been successfully introduced to simulate the natural LH surge and lead to oocyte maturation. When three follicles reach at least 18 mm in diameter, hCG is administered to induce oocyte maturation. Transvaginal egg retrieval is performed approximately 36–37 h after hCG injection, and retrieved oocytes can be fertilized by intracytoplasmic sperm injection (ICSI). hCG has a significantly longer half-life and will provide support to the multiple corpora lutea for 7–10 days, after which time hCG is cleared from circulation [30, 31], allowing time for egg retrieval However, the longer half-life of hCG in comparison to endogenous LH also results in a prolonged luteotrophic effect and an increased risk of ovarian hyperstimulation syndrome [32]. As a result alternative trigger agents have been investigated and developed because of this complication associated with the use of hCG.

Such an alternative are GnRH agonists, which can also promote oocyte maturation by inducing a surge in gonadotrophin secretion (flare-up effect), similar to the surge that occurs in the physiological cycle [33, 34]. The GnRH agonist-induced LH surge consists of two phases; a short ascending phase lasting >4 h and a long descending phase lasting >20 h and has a total duration between 24 and 36 h [34].

In breast cancer patients undergoing fertility preservation treatment, the use of a GnRH agonist oocyte maturation trigger has been associated with higher oocyte maturation and fertilization rates, increased numbers of available cryopreserved embryos and significantly decreased rates of ovarian hyperstimulation syndrome [35, 36].

## The Use of Aromatase Inhibitors: A Clinical Conundrum

A significant concern of patients and doctors is the potential effect that elevated serum estradiol concentrations can exert on cancer cell proliferation in estrogen sensitive breast cancer during IVF treatment. Letrozole is the most widely used aromatase inhibitor during fertility preservation treatment [37, 38]. Letrozole can selectively inhibit aromatization and decrease the serum levels of estradiol, estrone and estrone sulfate during the phase of ovarian stimulation. Furthermore, the elevated intrafollicular androgen levels, which result from the diminished aromatase activity, can increase follicular sensitivity to exogenous FSH stimulation [39, 40].

Unlike letrozole, anastrozole only exerts minimal suppression on estradiol concentrations during ovarian stimulation [38]. Consequently, breast cancer patients undergoing ovarian stimulation with anastrozole showed significantly higher serum estradiol levels than patients using letrozole. Combining gonadotrophins with aromatase inhibitors would augment the stimulation effect of these drugs, with a lower increase in serum concentrations of estradiol.

To date there are no randomized controlled trials studying the safety of fertility preservation regimens in breast cancer patients, particularly focusing on the use of aromatase inhibitors. The ethical considerations behind such studies would be considerable. In a prospective non-randomized trial of breast cancer patients having fertility preservation treatment prior to chemotherapy [41], women underwent ovarian stimulation cycles either with tamoxifen 60 mg/day alone or in combination with low-dose FSH or letrozole 5 mg in combination with FSH. Patients treated with FSH and tamoxifen or FSH and letrozole had significantly greater numbers of follicles, mature oocytes and embryos compared to patients treated with tamoxifen alone. Peak estradiol concentrations were lower in patients treated with letrozole and FSH. Recurrence rates after a mean follow-up of $554 \pm 31$ days was similar between IVF and control patients, and this was not affected by cancer stage. Notably there was no recurrence in the letrozole IVF group.

In a retrospective study of breast cancer patients by the same authors [42] the efficacy of aromatase inhibitors plus FSH in breast cancer patients was compared with a routine IVF protocol in age-matched controls without cancer. Total oocytes, mature oocytes, fertilization rate, the number of embryos and length of stimulation were similar between the two groups. Peak estradiol concentrations were significantly lower in the letrozole plus FSH group. Finally in a prospective, cohort study of breast cancer patients undergoing ovarian stimulation with FSH and letrozole or no stimulation before adjuvant chemotherapy, Azim et al. (2008) [43] reported no statistically significant survival difference between the two groups after a median follow-up of 23 months for the study group and 33 months for the control group.

The oocytes collected after the phase of ovarian stimulation can undergo fertilization with intracytoplasmic sperm injection (ICSI) and the resulting embryos can then be cryopreserved. Alternatively oocyte cryopreservation is an option for women who do not have a partner and do not want to use donor sperm.

## *Cryopreservation of Oocytes*

Since the first live birth from cryopreserved oocytes was reported in 1986, more than 900 healthy babies have been born worldwide [44]. Current live birth rates from series of frozen oocytes compare well to live birth rates in frozen embryo replacement cycles. Importantly there is no increase in the risk of congenital anomalies compared with national statistics for spontaneous conceptions as reported by the Center for Disease Control [44].

Human oocytes can be cryopreserved at the metaphase II stage by the slow freezing method or by vitrification. Oocyte cryopreservation remains challenging because the metaphase II stage, mature oocytes are very sensitive to temperature changes. The use of cryoprotectants and the formation of intracellular ice during a freeze-thaw procedure can potentially lead to depolymerization of the meiotic spindle [45, 46].

The method of vitrification, which is a form of ultra-rapid cooling, utilizes high concentrations of the cryoprotectant, which becomes an extremely viscous fluid without the formation of intracellular ice crystals. Vitrification can potentially increase oocyte survival and minimize damage to the meiotic spindle. In a prospective, randomized trial of patients undergoing oocyte cryopreservation, Smith et al. [47] reported that embryos resulting from vitrified oocytes had better clinical pregnancy rates compared with embryos resulting from slow-rate frozen oocytes (38 % vs 13 %).

Cryopreservation of immature oocytes germinal vesicle (GV) stage has been considered as an alternative for breast cancer patients, since it does not require a full ovarian stimulation cycle. Unfortunately the cryopreservation of immature oocytes at the GV stage has not been associated with favorable outcomes. It appears that immature oocytes are also vulnerable to cryoinjury resulting in a decreased capacity for maturation and fertilization.

## *Cryopreservation of Ovarian Tissue*

Ovarian tissue cryopreservation could have the potential to become a primary option for fertility preservation in breast cancer patients, particularly in patients with rapid disease progression or patients who do not wish to undergo ovarian stimulation in the future. The ovarian cortex is endowed with a large number of primordial follicles, which can be harvested by laparoscopy. The ovarian, cortical tissue obtained can then be cryopreserved in the form of thin slices. Initial results of xenografting frozen-thawed human ovarian tissue in animals showed encouraging results as 50–80 % of follicles survived the procedure [48]. The first livebirth after transplantation of cryopreserved ovarian tissue [49] was reported in 2004. Since then at least 13 babies have been born worldwide after transplantation of ovarian tissue.

The autotransplantation of frozen-thawed ovarian tissue can be orthotopic or heterotopic. During orthotopic autotransplantation, the ovarian tissue is transplanted on the remaining ovary or beneath the peritoneum of the ovarian fossa. Heterotopic autotransplantation has been performed to the subcutaneous tissue of the forearm [50], beneath the rectus sheath [50, 51] and the breast [50]. Although heterotopic sites are more practical because of the short lifespan of the frozen-thawed ovarian grafts, only orthotopic transplantation can potentially lead to a natural conception.

The main safety concern behind this promising fertility preservation technique refers to the risk of reintroduction of ovarian tissue with occult metastases in patients with breast cancer. Ovarian metastases are generally rare in breast cancer patients and they are more commonly associated with invasive lobular carcinomas. We need to acknowledge that the current experience of ovarian tissue transplantation in cancer patients remains limited. However, to date no case of cancer cell introduction has been reported with ovarian autotransplantation in such patients with breast cancer, Hodgkin's and non-Hodgkin's lymphoma and Ewing sarcoma.

## Pregnancy After Breast Cancer

Women aiming for a pregnancy after breast cancer treatment should consult their medical oncologist, breast surgeon and obstetrician. Patients on tamoxifen are generally advised to stop this treatment for 3 months before trying to conceive in view of the long half-life of this agent. Animal studies have confirmed the potential teratogenic effects of tamoxifen on the fetus. In the mouse and rat models, epithelial changes similar to those seen after administration of diethylstilbestrol (DES) have been observed. Vaginal adenosis, in particular, has been reported, which is comparable with the condition observed in young women exposed to DES in utero.

Women are normally advised to restart tamoxifen after pregnancy (and thus limit the duration of breast feeding) so that the duration of recommended endocrine treatment is completed, albeit 5 years or more recently 10 years. In the worldwide Adjuvant Tamoxifen: Longer Against Shorter (ATLAS) trial [52], 12,894 women with early breast cancer who had completed 5 years of treatment with tamoxifen were randomized to continue tamoxifen to 10 years or stop at 5 years. For women with ER-positive disease, the continuation of tamoxifen administration was associated with a reduced risk of recurrence ($p=0{\cdot}002$), reduced breast cancer mortality ($p=0{\cdot}01$), and reduced overall mortality ($p=0{\cdot}01$).

Women should wait at least 7 months after administration of HER2 targeted agents such as trastuzumab due to the reported risk of oligohydramnios [53] and longer if pertuzumab has been used in the neoadjuvant setting.

It has been typical practice to advise delaying pregnancy for at least 2 years after a diagnosis of breast cancer for a number of reasons. This delay could theoretically decrease potential risks to the fetus from exposure to chemotherapy, which could have possible, mutagenic effects on oocytes. For women with endocrine sensitive breast cancer, 2 years of tamoxifen significantly reduces breast cancer risk. On the other hand, this also provides some increased reassurance for women that their breast cancer has not relapsed and that the possibility of long term remission is possible.

The majority of pregnancies after breast cancer treatment will proceed to live birth. In a series of 465 breast cancer survivors who became pregnant after treatment [54], 51 % had a live birth at term, 8 % had a spontaneous miscarriage and 41 % of women proceeded to terminate the pregnancy. Reports on pregnancy outcomes after completion of breast cancer treatment remain conflicting. A large study from the Danish registry reported no increase in congenital anomalies, the incidence of stillbirth, low birth weight or preterm birth [55]. Conversely the Swedish registry data [56] showed an increased risk of malformations (OR 2.1, 95 % CI 1.2–3.7), birth before 32 weeks of gestation (OR 3.2, 95 % CI 1.7–6.0) and birth weight below 1500 g (OR 2.9, 95 % CI 1.4–5.8).

Evidence from epidemiological studies suggests that pregnancy after breast cancer does not have an adverse effect to breast cancer outcomes, regardless of the endocrine sensitivity of the diagnosed tumor. The "healthy mother effect" confounded many of these retrospective studies (i.e. only those who were very fit and well went on to become pregnant). However, in a large meta-analysis [57] of 14 studies in which 1244 cases of pregnancy after breast cancer were compared to 18,145 controls, no significant differences in survival were found. Hence, it appears safe and possible for many women to consider pregnancy and a family after a diagnosis of early breast cancer.

## References

1. Kim S, Klemp J, Fabian C. Breast cancer and fertility preservation. Fertil Steril. 2011; 95(5):1535–43.
2. Partridge AH, Gelber S, Peppercorn J, Sampson E, Knudsen K, Laufer M, Rosenberg R, Przypyszny M, Rein A, Winer EP. Web-based survey of fertility issues in young women with breast cancer. J Clin Oncol. 2004;22(20):4174–83.
3. Bines J, Oleske D, Cobleigh M. Ovarian function in premenopausal women treated with adjuvant chemotherapy for breast cancer. J Clin Oncol. 1996;14:1718–29.
4. Chapman R. Effect of cytotoxic therapy on sexuality and gonadal function. Semin Oncol. 1982;9:84–94.
5. De Vos M, Devroey P, Fauser B. Primary ovarian insufficiency. Lancet. 2010;376:911–21.
6. Meirow D, Biederman H, Anderson R, Wallace W. Toxicity of chemotherapy and radiation on female reproduction. Clin Obstet Gynecol. 2010;53:727–9.
7. Meirow D. Reproduction post-chemotherapy in young cancer patients. Mol Cell Endocrinol. 2000;169:123–31.
8. Walshe J, Denduluri N, Swain S. Amenorrhea in pre-menopausal women after adjuvant chemotherapy for breast cancer. J Clin Oncol. 2006;24:5769–79.

9. Di Cosimo S, Alimonti A, Ferretti G. Incidence of chemotherapy-induced amenorrhea depending on the timing of treatment by menstrual cycle phase in women with early breast cancer. Ann Oncol. 2004;15:1065–71.
10. Goodwin P, Ennis M, Pritchard K, Trudeau M, Hood N. Risk of menopause during the first year after breast cancer diagnosis. J Clin Oncol. 1999;17:2365–70.
11. Del Mastro L, Venturini M, Sertoli M, Rosso R. Amenorrhea induced by adjuvant chemotherapy in early breast cancer patients: prognostic role and clinical implications. Breast Cancer Res Treat. 1997;43:183–90.
12. Sonmezer M, Oktay K. Fertility preservation in young women undergoing breast cancer therapy. Oncologist. 2006;11:422–34.
13. Tham Y, Sexton K, Weiss H, Elledge R, Friedman L, Kramer R. The rates of chemotherapy induced amenorrhea in patients treated with adjuvant doxorubicin and cyclophosphamide followed by a taxane. Am J Clin Oncol. 2007;30:126–32.
14. Han H, Ro J, Lee K, et al. Analysis of chemotherapy-induced amenorrhea rates by three different anthracycline and taxane containing regimens for early breast cancer. Breast Cancer Res Treat. 2009;115:335–42.
15. Martin M, Pienkowski T, Mackey J, et al. Adjuvant docetaxel for node-positive breast cancer. N Eng J Med. 2005;352:2302–13.
16. Najafi S, Djavid G, Mehrdad N, et al. Taxane-based regimens as a risk factor for chemotherapy-induced amenorrhea. Menopause. 2011;18:208–12.
17. Fornier M, Modi S, Panageas K, Norton L, Hudis C. Incidence of chemotherapy-induced, long-term amenorrhea in patients with breast carcinoma age 40 years and younger after adjuvant anthracycline and taxane. Cancer. 2005;104:1575–9.
18. Zhou W, Yin H, Liu X, et al. Incidence of chemotherapy-induced amenorrhea associated with epirubicin, docetaxel and navelbine in younger breast cancer patients. BMC Cancer. 2010;10:281.
19. Del Mastro L, Boni L, Michelotti A, Gamucci T, Olmeo N, Gori S, Giordano M, Garrone O, Pronzato P, Bighin C, Levaggi A, Giraudi S, Cresti N, Magnolfi E, Scotto T, Vecchio C, Venturini M. Effect of the gonadotropin-releasing hormone analogue triptorelin on the occurrence of chemotherapy-induced early menopause in premenopausal women with breast cancer: a randomized trial. JAMA. 2011;306(3):269–76.
20. Moore HC, Unger JM, Phillips KA, Boyle F, Hitre E, Porter D, Francis PA, Goldstein LJ, Gomez HL, Vallejos CS, Partridge AH, Dakhil SR, Garcia AA, Gralow J, Lombard JM, Forbes JF, Martino S, Barlow WE, Fabian CJ, Minasian L, Meyskens FL, Gelber RD, Hortobagyi GN, Albain KS, POEMS/S0230 Investigators. Goserelin for ovarian protection during breast-cancer adjuvant chemotherapy. N Engl J Med. 2015;372(10):923–32.
21. Lambertini M, Ceppi M, Poggio F, Peccatori FA, Azim HA, Ugolini D, Pronzato P, Loibl S, Moore HC, Partridge AH, Bruzzi P, Del Mastro L. Ovarian suppression using luteinizing hormone-releasing hormone agonists during chemotherapy to preserve ovarian function and fertility of breast cancer patients: a meta-analysis of randomized studies. Ann Oncol. 2015;26(12):2408–19.
22. Nelson SM, Yates RW, Fleming R. Serum anti-Müllerian hormone and FSH: prediction of live birth and extremes of response in stimulated cycles--implications for individualization of therapy. Hum Reprod. 2007;22(9):2414–21.
23. Al-Azemi M, Killick SR, Duffy S, Pye C, Refaat B, Hill N, Ledger W. Multi-marker assessment of ovarian reserve predicts oocyte yield after ovulation induction. Hum Reprod. 2011;26(2):414–22.
24. Chang MY, Chiang CH, Hsieh TT, Soong YK, Hsu KH. Use of the antral follicle count to predict the outcome of assisted reproductive technologies. Fertil Steril. 1998;69(3): 505–10.
25. Melo MA, Garrido N, Alvarez C, Bellver J, Meseguer M, Pellicer A, Remohí J. Antral follicle count (AFC) can be used in the prediction of ovarian response but cannot predict the oocyte/embryo quality or the in vitro fertilization outcome in an egg donation program. Fertil Steril. 2009;91(1):148–56.

26. Frattarelli JL, Levi AJ, Miller BT, Segars JH. A prospective assessment of the predictive value of basal antral follicles in in vitro fertilization cycles. Fertil Steril. 2003;80(2):350–5.
27. Jayaprakasan K, Campbell B, Hopkisson J, Johnson I, Raine-Fenning N. A prospective, comparative analysis of anti-Müllerian hormone, inhibin-B, and three-dimensional ultrasound determinants of ovarian reserve in the prediction of poor response to controlled ovarian stimulation. Fertil Steril. 2010;93(3):855–64.
28. Huirne JA, Homburg R, Lambalk CB. Are GnRH antagonists comparable to agonists for use in IVF? Hum Reprod. 2007;22(11):2805–13.
29. Kasum M, Beketić-Orešković L, Peddi PF, et al. Fertility after breast cancer treatment. Eur J Obstet Gynecol Reprod Biol. 2014;173:13–8.
30. Damewood M, Shen W, Zacur H, Schlaff W, Rock J, Wallach E. Disappearance of exogenously administered human chorionic gonadotropin. Fertil Steril. 1989;52:398–400.
31. Mannaerts BM, Geurts TB, Odink J. A randomized three-way crossover study in healthy pituitary-suppressed women to compare the bioavailability of human chorionic gonadotrophin (Pregnyl) after intramuscular and subcutaneous administration. Hum Reprod. 1998;13:1461–4.
32. Haning R, Strawn E, Nolten W. Pathophysiology of the ovarian hyperstimulation syndrome. Obstet Gynecol. 1985;66:220–4.
33. Gonen Y, Balakier H, Powell W, Casper R. Use of GnRH agonist to trigger follicular maturation for in vitro fertilization. J Clin Endocrinol Metab. 1990;71:918–22.
34. Itskovitz J, Boldes R, Levron J, Erlik Y, Kahana L, Brandes J. Induction of preovulatory luteinizing hormone surge and prevention of ovarian hyperstimulation syndrome by gonadotropin-releasing hormone agonist. Fertil Steril. 1991;56:213–20.
35. Reddy J, Turan V, Bedoschi G, Moy F, Oktay K. Triggering final oocyte maturation with gonadotropin-releasing hormone agonist (GnRHa) versus human chorionic gonadotropin (hCG) in breast cancer patients undergoing fertility preservation: an extended experience. J Assist Reprod Genet. 2014;31(7):927–32.
36. Oktay K, Türkçüoğlu I, Rodriguez-Wallberg KA. GnRH agonist trigger for women with breast cancer undergoing fertility preservation by aromatase inhibitor/FSH stimulation. Reprod Biomed Online. 2010;20(6):783–8.
37. Requena A, Herrero J, Landeras J, Navarro E, Neyro JL, Salvador C, Tur R, Callejo J, Checa MA, Farré M, Espinós JJ, Fábregues F, Graña-Barcia M. Use of letrozole in assisted reproduction: a systematic review and meta-analysis. Hum Reprod Update. 2008;14(6):571–82.
38. Azim A, Costantini-Ferrando M, Lostritto K, Oktay K. Relative potencies of anastrozole and letrozole to suppress estradiol in breast cancer patients undergoing ovarian stimulation before in vitro fertilization. J Clin Endocrinol Metab. 2007;92(6):2197–200.
39. Holzer H, Casper R, Tulandi T. A new era in ovulation induction. Fertil Steril. 2006;85(2):277–84.
40. Mitwally MF, Casper RF, Diamond MP. The role of aromatase inhibitors in ameliorating deleterious effects of ovarian stimulation on outcome of infertility treatment. Reprod Biol Endocrinol. 2005;3:54.
41. Oktay K, Buyuk E, Libertella N, Akar M, Rosenwaks Z. Fertility preservation in breast cancer patients: a prospective controlled comparison of ovarian stimulation with tamoxifen and letrozole for embryo cryopreservation. J Clin Oncol. 2005;23(19):4347–53.
42. Oktay K, Rodriguez-Wallberg K, Schover L. Preservation of fertility in patients with cancer. N Engl J Med. 2009;360(25):2681.
43. Azim AA, Costantini-Ferrando M, Oktay K. Safety of fertility preservation by ovarian stimulation with letrozole and gonadotropins in patients with breast cancer: a prospective controlled study. J Clin Oncol. 2008;26(16):2630–5.
44. Noyes N, Porcu E, Borini A. Over 900 oocyte cryo-preservation babies born with no apparent increase in congenital anomalies. Reprod Biomed Online. 2009;18:769–76.
45. Baka SG, Toth TL, Veeck LL, Jones Jr HW, Muasher SJ, Lanzendorf SE. Evaluation of the spindle apparatus of in-vitro matured human oocytes following cryopreservation. Hum Reprod. 1995;10:1816–20.
46. Pickering SJ, Braude PR, Johnson MH, Cant A, Currie J. Transient cooling to room temperature can cause irreversible disruption of the meiotic spindle in the human oocyte. Fertil Steril. 1990;54:102–8.

47. Smith GD, Serafini PC, Fioravanti J, Yadid I, Coslovsky M, Hassun P, et al. Prospective randomized comparison of human oocyte cryopreservation with slow-rate freezing or vitrification. Fertil Steril. 2010;94:2088–95.
48. Newton H, Aubard Y, Rutherford A, Sharma V, Gosden R. Low temperature storage and grafting of human ovarian tissue. Hum Reprod. 1996;11(7):1487–91.
49. Donnez J, Dolmans MM, Demylle D, Jadoul P, Pirard C, Squifflet J, Martinez-Madrid B, van Langendonckt A. Livebirth after orthotopic transplantation of cryopreserved ovarian tissue. Lancet. 2004;364(9443):1405–10.
50. Oktay K, Economos K, Kan M, Rucinski J, Veeck L, Rosenwaks Z. Endocrine function and oocyte retrieval after autologous transplantation of ovarian cortical strips to the forearm. JAMA. 2001;286:1490–3.
51. Kim SS, Hwang IT, Lee HC. Heterotopic autotransplantation of cryobanked human ovarian tissue as a strategy to restore ovarian function. Fertil Steril. 2004;82:930–2.
52. Davies C, Pan H, Godwin J, Gray R, Arriagada R, Raina V, Adjuvant Tamoxifen: Longer Against Shorter (ATLAS) Collaborative Group, et al. Long-term effects of continuing adjuvant tamoxifen to 10 years versus stopping at 5 years after diagnosis of oestrogen receptor-positive breast cancer: ATLAS, a randomised trial. Lancet. 2013;381(9869):805–16. Erratum in: Lancet. 2013 Mar 9;381(9869):804.
53. Bader AA, Schlembach D, Tamussino KF, Pristauz G, Petru E. Anhydramnios associated with administration of trastuzumab and paclitaxel for metastatic breast cancer during pregnancy. Lancet Oncol. 2007;8(1):79–81.
54. Mueller BA, Simon MS, Deapen D, Kamineni A, Malone KE, Daling JR. Childbearing and survival after breast carcinoma in young women. Cancer. 2003;98:1131–40.
55. Langagergaard V, Gislum M, Skriver MV, Nørgård B, Lash TL, Rothman KJ, et al. Birth outcome in women with breast cancer. Br J Cancer. 2006;94:142–6.
56. Dalberg K, Eriksson J, Holmberg L. Birth outcome in women with previously treated breast cancer – a population-based cohort study from Sweden. PLoS Med. 2006;9:e336.
57. Azim HA, Santoro L, Pavlidis N, Gelber S, Kroman N, Azim H, Peccatori FA. Safety of pregnancy following breast cancer diagnosis: a meta-analysis of 14 studies. Eur J Cancer. 2011;47(1):74–83.

# Chapter 16
# Cardiotoxicity in Breast Cancer Survivors

**Nilesh Pareek, Susannah Stanway, Anna M. Kirby, and Alexander Lyon**

**Abstract** Breast cancer is the most common cancer in females globally and, with earlier detection and improvements in treatment, increasing numbers of women are surviving and living free of disease for many decades. However, several breast cancer treatment modalities are associated with a significant risk of toxicity to the heart both at the time of treatment and many years afterwards. This chapter will discuss the risks, pathogenesis, diagnosis and treatment of cardiotoxicity secondary to Anthracyclines, Trastuzumab and radiotherapy, in breast cancer patients. Approaches to risk stratification, surveillance, prevention and treatment of cardiotoxicity in these patients will also be discussed.

**Keywords** Breast cancer • Cardiotoxicity • Anthracyclines • Trastuzumab • Heart Failure

## Background

Breast cancer is the most prevalent cancer in females globally and with improved modern treatment programs, increasing numbers of patients are surviving free of recurrence or living with the disease [1–4]. Pharmacological treatments for breast

---

N. Pareek, MA (Hons) Cantab, MBBS, MRCP (✉)
Department of Cardiology, Royal Brompton and Harefield Foundation NHS Trust, Sydney Street, London, UK
e-mail: n.pareek@rbht.nhs.uk

S. Stanway, MBChB, MD, MRCP, MSc
The Breast Unit, The Royal Marsden NHS Foundation Trust, Surrey, UK

A.M. Kirby, BA, MB, BChir, MA, MRCP, FRCR, MD
Royal Marsden NHS Foundation Trust & Institute of Cancer Research, Surrey, UK

A. Lyon, MA, BM, BCh, PhD, FRCP
NIHR Cardiovascular Biomedical Research Unit, Royal Brompton Hospital, Sydney Street, London, UK



A. Ring, M. Parton (eds.), *Breast Cancer Survivorship*,
DOI 10.1007/978-3-319-41858-2_16

cancer have diversified over the past 20 years and whilst these have improved survival, several have been associated with significant cardiovascular toxicity. The three main cardiotoxic therapies used in the management of early breast cancer are anthracyclines, anti-HER2 therapies and radiotherapy; and the toxicity of these treatments is synergistic [5]. A further treatment which may influence long-term cardiovascular risk is the use of endocrine therapy, though the risk is less well established [6, 7].

The risk from these therapies is compounded by the fact that breast cancer is most commonly diagnosed in the over 65 year age group [8], who have a higher rate of cardiovascular co-morbidities and are more predisposed to treatment related toxicities [9]. It is important to recognize that 9–10 years after a breast cancer diagnosis, cardiovascular causes for death overtake those from the cancer in the survivors [10]. This may be a reflection of a higher prevalence of cardiac co-morbidities, the impact of cardiotoxicity of some treatments, and also the increasing age of the breast cancer population.

## Cardiac Complications of Radiotherapy

### *Risks of Radiation-Induced Heart Disease (RIHD)*

The Early Breast Cancer Trialists' Collaborative Group (EBCTCG) meta-analysis of randomized studies testing the benefits of adding radiotherapy to breast conservation surgery, demonstrated that breast radiotherapy halves the risk of local breast cancer recurrence, and reduces breast cancer mortality by around 5 % at 15 years [11]. However, this meta-analysis also demonstrates that the use of radiotherapy is associated with a 1 % increase in non-breast-cancer-related deaths, 90 % of which are cardiovascular in origin [11].

Radiotherapy techniques have improved since the women in these studies were treated, leading to lower radiation doses to the heart, and correlating with reductions in mortality from cardiovascular disease [12, 13]. However, even using modern breast radiotherapy techniques, mean doses to the heart have been measured at around 2Gy [14]. A recent population-based case–control study of major coronary events (death from ischaemic heart disease, myocardial infarction, and/or coronary revascularization procedures) in women treated between 1958 and 2001 revealed two important findings. The first was that the mean radiation dose to the heart is linearly related to the risk of major coronary events and, secondly, that there is no threshold mean heart dose below which a woman is at *no* risk of radiation-induced heart disease [15].

RIHD develops 5–30 years after the delivery of radiotherapy [15]. Risk factors for RIHD in breast cancer patients include treatment of left breast cancer, prior history of coronary artery disease, other circulatory diseases, diabetes mellitus, chronic obstructive pulmonary disease, smoking history, high body-mass index, and a history of regular analgesic use [15].

## *Pathogenesis of Radiation-Induced Heart Disease (RIHD)*

Irradiation of segments of coronary arteries is thought to be atherogenic [16]. The left anterior descending coronary artery (LAD) is the cardiac structure most proximal to the chest wall and therefore most likely to be encompassed in a breast or chest-wall radiotherapy field [13, 17]. Radiation-induced atherosclerosis in the LAD is thought to be a major contributor to the increase in cardiac mortality after radiotherapy for breast cancer [18]. A study using myocardial perfusion imaging to assess coronary artery damage found that left-sided tangential breast radiotherapy was associated with quantifiable perfusion deficits which, in around one third of cases, correlated with later development of ischaemic symptoms [19]. Single photon emission computerized tomography (SPECT) myocardial perfusion imaging has demonstrated more perfusion deficits in left- as opposed to right-breast irradiated patients up to 5 years following radiotherapy [20]. A significantly higher prevalence of cardiac stress test abnormalities has also been demonstrated amongst left- versus right-side-irradiated patients, with 70 % of abnormalities in left-side-irradiated patients being found in the LAD [21]. Furthermore, a study of thirteen left-sided irradiated patients who had undergone coronary angiography, found that 12/13 had coronary stenoses, eight of which were solely in the LAD [22]. The same authors found, in symptomatic left-side-irradiated patients, a higher than expected incidence of late cardiac diagnostic test abnormalities (myocardial perfusion imaging and echocardiograms), the majority of which were again localizable to the LAD.

Coronary artery disease alone however may not fully explain the increased risk of other types of RIHD including congestive cardiac failure and valvular abnormalities [12, 23]. The location and characteristics of perfusion deficits in one study [20], suggests that deficits are likely to be due to a combination of macrovascular and microvascular effects, the latter occurring as a result of the direct effects of radiation on endothelial cells of myocardial capillaries, causing capillary swelling and progressive obstruction of the vessel lumen, and leading to pericardial and myocardial fibrosis. A prospective SPECT study following conventional tangential-beam breast RT found localized myocardial perfusion defects compatible with transmural microvascular damage, resulting in segmental wall motion abnormalities [24]. Although a high percentage of perfusion defects persisted at 3–6 years, no reduction in ejection fraction was found and follow-up continues to determine their clinical significance [25].

## *Methods for Reducing Risks of RIHD*

For most women undergoing radiotherapy for breast cancer, the risk of RIHD from modern radiotherapy techniques is very low and is outweighed by the benefits [26]. However, since the numbers of patients living for many decades after breast cancer treatment is increasing [3], the potential population benefits from reducing radiation doses to the heart, even by a small amount are substantial

Simple methods of minimizing heart dose include optimization of tangential beam angles and the use of multileaf collimator lead shielding. However, where disease was present in the lower aspect of the breast, these methods are less suitable as they may compromise the radiation dose to the tumor bed.

Deep breath-holding techniques move the heart medially, inferiorly and posteriorly away from the chest wall and have been shown to halve radiation exposure to the heart [27–30], as well as being simple to deliver [30].

Prone positioning (in which patients are treated lying on their fronts rather than on their backs) can reduce doses to the heart particularly in women with larger breasts [31] in whom breast tissue falls away from the chest wall under gravity. However, the position can be difficult to reproduce on a daily basis [30] and recent work suggests that the heart-sparing effects are comparable to those of breath-hold even in larger-breasted women [30].

Intensity-modulated radiotherapy (IMRT) techniques including arc therapies can reduce high-dose irradiation of the heart but may also increase the volume of normal tissues irradiated to lower doses such that may need to be combined with breath-holding techniques in order to reduce the mean heart dose [32].

Proton beam therapy (PBT) is not yet widely available in the UK but can reduce the mean heart dose in women undergoing locoregional lymph node irradiation including the internal mammary chain [33]. It is not yet clear whether or not PBT offers significant advantages over simpler techniques such as breath-hold. There are also concerns about reports of increased rates of skin telangiectasia and pigmentation [34]. The use of radiation should be tailored carefully to the patient's individualized risk. While many patients obtain benefit from radiotherapy, omission of radiotherapy in patients with low risk breast cancer and risk factors for RIHD may be considered [35].

### *Surveillance of Patients Receiving Left Breast and Chest Wall Radiotherapy*

No specific guidelines currently exist for cardiac screening for breast cancer patients who have received previous breast or chest wall radiotherapy. Prior left breast radiotherapy should be considered a risk factor for coronary artery disease that should be managed in a routine manner, particularly at longer follow-ups (level of evidence Class III, B).

## Anthracycline Induced Cardiotoxicity (AIC)

The role of anthracyclines in the treatment of breast cancer is well-established [36, 37]. For the most part, the benefits in terms of disease outcomes outweigh the risks, but the risk of myocardial toxicity is an important potential sequelae in breast cancer survivors.

The most commonly used anthracyclines in the adjuvant and neo-adjuvant treatment of early breast cancer are Doxorubicin (total cumulative dose 240–300 mg/m$^2$) and Epirubicin (total cumulative dose 240–450 mg/m$^2$). The risk of myocardial toxicity from Doxorubicin is dose dependent although there are conflicting data on the levels at which this becomes significant. Initially, studies suggested a risk of 3 %, 7 % and 18 % of developing clinical heart failure at doses of 400 mg/m$^2$,500 mg/m$^2$ and 700 mg/m$^2$ respectively [9, 38]. However these rates reflect a range of malignancies and often in the metastatic setting, whereby long-term cardiotoxicity data was not available. These doses are much higher than the total cumulative doses currently used in adjuvant and neo-adjuvant protocols in the treatment of early breast cancer, but the rates of reported AIC remain high in real world registries [39]. A standard dose–response is exhibited but the curve is shifted depending on the presence of other risk factors and in particular age and prior exposure to radiotherapy. Although, histopathological changes have been reported in patients receiving as little as 200 mg/m$^2$ [40], cumulative doses of doxorubicin in clinical practice are usually limited to 450 mg/m$^2$, and rarely exceed 300 mg/m$^2$ in women receiving treatment for early breast cancer.

Epirubicin is also routinely used in the treatment of early breast cancer (the anthracycline component of "FEC" chemotherapy [41]). Epirubicin displays a similar dose dependent toxicity to Doxorubicin with a cumulative risk of developing clinical cardiac failure of 4 % at 600 mg/m$^2$, 9 % at doses of 800 mg/m$^2$ and 15 % at 1000 mg/m$^2$ [42]. Epirubicin is a less potent agent than Doxorubicin per milligram, but there is no evidence that Epirubicin is less cardiotoxic at equivalent doses [42].

Pre-existing cardiac disease, including prior left ventricular impairment, prior myocardial infarction or known cardiomyopathy identify the highest risk patients. Classical cardiovascular risk factors, including hypertension, diabetes mellitus, obesity and age are also important risk factors for the development of AIC [43]. They are all continuous variables and the absolute impact of each requires further studies. Other important and relevant risk factors are ethnicity, previous chest radiotherapy and concomitant use of Trastuzumab [39, 43].

## *Pathogenesis of Anthracycline Induced Cardiotoxicity*

Anthracyclines are cell cycle non-specific chemotherapy agents which act via several mechanisms, including inhibition of DNA transcription and RNA replication, inhibition of Topoisomerase II and free radical generation leading to DNA damage and DNA alkylation [44].

Two main models predominate to explain the mechanisms of AIC [45].

The first "off-target toxicity" is the production of reactive oxygen species by the formation of complexes between Anthracyclines and iron leading to direct electron exchange with oxygen molecules [46]. This oxidative stress has multiple toxic effects but, in particular, on mitochondrial signaling pathways mediating cell fate. The heart is particularly sensitive to this toxicity owing to presence of thousands of mitochondria in each myocytes [47]. Nonetheless, strategies employing anti-oxidants to prevent AIC have been disappointing [46].

The second pertains to the "on-target toxicity" of Anthracyclines on the Topoisomerase (Top) 2b enzyme. While the Top2a enzyme is expressed exclusively on cancer cells, Top2b enzymes are expressed in cardiac myocytes. Anthracyclines cause Top2b mediated DNA damage, mitochondrial dysfunction and generation of reactive oxygen species [48]. Mouse knockout models of Top2b are protected from developing AIC [49].

### *Clinical Manifestations*

AIC is classically described as permanent, exhibits a dose response and is irreversible [50]. However, there is evidence that with early detection more functional recovery is possible [51]. Early and Late AIC are classified as occurring within or after 1 year of treatment. Peak incidence of clinical cardiac events occurs at 1 year though the rate of late cardiotoxicity is unknown owing to a lack of large long-term follow-up studies [52, 53].

Early acute AIC presents with acute heart failure, ECG changes or arrhythmia. It is rare during treatment cycles in low risk patients [9, 53, 54]. Chronic AIC is the most common manifestation, usually with symptomatic congestive heart failure (CHF) and commonly occurs within the first 12 months of treatment but has been shown in survivors of pediatric cancer treated with Anthracyclines to occur up to 20 years after administration [55].

## Cardiac Complications of Anti-HER2 Therapy

Human epidermal growth factor receptor-2 (HER-2 or ErbB2) is expressed in 10–15 % of breast cancer cases and is associated with a more aggressive clinical course, poor response to therapy and reduced survival [56–58]. The advent of HER-2 directed therapies, including Trastuzumab (Herceptin®), Pertuzumab, which are recombinant, humanized monoclonal antibodies and Lapatinib (a small molecule Tyrosine Kinase Inhibitor) that, to differing extents, inhibit HER-2 mediated pathways, have significantly improved outcomes for patients with HER-2 positive early and metastatic breast cancer [59–62].

The cardiotoxicity of Trastuzumab was first identified in a pivotal trial in metastatic breast cancer, where Trastuzumab was associated with a significantly higher rate of CHF (~20 %) and Trastuzumab-induced cardiotoxicity [63]. Delaying trastuzumab until after Anthracycline treatment has been completed has significantly reduced rates in the subsequent adjuvant and neoadjuvant trials [61, 62]. Clinical rates of heart failure range from 1 to 16 % for symptomatic (NYHA class III or IV) CHF in the early studies when Trastuzumab was given concurrently with Anthracyclines [63], but the majority of contemporary clinical trials report lower rates (1–3 %) [61, 62]. However, surveillance strategies have detected earlier asymptomatic reductions in LVEF from 14 to 28 % when Trastuzumab was added to standard anthracycline based regimes [61–63]. Real world studies have suggested that rates of Trastuzumab-induced cardiotoxicity are higher, reaching 44 % of treated patients in one large study, but these are based on ICD-10 coding which may reflect asymptomatic LVEF reductions rather than clinical CHF [64]. The higher rates are likely to reflect older age, a higher rate of prior cardiovascular disease and secondary malignancies in the real world cohort than in clinical trials [64].

In addition to pre-existing heart disease, age and recent or previous Anthracycline treatment are the most important risk factors. Anthracycline treatment doubles rates of Trastuzumab cardiotoxicity at 5 years follow-up [39, 64, 65]. The impact of other cardiovascular risk factors including smoking, obesity and hypertension remain to be determined.

## *Pathogenesis of Cardiotoxicity Associated with Anti-HER2 Therapy*

The mechanism of HER-2 mediated cardiotoxicity is an area of considerable research interest. The HER-2 receptor plays an important role in cardiomyocyte (heart muscle cell) survival and, in particular, mediates effects of Neuregulin-1, which is released by the coronary vascular endothelium in response to cardiovascular stress. Trastuzumab binding to the HER-2 receptor prevents HER2-HER4 heterodimersiation and attenuates several downstream cell survival pathways including MAP kinase, ERK1/2, AKT and FAK dependent pathways [66].

These mechanisms are borne out by animal models with HER-2 knockout mice displaying features of dilated cardiomyopathy and impaired cardiac function [67]. HER-2 receptors are upregulated in animal models in response to cardiovascular stress [68] and in humans challenged with Anthracycline therapy [69]. Cardiac myocytes deficient in HER-2 activity are known to have increased susceptibility to Anthracycline toxicity and apoptosis [67]. Trastuzumab inhibition of intrinsic HER-2 mediated cellular protective mechanisms thus explains the potentiation of Anthracycline toxicity seen in real world clinical practice.

## *Clinical Manifestations*

In contrast to AIC, Trastuzumab-induced cardiotoxicity is usually considered to be a reversible, non-dose dependent process with no associated histopathological features [50]. Many patients (up to 95 % in some series [64]) who develop Trastuzumab-induced cardiotoxicity are asymptomatic. Trastuzumab-induced cardiotoxicity occurs primarily within the first 18 months of active treatment [70] and withdrawal of the drug is usually associated with a rapid recovery of LVEF (usually also within 18 months) even without medical therapy.

However, there is growing data which is challenging these traditional concepts. In the HERA study, 2 years of treatment with Trastuzumab were associated with almost a doubling of rates of LV dysfunction compared with 1 year (7.2 % vs. 4.1 %) [60]. In the NSABP (B31) trial, cumulative rates of Trastuzumab-induced cardiotoxicity were 3.8 % over 5 years in patients treated in the adjuvant setting [61]. Only 86 % of cases showed complete or partial resolution, confirming that not all cases are reversible [61].

## Modern Approaches to the Prevention and Treatment of Cardiotoxicity

The management of the long-term cardiac complications of modern breast cancer therapies in survivors is exemplified by an integrated multi-disciplinary approach to Oncology and Cardiac care which has been termed Cardio-Oncology. This approach incorporates a prompt diagnosis or baseline risk assessment; appropriately targeted echocardiographic and biomarker surveillance and early medical intervention of both clinical heart failure and asymptomatic left ventricular systolic dysfunction.

Guidelines to reduce cancer therapy related cardiovascular toxicity have been developed [71, 72] which emphasize the concepts of a thorough baseline risk assessment and a surveillance program. These guidelines are pragmatic and, whilst useful as clinical tools, they are limited by a lack of evidence base and are based largely on expert opinion.

### *Baseline Risk Assessment*

Identification and risk stratification of patients at risk of myocardial toxicity from cancer therapies are the cornerstone of managing these patients. This should involve a baseline clinical assessment of the patient's medical history for any symptoms and the presence of co-existing cardiovascular risk factors, such as hypertension, diabetes mellitus and prior cardiac disease. Routine physical examination including blood pressure measurement, 12 lead electrocardiogram and blood tests for lipid profile, renal function and cardiac biomarkers (where available) should also be performed. Any abnormalities in this baseline assessment should precipitate early referral to the Cardio-Oncology service for further evaluation and may guide treatment strategies and monitoring intervals whilst on cancer therapy.

#### Imaging for Baseline Risk Assessment

Cardiac imaging with LVEF measurement at baseline before neo-adjuvant or adjuvant treatment with Anthracyclines and/or Trastuzumab should be considered in all patients with early breast cancer as an important element of baseline risk assessment [71–73]. Transthoracic echocardiography (TTE) is the recommended modality for

LVEF screening, though multi-gated acquisition scanning (MUGA) and Magnetic resonance Imaging (MRI) have also been used. Advantages of TTE over MUGA include avoidance of radiation exposure, a wealth of other helpful anatomical and physiological information (hypertrophy, valvular function, and pulmonary artery pressure), assessment of more subtle parameters of left and right ventricular dysfunction, low cost and availability. Echocardiography is limited by poor acoustic windows in up to 30 % patients and due to operator-dependent measurement has variability of LVEF measurement which in clinical practice is up to 8 %. This is important to consider when reviewing serial measurements. MUGA has the advantage of less inter-observer variability and is more suitable if the patient has poor echocardiography windows. MRI is the gold-standard for imaging assessment but its clinical use is currently limited by availability [71, 72].

Baseline evaluation of Tissue Doppler Imaging and Global Longitudinal Strain (GLS) have both shown promise in predicting deterioration in LVEF in patients treated with Anthracycline and combination Anthracycline/Trastuzumab regimes [74–77]. However, the evidence of clinical utility originates from small scale studies and their routine use in this setting requires further evaluation [78].

#### Biomarkers for Baseline Risk Assessment

Cardiac biomarkers, B-type natriuretic peptide [BNP], N-terminal pro-BNP [NT-proBNP] and Toponins T and I, have assumed an increasingly important role in the baseline assessment of patients receiving cardiotoxic therapies.

Elevated Troponin I levels at baseline (pre-treatment) may predict the development of both clinical and subclinical reduction in LVEF in both Anthracycline and Trastuzumab treated patients [79–82]. However other observational studies have not corroborated these findings and other biomarkers have proved less useful [74, 83–86]. The threshold for defining abnormality of cardiac biomarkers, timing and use of appropriate assays remain unclear and an area of ongoing research but the use of biomarkers in the baseline assessment of patients has already been incorporated in some clinical practice guidelines [71, 72].

### *Surveillance*

The use of biomarkers and imaging also form the basis of surveillance of patients receiving cardiotoxic therapies.

#### Imaging for Surveillance

The European Society for Medical Oncology (ESMO) guidelines recommends screening at baseline, 3, 6, 9 and 12 months post-commencing Anthracycline or Trastuzumab therapy and a final screening TTE at 18 months post-treatment.

It raises the possibility of integrating biomarker screening but acknowledged that evidence for this is currently lacking [71].

The combined guidelines from the American Society of Echocardiography (ASE) and the European Association of Cardiovascular Imaging (EACVI) recommend similar screening intervals (baseline, 3, 6, 9, 12 months). The UK guidelines for patients treated with Trastuzumab advocate echocardiographic surveillance at 4, 8 and 12 months (in addition to baseline and post-chemotherapy assessments) in low risk individuals who do not show abnormalities of LV function on screening. It is important to consider baseline risk as this may guide increasing monitoring frequency intervals [73].

Owing to a lack of evidence base, several differences exist between the guidelines. In particular, the ASE recommends continued echocardiographic monitoring 6 months post-treatment with Anthracyclines, baseline TTE screening in Trastuzumab therapy is only recommended in those previously treated with Anthracycline therapy and the routine use of GLS is also recommended [71, 72].

Our opinion is that baseline risk assessment including LVEF measurement and biomarkers is most important as this can guide surveillance strategy. Low risk patients can be reviewed with cardiac imaging at 4 monthly intervals, whereas higher risk individuals require more frequent monitoring. The same imaging modality should be used during surveillance, and our preference is echocardiography, where available, from an accredited service.

## Biomarkers for Surveillance

There is considerable interest in the use of cardiac biomarkers for surveillance of cardiotoxicity since they are non-invasive and significantly cheaper than imaging modalities. Early rises in Troponin I can predict the development of reduction in LVEF in breast cancer patients treated with Anthracycline and Trastuzumab therapy [87, 88]. Rises in Troponin I also correlate with the magnitude of LV impairment [89–91] and persistence of raised Troponin levels is an important marker of the extent of LVEF impairment [80, 81, 92]. The positive predictive value for Troponin for prediction of deterioration in LVEF was 65 % and negative predictive value for was 100 % [79].

It is important to note that the role of cardiac biomarkers in surveillance of lower doses of Anthracycline therapy appears limited [93–95], and the association between troponin and cardiotoxicity is not universal, with several studies failing to show a link [96–98]. Many of these studies were not in patients with breast cancer, did not use modern high-sensitivity Troponin assays and varied in terms of cut-offs [96–98].

A further critical issue is the timing of biomarker measurement. The studies reporting benefit have generally measured Troponin in the 12–72 h period following Anthracycline or Trastuzumab dosing, which raises a number of practical challenges for patients receiving ambulatory outpatient treatment.

## Treatment Strategies: A Modern Approach

### *Prevention of Myocardial Cardiotoxicity*

#### Prevention of Anthracycline Induced Cardiotoxicity

Heart failure treatments used at baseline may have a role in preventing the development of cardiotoxicity. Beta-blockers may limit the development of AIC in breast cancer patients although current evidence is limited to small clinical trials and registry data. Evidence supporting the notion that beta-blockers may have a protective effect on AIC and Trastuzumab induced cardiotoxicity came from a real world registry of 920 patients with incidental beta-blocker use. Patients already on beta-blockers had a significantly lower rate of reduction in LVEF (though with no difference observed in mortality) [99]. Furthermore, larger clinical trials in non-breast cancer patients have suggested benefit in terms of symptomatic heart failure, reduction in LVEF and all-cause mortality [100–102]. Only one relatively small randomized controlled trial has been carried out in a breast cancer cohort to date, which showed that Nebivolol was associated with lower rates of reduction in LVEF compared with placebo in patients treated with adjuvant Anthracycline [103]. Several studies in non-breast cancer populations have reported the protective effects of Carvedilol against AIC. The efficacy of beta-blockers has been called into question by the recently published PRADA trial which reported benefit from Candesartan but not Metoprolol in patients treated with early breast cancer receiving adjuvant Anthracyclines with or without Trastuzumab in preventing LVEF reduction [104]. This was a relatively small trial with a short follow-up duration and may reflect the specific limitations of Metoprolol rather than a class effect.

Several pre-clinical studies have also provided a rationale for the role of ACE-inhibitors or Angiotensin II receptor blockers in preventing AIC, though evidence in clinical practice is limited [105–107]. Relatively small randomized controlled trials in non-breast cancer patients have shown a reduction in AIC compared with placebo [108]. The PRADA trial is the largest such study (120 breast cancer patients treated adjuvant Anthracycline-containing chemotherapy with or without Trastuzumab), in which Candesartan prevented deterioration in LVEF compared with placebo [104].

Although Spironolactone has anti-androgen properties, one randomized controlled trial has evaluated its use in preventing AIC in breast cancer patients treated with adjuvant Anthracyclines [109]. This study showed that Spironolactone significantly improved asymptomatic reductions in LVEF compared with placebo. There may be logical reasons to consider usage of the more selective aldosterone antagonist Eplerenone as opposed to Spironolactone in this setting, particularly in estrogen receptor positive patients, but this requires further evaluation and is currently based on expert opinion.

### Prevention of Trastuzumab Induced Cardiotoxicity

There is no randomized controlled trial data assessing the role of beta-blockade in prevention of trastuzumab-induced cardiotoxicity, although observational non-randomized data has suggested that this may be useful in preventing asymptomatic reductions in LVEF [110, 111]. There is also currently no clinical data assessing the role of ACE-inhibitors or Angiotensin II receptor blockers in the prevention of TIC but this is the subject of ongoing controlled clinical trials. It should also be recognized that a number of ongoing clinical trials are examining durations of Trastuzumab of less than the standard 1 year, in the hope that shorter durations may be equally efficacious but with lower risks of long-term cardiac toxicity.

## *Treatment of Established Myocardial Cardiotoxicity*

### Treatment of Anthracycline Induced Cardiotoxicity

The goals of treatment are to normalize LVEF, to minimize morbidity and mortality from CHF and to improve optimal cancer therapy adherence free of drug interruptions.

Prompt detection of asymptomatic reductions in LVEF (>10 % reduction in LVEF, especially to LVEF <50 %) and institution of beta-blockade and/or ACE-inhibitor therapy are widely accepted as optimal approaches to treatment of cardiotoxicity. Although it is recognized that there is limited randomized controlled trial evidence to support this approach for the treatment of AIC which is currently mainly limited to small prospective studies in a non-breast cancer cohort [92, 112]. There is a signal that LVEF is more likely to respond and improve if heart failure treatments are instituted early in breast cancer patients, but it should be noted that this study did not include a control arm [51]. One small clinical trial used a rise in Troponin I at 72 h to guide treatment with ACE-inhibitors, showing benefit from treatment with Enalapril compared with placebo [92]. Anthracycline containing chemotherapy is contra-indicated in patients with an LVEF<40 % at baseline. Should the LVEF drop to <40 % on treatment, Anthracyclines should be temporarily discontinued, heart failure treatments (ACE-I, beta-blockers, Mineralocorticoid Antagonists) initiated and then the patient should either be re-challenged when the LVEF has improved or commenced on a different cancer drug [71, 72] (Class II, B).

### Treatment of Trastuzumab Induced Cardiotoxicity

Treatment of trastuzumab-induced cardiotoxicity (>10 % reduction in LVEF, particularly to LVEF <50 %) with ACE inhibitors or beta-blockade is currently recommended though this is also supported by a limited evidence base [71, 113] (level of evidence Class II, B). It is recommended that Trastuzumab be withheld temporarily if the LVEF drops to less than 40 % [114]. However, this is based on limited evidence and with integrated Cardio-Oncology care and early institution of heart failure treatments, recovery or stabilization of LVEF is possible. This is important as early data suggests cancer recurrence rates are higher in patients with interruptions [115], and therefore increasing efforts to minimize the number and duration of interruptions of Trastuzumab are important. Treatment with ACE inhibitors and/or beta-blockers with rapid uptitration protocols and imaging evaluation, ideally at 2–3 weeks, should be performed. A repeat challenge of Trastuzumab with further follow-up at 4 weeks with clinical biomarker and imaging assessment is recommended [71, 113]. In the event of persistent symptoms and/or reduction in LVEF, a multi-disciplinary decision on the implications of discontinuing Trastuzumab should be made.

Treatment of symptomatic CHF should be managed in accordance with evidence-based guidelines with diuretics for symptoms and ACE-I/beta-blockers/Mineralocorticoid Antagonists [116].

## Long-Term Follow Up

The strategy for long-term follow up of breast cancer survivors who have been treated with cardiotoxic therapy remains to be clarified. Low risk patients at baseline with no evidence of cardiotoxicity during surveillance may be reassured that the absolute risk of long-term problems is low and no follow up is required. Those patients with higher baseline risk and/or detectable cardiotoxicity during surveillance may require further cardiac review. One specific group are those who started cardioprotective medications before or during breast cancer treatment. Cautious withdrawal of cardiac medication with review following cessation is usually appropriate for asymptomatic individuals with normal cardiac imaging and biomarkers. In other patients with evidence of persisting abnormalities a risk-benefit balance is required to guide long-term cardiology management.

Long-term follow up for patients who have been treated with left sided radiotherapy remains to be determined. Absolute estimated cardiac radiation dose received should help risk stratify, and those with higher total cardiac dose (>2Gy) may be considered for long-term (for example 5 yearly) surveillance.

Similar to selection of surveillance strategies, follow up strategies should be personalized to the patient and their situation.

## Conclusions

With improved rates of breast cancer survival, the lifetime burden of cardiotoxicity from cancer therapies is potentially substantial. Equally, the benefit of treatments directed towards prevention and prompt treatment of cardiotoxicity may have a profound impact on breast cancer survivors. While treating these issues is currently limited by a lack of evidence, a modern approach with an integrated multidisciplinary Cardio-Oncology service will enable more effective prevention and treatment of cardiotoxicity. Effective baseline risk assessment followed by personalized surveillance, early intervention with cardioprotective treatments to prevent interruption of effective cancer treatments, and personalized long-term follow up are the new clinical paradigm for this patient group. With an improved understanding of the clinical problem and with broadening of the evidence base and treatment developments in this area, both cancer and cardiovascular outcomes are likely to improve for breast cancer survivors.

## References


1. Siegel R, Naishadham D, Jemal A. Cancer statistics, 2012. CA Cancer J Clin. 2012;62(1): 10–29.
2. Effects of radiotherapy and surgery in early breast cancer. An overview of the randomized trials. Early Breast Cancer Trialists' Collaborative Group. N Engl J Med. 1995;333(22): 1444–55.
3. Maddams J, Utley M, Moller H. Projections of cancer prevalence in the United Kingdom, 2010-2040. Br J Cancer. 2012;107(7):1195–202.
4. Coombes RC, Kilburn LS, Snowdon CF, Paridaens R, Coleman RE, Jones SE, et al. Survival and safety of exemestane versus tamoxifen after 2-3 years' tamoxifen treatment (Intergroup Exemestane Study): a randomised controlled trial. Lancet. 2007;369(9561):559–70.
5. Seidman A, Hudis C, Pierri MK, Shak S, Paton V, Ashby M, et al. Cardiac dysfunction in the trastuzumab clinical trials experience. J Clin Oncol. 2002;20(5):1215–21.
6. Cuppone F, Bria E, Verma S, Pritchard KI, Gandhi S, Carlini P, et al. Do adjuvant aromatase inhibitors increase the cardiovascular risk in postmenopausal women with early breast cancer? Meta-analysis of randomized trials. Cancer. 2008;112(2):260–7.
7. McDonald CC, Alexander FE, Whyte BW, Forrest AP, Stewart HJ. Cardiac and vascular morbidity in women receiving adjuvant tamoxifen for breast cancer in a randomised trial. The Scottish Cancer Trials Breast Group. BMJ. 1995;311(7011):977–80.
8. United States Cancer Statistics. National cancer institute and centers for disease control and prevention; 2013.
9. Von Hoff DD, Layard MW, Basa P, Davis Jr HL, Von Hoff AL, Rozencweig M, et al. Risk factors for doxorubicin-induced congestive heart failure. Ann Intern Med. 1979;91(5):710–7.
10. Patnaik JL, Byers T, DiGuiseppi C, Dabelea D, Denberg TD. Cardiovascular disease competes with breast cancer as the leading cause of death for older females diagnosed with breast cancer: a retrospective cohort study. Breast Cancer Res. 2011;13(3):R64.
11. Early Breast Cancer Trialists' Collaborative Group; Darby S, McGale P, Correa C, Taylor C, Arriagada R, et al. Effect of radiotherapy after breast-conserving surgery on 10-year recurrence and 15-year breast cancer death: meta-analysis of individual patient data for 10,801 women in 17 randomised trials. Lancet. 2011;378(9804):1707–16.
12. Darby SC, McGale P, Taylor CW, Peto R. Long-term mortality from heart disease and lung cancer after radiotherapy for early breast cancer: prospective cohort study of about 300,000 women in US SEER cancer registries. Lancet Oncol. 2005;6(8):557–65.
13. Taylor CW, Nisbet A, McGale P, Darby SC. Cardiac exposures in breast cancer radiotherapy: 1950s-1990s. Int J Radiat Oncol Biol Phys. 2007;69(5):1484–95.
14. Taylor CW, Povall JM, McGale P, Nisbet A, Dodwell D, Smith JT, et al. Cardiac dose from tangential breast cancer radiotherapy in the year 2006. Int J Radiat Oncol Biol Phys. 2008; 72(2):501–7.

15. Darby SC, Ewertz M, McGale P, Bennet AM, Blom-Goldman U, Bronnum D, et al. Risk of ischemic heart disease in women after radiotherapy for breast cancer. N Engl J Med. 2013;368(11):987–98.
16. Artom C, Lofland Jr HB, Clarkson TB. Ionizing radiation, atherosclerosis, and lipid metabolism in pigeons. Radiat Res. 1965;26(2):165–77.
17. Fuller SA, Haybittle JL, Smith RE, Dobbs HJ. Cardiac doses in post-operative breast irradiation. Radiother Oncol. 1992;25(1):19–24.
18. Gyenes G, Fornander T, Carlens P, Rutqvist LE. Morbidity of ischemic heart disease in early breast cancer 15-20 years after adjuvant radiotherapy. Int J Radiat Oncol Biol Phys. 1994; 28(5):1235–41.
19. Yu X, Prosnitz RR, Zhou S, Hardenberg PH, Tisch A, Blazing MA, et al. Symptomatic cardiac events following radiation therapy for left-sided breast cancer: possible association with radiation therapy-induced changes in regional perfusion. Clin Breast Cancer. 2003;4(3): 193–7.
20. Seddon B, Cook A, Gothard L, Salmon E, Latus K, Underwood SR, et al. Detection of defects in myocardial perfusion imaging in patients with early breast cancer treated with radiotherapy. Radiother Oncol. 2002;64(1):53–63.
21. Correa CR, Das IJ, Litt HI, Ferrari V, Hwang WT, Solin LJ, et al. Association between tangential beam treatment parameters and cardiac abnormalities after definitive radiation treatment for left-sided breast cancer. Int J Radiat Oncol Biol Phys. 2008;72(2):508–16.
22. Correa CR, Litt HI, Hwang WT, Ferrari VA, Solin LJ, Harris EE. Coronary artery findings after left-sided compared with right-sided radiation treatment for early-stage breast cancer. J Clin Oncol. 2007;25(21):3031–7.
23. Borger JH, Hooning MJ, Boersma LJ, Snijders-Keilholz A, Aleman BM, Lintzen E, et al. Cardiotoxic effects of tangential breast irradiation in early breast cancer patients: the role of irradiated heart volume. Int J Radiat Oncol Biol Phys. 2007;69(4):1131–8.
24. Marks LB, Yu X, Prosnitz RG, Zhou SM, Hardenbergh PH, Blazing M, et al. The incidence and functional consequences of RT-associated cardiac perfusion defects. Int J Radiat Oncol Biol Phys. 2005;63(1):214–23.
25. Prosnitz RG, Hubbs JL, Evans ES, Zhou SM, Yu X, Blazing MA, et al. Prospective assessment of radiotherapy-associated cardiac toxicity in breast cancer patients: analysis of data 3 to 6 years after treatment. Cancer. 2007;110(8):1840–50.
26. Taylor CW, Kirby AM. Cardiac side-effects from breast cancer radiotherapy. Clin Oncol (R Coll Radiol). 2015;27(11):621–9.
27. Hjelstuen MH, Mjaaland I, Vikstrom J, Dybvik KI. Radiation during deep inspiration allows loco-regional treatment of left breast and axillary-, supraclavicular- and internal mammary lymph nodes without compromising target coverage or dose restrictions to organs at risk. Acta Oncol. 2012;51(3):333–44.
28. Nissen HD, Appelt AL. Improved heart, lung and target dose with deep inspiration breath hold in a large clinical series of breast cancer patients. Radiother Oncol. 2013;106(1):28–32.
29. Wang W, Purdie TG, Rahman M, Marshall A, Liu FF, Fyles A. Rapid automated treatment planning process to select breast cancer patients for active breathing control to achieve cardiac dose reduction. Int J Radiat Oncol Biol Phys. 2012;82(1):386–93.
30. Bartlett FR, Colgan RM, Carr K, Donovan EM, McNair HA, Locke I, et al. The UK HeartSpare Study: randomised evaluation of voluntary deep-inspiratory breath-hold in women undergoing breast radiotherapy. Radiother Oncol. 2013;108(2):242–7.
31. Buijsen J, Jager JJ, Bovendeerd J, Voncken R, Borger JH, Boersma LJ, et al. Prone breast irradiation for pendulous breasts. Radiother Oncol. 2007;82(3):337–40.
32. Osman SO, Hol S, Poortmans PM, Essers M. Volumetric modulated arc therapy and breath-hold in image-guided locoregional left-sided breast irradiation. Radiother Oncol. 2014; 112(1):17–22.
33. MacDonald SM, Jimenez R, Paetzold P, Adams J, Beatty J, DeLaney TF, et al. Proton radiotherapy for chest wall and regional lymphatic radiation; dose comparisons and treatment delivery. Radiat Oncol. 2013;8:71.

34. Galland-Girodet S, Pashtan I, MacDonald SM, Ancukiewicz M, Hirsch AE, Kachnic LA, et al. Long-term cosmetic outcomes and toxicities of proton beam therapy compared with photon-based 3-dimensional conformal accelerated partial-breast irradiation: a phase 1 trial. Int J Radiat Oncol Biol Phys. 2014;90(3):493–500.
35. Kunkler IH, Williams LJ, Jack WJ, Cameron DA, Dixon JM, investigators PI. Breast-conserving surgery with or without irradiation in women aged 65 years or older with early breast cancer (PRIME II): a randomised controlled trial. Lancet Oncol. 2015;16(3):266–73.
36. Laufs U, La Fata V, Plutzky J, Liao JK. Upregulation of endothelial nitric oxide synthase by HMG CoA reductase inhibitors. Circulation. 1998;97(12):1129–35.
37. A'Hern RP, Smith IE, Ebbs SR. Chemotherapy and survival in advanced breast cancer: the inclusion of doxorubicin in Cooper type regimens. Br J Cancer. 1993;67(4):801–5.
38. Vejpongsa P, Yeh ET. Prevention of anthracycline-induced cardiotoxicity: challenges and opportunities. J Am Coll Cardiol. 2014;64(9):938–45.
39. Bowles EJ, Wellman R, Feigelson HS, Onitilo AA, Freedman AN, Delate T, et al. Risk of heart failure in breast cancer patients after anthracycline and trastuzumab treatment: a retrospective cohort study. J Natl Cancer Inst. 2012;104(17):1293–305.
40. Ewer MS, Ali MK, Mackay B, Wallace S, Valdivieso M, Legha SS, et al. A comparison of cardiac biopsy grades and ejection fraction estimations in patients receiving Adriamycin. J Clin Oncol. 1984;2(2):112–7.
41. Levine MN, Bramwell VH, Pritchard KI, Norris BD, Shepherd LE, Abu-Zahra H, et al. Randomized trial of intensive cyclophosphamide, epirubicin, and fluorouracil chemotherapy compared with cyclophosphamide, methotrexate, and fluorouracil in premenopausal women with node-positive breast cancer. National Cancer Institute of Canada Clinical Trials Group. J Clin Oncol. 1998;16(8):2651–8.
42. Ryberg M, Nielsen D, Skovsgaard T, Hansen J, Jensen BV, Dombernowsky P. Epirubicin cardiotoxicity: an analysis of 469 patients with metastatic breast cancer. J Clin Oncol. 1998; 16(11):3502–8.
43. Yeh ET, Bickford CL. Cardiovascular complications of cancer therapy: incidence, pathogenesis, diagnosis, and management. J Am Coll Cardiol. 2009;53(24):2231–47.
44. Gewirtz DA. A critical evaluation of the mechanisms of action proposed for the antitumor effects of the anthracycline antibiotics adriamycin and daunorubicin. Biochem Pharmacol. 1999;57(7):727–41.
45. Sawyer DB. Anthracyclines and heart failure. N Engl J Med. 2013;368(12):1154–6.
46. Ladas EJ, Jacobson JS, Kennedy DD, Teel K, Fleischauer A, Kelly KM. Antioxidants and cancer therapy: a systematic review. J Clin Oncol. 2004;22(3):517–28.
47. Sawyer DB, Peng X, Chen B, Pentassuglia L, Lim CC. Mechanisms of anthracycline cardiac injury: can we identify strategies for cardioprotection? Prog Cardiovasc Dis. 2010;53(2): 105–13.
48. Zhang S, Liu X, Bawa-Khalfe T, Lu LS, Lyu YL, Liu LF, et al. Identification of the molecular basis of doxorubicin-induced cardiotoxicity. Nat Med. 2012;18(11):1639–42.
49. Deng S, Yan T, Jendrny C, Nemecek A, Vincetic M, Godtel-Armbrust U, et al. Dexrazoxane may prevent doxorubicin-induced DNA damage via depleting both topoisomerase II isoforms. BMC Cancer. 2014;14:842.
50. Suter TM, Ewer MS. Cancer drugs and the heart: importance and management. Eur Heart J. 2013;34(15):1102–11.
51. Cardinale D, Colombo A, Bacchiani G, Tedeschi I, Meroni CA, Veglia F, et al. Early detection of anthracycline cardiotoxicity and improvement with heart failure therapy. Circulation. 2015;131(22):1981–8.
52. Perez EA, Suman VJ, Davidson NE, Sledge GW, Kaufman PA, Hudis CA, et al. Cardiac safety analysis of doxorubicin and cyclophosphamide followed by paclitaxel with or without trastuzumab in the North Central Cancer Treatment Group N9831 adjuvant breast cancer trial. J Clin Oncol. 2008;26(8):1231–8.
53. Steinherz LJ, Steinherz PG, Tan CT, Heller G, Murphy ML. Cardiac toxicity 4 to 20 years after completing anthracycline therapy. JAMA. 1991;266(12):1672–7.

54. Lefrak EA, Pitha J, Rosenheim S, Gottlieb JA. A clinicopathologic analysis of adriamycin cardiotoxicity. Cancer. 1973;32(2):302–14.
55. Kremer LC, van Dalen EC, Offringa M, Ottenkamp J, Voute PA. Anthracycline-induced clinical heart failure in a cohort of 607 children: long-term follow-up study. J Clin Oncol. 2001;19(1):191–6.
56. Slamon DJ, Clark GM, Wong SG, Levin WJ, Ullrich A, McGuire WL. Human breast cancer: correlation of relapse and survival with amplification of the HER-2/neu oncogene. Science. 1987;235(4785):177–82.
57. Owens MA, Horten BC, Da Silva MM. HER2 amplification ratios by fluorescence in situ hybridization and correlation with immunohistochemistry in a cohort of 6556 breast cancer tissues. Clin Breast Cancer. 2004;5(1):63–9.
58. Kallioniemi OP, Holli K, Visakorpi T, Koivula T, Helin HH, Isola JJ. Association of c-erbB-2 protein over-expression with high rate of cell proliferation, increased risk of visceral metastasis and poor long-term survival in breast cancer. Int J Cancer. 1991;49(5):650–5.
59. Geyer CE, Forster J, Lindquist D, Chan S, Romieu CG, Pienkowski T, et al. Lapatinib plus capecitabine for HER2-positive advanced breast cancer. N Engl J Med. 2006;355(26): 2733–43.
60. Goldhirsch A, Gelber RD, Piccart-Gebhart MJ, de Azambuja E, Procter M, Suter TM, et al. 2 years versus 1 year of adjuvant trastuzumab for HER2-positive breast cancer (HERA): an open-label, randomised controlled trial. Lancet. 2013;382(9897):1021–8.
61. Perez EA, Romond EH, Suman VJ, Jeong JH, Davidson NE, Geyer Jr CE, et al. Four-year follow-up of trastuzumab plus adjuvant chemotherapy for operable human epidermal growth factor receptor 2-positive breast cancer: joint analysis of data from NCCTG N9831 and NSABP B-31. J Clin Oncol. 2011;29(25):3366–73.
62. Slamon D, Eiermann W, Robert N, Pienkowski T, Martin M, Press M, et al. Adjuvant trastuzumab in HER2-positive breast cancer. N Engl J Med. 2011;365(14):1273–83.
63. Slamon DJ, Leyland-Jones B, Shak S, Fuchs H, Paton V, Bajamonde A, et al. Use of chemotherapy plus a monoclonal antibody against HER2 for metastatic breast cancer that overexpresses HER2. N Engl J Med. 2001;344(11):783–92.
64. Farolfi A, Melegari E, Aquilina M, Scarpi E, Ibrahim T, Maltoni R, et al. Trastuzumab-induced cardiotoxicity in early breast cancer patients: a retrospective study of possible risk and protective factors. Heart. 2013;99(9):634–9.
65. Naumann D, Rusius V, Margiotta C, Nevill A, Carmichael A, Rea D, et al. Factors predicting trastuzumab-related cardiotoxicity in a real-world population of women with HER2+ breast cancer. Anticancer Res. 2013;33(4):1717–20.
66. De Keulenaer GW, Doggen K, Lemmens K. The vulnerability of the heart as a pluricellular paracrine organ: lessons from unexpected triggers of heart failure in targeted ErbB2 anticancer therapy. Circ Res. 2010;106(1):35–46.
67. Crone SA, Zhao YY, Fan L, Gu Y, Minamisawa S, Liu Y, et al. ErbB2 is essential in the prevention of dilated cardiomyopathy. Nat Med. 2002;8(5):459–65.
68. Gabrielson K, Bedja D, Pin S, Tsao A, Gama L, Yuan B, et al. Heat shock protein 90 and ErbB2 in the cardiac response to doxorubicin injury. Cancer Res. 2007;67(4):1436–41.
69. de Korte MA, de Vries EG, Lub-de Hooge MN, Jager PL, Gietema JA, van der Graaf WT, et al. 111Indium-trastuzumab visualises myocardial human epidermal growth factor receptor 2 expression shortly after anthracycline treatment but not during heart failure: a clue to uncover the mechanisms of trastuzumab-related cardiotoxicity. Eur J Cancer. 2007;43(14):2046–51.
70. Goldhar HA, Yan AT, Ko DT, Earle CC, Tomlinson GA, Trudeau ME, et al. The Temporal Risk of Heart Failure Associated With Adjuvant Trastuzumab in Breast Cancer Patients: A Population Study. J Natl Cancer Inst. 2016;108(1):djv301. doi:10.1093/jnci/djv301. Accessed 13th November 2016.
71. Curigliano G, Cardinale D, Suter T, Plataniotis G, de Azambuja E, Sandri MT, et al. Cardiovascular toxicity induced by chemotherapy, targeted agents and radiotherapy: ESMO Clinical Practice Guidelines. Ann Oncol. 2012;23 Suppl 7:vii155–66.

72. Plana JC, Galderisi M, Barac A, Ewer MS, Ky B, Scherrer-Crosbie M, et al. Expert consensus for multimodality imaging evaluation of adult patients during and after cancer therapy: a report from the American Society of Echocardiography and the European Association of Cardiovascular Imaging. Eur Heart J Cardiovasc Imaging. 2014;15(10):1063–93.
73. Jones AL, Barlow M, Barrett-Lee PJ, Canney PA, Gilmour IM, Robb SD, et al. Management of cardiac health in trastuzumab-treated patients with breast cancer: updated United Kingdom National Cancer Research Institute recommendations for monitoring. Br J Cancer. 2009;100(5):684–92.
74. Erven K, Jurcut R, Weltens C, Giusca S, Ector J, Wildiers H, et al. Acute radiation effects on cardiac function detected by strain rate imaging in breast cancer patients. Int J Radiat Oncol Biol Phys. 2011;79(5):1444–51.
75. Fallah-Rad N, Walker JR, Wassef A, Lytwyn M, Bohonis S, Fang T, et al. The utility of cardiac biomarkers, tissue velocity and strain imaging, and cardiac magnetic resonance imaging in predicting early left ventricular dysfunction in patients with human epidermal growth factor receptor II-positive breast cancer treated with adjuvant trastuzumab therapy. J Am Coll Cardiol. 2011;57(22):2263–70.
76. Hare JL, Brown JK, Leano R, Jenkins C, Woodward N, Marwick TH. Use of myocardial deformation imaging to detect preclinical myocardial dysfunction before conventional measures in patients undergoing breast cancer treatment with trastuzumab. Am Heart J. 2009;158(2):294–301.
77. Jurcut R, Wildiers H, Ganame J, D'Hooge J, De Backer J, Denys H, et al. Strain rate imaging detects early cardiac effects of pegylated liposomal Doxorubicin as adjuvant therapy in elderly patients with breast cancer. J Am Soc Echocardiogr. 2008;21(12):1283–9.
78. Stoodley PW, Richards DA, Boyd A, Hui R, Harnett PR, Meikle SR, et al. Altered left ventricular longitudinal diastolic function correlates with reduced systolic function immediately after anthracycline chemotherapy. Eur Heart J Cardiovasc Imaging. 2013;14(3):228–34.
79. Cardinale D, Colombo A, Torrisi R, Sandri MT, Civelli M, Salvatici M, et al. Trastuzumab-induced cardiotoxicity: clinical and prognostic implications of troponin I evaluation. J Clin Oncol. 2010;28(25):3910–6.
80. Cardinale D, Sandri MT, Colombo A, Colombo N, Boeri M, Lamantia G, et al. Prognostic value of troponin I in cardiac risk stratification of cancer patients undergoing high-dose chemotherapy. Circulation. 2004;109(22):2749–54.
81. Sawaya H, Sebag IA, Plana JC, Januzzi JL, Ky B, Cohen V, et al. Early detection and prediction of cardiotoxicity in chemotherapy-treated patients. Am J Cardiol. 2011;107(9):1375–80.
82. Sawaya H, Sebag IA, Plana JC, Januzzi JL, Ky B, Tan TC, et al. Assessment of echocardiography and biomarkers for the extended prediction of cardiotoxicity in patients treated with anthracyclines, taxanes, and trastuzumab. Circ Cardiovasc Imaging. 2012;5(5):596–603.
83. Dodos F, Halbsguth T, Erdmann E, Hoppe UC. Usefulness of myocardial performance index and biochemical markers for early detection of anthracycline-induced cardiotoxicity in adults. Clin Res Cardiol. 2008;97(5):318–26.
84. Knobloch K, Tepe J, Lichtinghagen R, Luck HJ, Vogt PM. Monitoring of cardiotoxicity during immunotherapy with Herceptin using simultaneous continuous wave Doppler depending on N-terminal pro-brain natriuretic peptide. Clin Med. 2007;7(1):88–9; author reply 9.
85. Knobloch K, Tepe J, Rossner D, Lichtinghagen R, Luck HJ, Busch KH, et al. Combined NT-pro-BNP and CW-Doppler ultrasound cardiac output monitoring (USCOM) in epirubicin and liposomal doxorubicin therapy. Int J Cardiol. 2008;128(3):316–25.
86. Raderer M, Kornek G, Weinlander G, Kastner J. Serum troponin T levels in adults undergoing anthracycline therapy. J Natl Cancer Inst. 1997;89(2):171.
87. Ky B, Putt M, Sawaya H, French B, Januzzi Jr JL, Sebag IA, et al. Early increases in multiple biomarkers predict subsequent cardiotoxicity in patients with breast cancer treated with doxorubicin, taxanes, and trastuzumab. J Am Coll Cardiol. 2014;63(8):809–16.
88. Dolci A, Dominici R, Cardinale D, Sandri MT, Panteghini M. Biochemical markers for prediction of chemotherapy-induced cardiotoxicity: systematic review of the literature and recommendations for use. Am J Clin Pathol. 2008;130(5):688–95.

89. Cardinale D, Sandri MT, Martinoni A, Borghini E, Civelli M, Lamantia G, et al. Myocardial injury revealed by plasma troponin I in breast cancer treated with high-dose chemotherapy. Ann Oncol. 2002;13(5):710–5.
90. Garrone O, Crosetto N, Lo Nigro C, Catzeddu T, Vivenza D, Monteverde M, et al. Prediction of anthracycline cardiotoxicity after chemotherapy by biomarkers kinetic analysis. Cardiovasc Toxicol. 2012;12(2):135–42.
91. Mornos C, Petrescu L. Early detection of anthracycline-mediated cardiotoxicity: the value of considering both global longitudinal left ventricular strain and twist. Can J Physiol Pharmacol. 2013;91(8):601–7.
92. Cardinale D, Colombo A, Sandri MT, Lamantia G, Colombo N, Civelli M, et al. Prevention of high-dose chemotherapy-induced cardiotoxicity in high-risk patients by angiotensin-converting enzyme inhibition. Circulation. 2006;114(23):2474–81.
93. Erkus B, Demirtas S, Yarpuzlu AA, Can M, Genc Y, Karaca L. Early prediction of anthracycline induced cardiotoxicity. Acta Paediatr. 2007;96(4):506–9.
94. Feola M, Garrone O, Occelli M, Francini A, Biggi A, Visconti G, et al. Cardiotoxicity after anthracycline chemotherapy in breast carcinoma: effects on left ventricular ejection fraction, troponin I and brain natriuretic peptide. Int J Cardiol. 2011;148(2):194–8.
95. Romano S, Fratini S, Ricevuto E, Procaccini V, Stifano G, Mancini M, et al. Serial measurements of NT-proBNP are predictive of not-high-dose anthracycline cardiotoxicity in breast cancer patients. Br J Cancer. 2011;105(11):1663–8.
96. Grover S, Leong DP, Chakrabarty A, Joerg L, Kotasek D, Cheong K, et al. Left and right ventricular effects of anthracycline and trastuzumab chemotherapy: a prospective study using novel cardiac imaging and biochemical markers. Int J Cardiol. 2013;168(6):5465–7.
97. Kismet E, Varan A, Ayabakan C, Alehan D, Portakal O, Buyukpamukcu M. Serum troponin T levels and echocardiographic evaluation in children treated with doxorubicin. Pediatr Blood Cancer. 2004;42(3):220–4.
98. Kremer LC, Bastiaansen BA, Offringa M, Lam J, van Straalen JP, de Winter RJ, et al. Troponin T in the first 24 hours after the administration of chemotherapy and the detection of myocardial damage in children. Eur J Cancer. 2002;38(5):686–9.
99. Seicean S, Seicean A, Alan N, Plana JC, Budd GT, Marwick TH. Cardioprotective effect of beta-adrenoceptor blockade in patients with breast cancer undergoing chemotherapy: follow-up study of heart failure. Circ Heart Fail. 2013;6(3):420–6.
100. Kalay N, Basar E, Ozdogru I, Er O, Cetinkaya Y, Dogan A, et al. Protective effects of carvedilol against anthracycline-induced cardiomyopathy. J Am Coll Cardiol. 2006;48(11):2258–62.
101. Georgakopoulos P, Roussou P, Matsakas E, Karavidas A, Anagnostopoulos N, Marinakis T, et al. Cardioprotective effect of metoprolol and enalapril in doxorubicin-treated lymphoma patients: a prospective, parallel-group, randomized, controlled study with 36-month follow-up. Am J Hematol. 2010;85(11):894–6.
102. Bosch X, Rovira M, Sitges M, Domenech A, Ortiz-Perez JT, de Caralt TM, et al. Enalapril and carvedilol for preventing chemotherapy-induced left ventricular systolic dysfunction in patients with malignant hemopathies: the OVERCOME trial (preventiOn of left Ventricular dysfunction with Enalapril and caRvedilol in patients submitted to intensive ChemOtherapy for the treatment of Malignant hEmopathies). J Am Coll Cardiol. 2013;61(23):2355–62.
103. Kaya MG, Ozkan M, Gunebakmaz O, Akkaya H, Kaya EG, Akpek M, et al. Protective effects of nebivolol against anthracycline-induced cardiomyopathy: a randomized control study. Int J Cardiol. 2013;167(5):2306–10.
104. Gulati G, Heck SL, Ree AH, Hoffmann P, Schulz-Menger J, Fagerland MW, et al. Prevention of cardiac dysfunction during adjuvant breast cancer therapy (PRADA): a 2 x 2 factorial, randomized, placebo-controlled, double-blind clinical trial of candesartan and metoprolol. Eur Heart J. 2016;37(21):1671–80.
105. Abd El-Aziz MA, Othman AI, Amer M, El-Missiry MA. Potential protective role of angiotensin-converting enzyme inhibitors captopril and enalapril against adriamycin-induced acute cardiac and hepatic toxicity in rats. J Appl Toxicol. 2001;21(6):469–73.

106. Lemmens K, Segers VF, Demolder M, De Keulenaer GW. Role of neuregulin-1/ErbB2 signaling in endothelium-cardiomyocyte cross-talk. J Biol Chem. 2006;281(28):19469–77.
107. Tokudome T, Mizushige K, Noma T, Manabe K, Murakami K, Tsuji T, et al. Prevention of doxorubicin (adriamycin)-induced cardiomyopathy by simultaneous administration of angiotensin-converting enzyme inhibitor assessed by acoustic densitometry. J Cardiovasc Pharmacol. 2000;36(3):361–8.
108. Dessi M, Madeddu C, Piras A, Cadeddu C, Antoni G, Mercuro G, et al. Long-term, up to 18 months, protective effects of the angiotensin II receptor blocker telmisartan on Epirubin-induced inflammation and oxidative stress assessed by serial strain rate. Springerplus. 2013;2(1):198.
109. Akpek M, Ozdogru I, Sahin O, Inanc M, Dogan A, Yazici C, et al. Protective effects of spironolactone against anthracycline-induced cardiomyopathy. Eur J Heart Fail. 2015;17(1):81–9.
110. Ewer MS, Vooletich MT, Durand JB, Woods ML, Davis JR, Valero V, et al. Reversibility of trastuzumab-related cardiotoxicity: new insights based on clinical course and response to medical treatment. J Clin Oncol. 2005;23(31):7820–6.
111. Oliva S, Cioffi G, Frattini S, Simoncini EL, Faggiano P, Boccardi L, et al. Administration of angiotensin-converting enzyme inhibitors and beta-blockers during adjuvant trastuzumab chemotherapy for nonmetastatic breast cancer: marker of risk or cardioprotection in the real world? Oncologist. 2012;17(7):917–24.
112. Cardinale D, Colombo A, Lamantia G, Colombo N, Civelli M, De Giacomi G, et al. Anthracycline-induced cardiomyopathy: clinical relevance and response to pharmacologic therapy. J Am Coll Cardiol. 2010;55(3):213–20.
113. Tocchetti CG, Ragone G, Coppola C, Rea D, Piscopo G, Scala S, et al. Detection, monitoring, and management of trastuzumab-induced left ventricular dysfunction: an actual challenge. Eur J Heart Fail. 2012;14(2):130–7.
114. Suter TM, Procter M, van Veldhuisen DJ, Muscholl M, Bergh J, Carlomagno C, et al. Trastuzumab-associated cardiac adverse effects in the herceptin adjuvant trial. J Clin Oncol. 2007;25(25):3859–65.
115. Steingart. Impact of trastuzumab-induced cardiotoxicity and subsequent trastuzumab interruption on breast cancer outcome. American College of Cardiology Annual Congress; 2013.
116. McMurray JJ, Adamopoulos S, Anker SD, Auricchio A, Bohm M, Dickstein K, et al. ESC Guidelines for the diagnosis and treatment of acute and chronic heart failure 2012: the Task Force for the Diagnosis and Treatment of Acute and Chronic Heart Failure 2012 of the European Society of Cardiology. Developed in collaboration with the Heart Failure Association (HFA) of the ESC. Eur Heart J. 2012;33(14):1787–847.

# Chapter 17
# Second Primary Neoplasms Following a Diagnosis of Breast Cancer

**Felicity Paterson, Susannah Stanway, Lone Gothard, and Navita Somaiah**

**Abstract** Many women diagnosed with early breast cancer will be cured and survive for many years after their initial diagnosis. Therefore it is important to take into account the risk of the development of new primary malignancies in such patients. Patients may be predisposed to develop new primary cancers as a result of genetic predisposition, environmental factors, or as a result of the adjuvant therapies used to treat early breast cancer. Treatment-related second primary cancers include an increased risk of breast and lung cancers following adjuvant radiotherapy, hematological malignancies following adjuvant chemotherapy, and endometrial cancer following tamoxifen. As a result of confounding factors the increased risk of these events differs between analyses, but the overall absolute risk of treatment-related second primary cancers remains low. Nonetheless it is important that patients are informed of these risks, modifiable risk factors are addressed and measures to minimize risks are undertaken, particularly when considering adjuvant therapies in women at low risks of recurrence.

**Keywords** Second cancers • Radiation induced cancers • Leukemia • Anthracycline • Tamoxifen • Endometrial

F. Paterson, MBBS, BSc
Department of Clinical Oncology, The Royal Marsden NHS Foundation Trust, Sutton, Surrey, UK

S. Stanway, MBChB, MD, MRCP, MSc
The Breast Unit, The Royal Marsden NHS Foundation Trust, Sutton, Surrey, UK

L. Gothard, HND
Division of Radiotherapy and Imaging, The Institute of Cancer Research, London, UK

N. Somaiah, DPhil, FRCR, MD, MBBS (✉)
Division of Radiotherapy and Imaging, The Institute of Cancer Research and The Royal Marsden NHS Foundation Trust, London, UK
e-mail: navita.somaiah@icr.ac.uk


A. Ring, M. Parton (eds.), *Breast Cancer Survivorship*,
DOI 10.1007/978-3-319-41858-2_17

## Introduction

Breast cancer is the commonest malignancy affecting women in the UK. With earlier detection and improved multi-modality treatment increasing numbers of women are surviving early breast cancer (EBC) and therefore the risk of developing second primary neoplasms needs to be considered.

Much of the data on sequelae following cancer treatment comes from the USA Survival epidemiology end results (SEER) data 1975–2010 [1]. This estimates that 18 % of all incident malignancies are second primary tumors. Second primary malignancies can be induced by many forms of non-surgical cancer therapy. The effect of these treatments can be compounded by host related factors such as germline mutations or environmental factors such as smoking. Second cancers may also be "sporadic" and not related to these factors. These factors and their interactions, along with patient age, contribute to the overall risk of developing a second primary neoplasm.

Following a diagnosis of a primary breast cancer, a second primary breast cancer, either in the same breast or in the contralateral breast is the most likely second primary cancer to be diagnosed, with between 2 and 11 % of women developing a second contralateral cancer [2–4]. Women with a history of breast cancer have a two to six fold increased risk of developing a second breast cancer, which accounts for between 30 and 50 % of all second tumors [5]. Over time, there has been a documented reduction in subsequent contralateral breast cancers diagnosed, which has been attributed to the use of adjuvant endocrine therapy [6, 7].

Analyses of cancer registries have reported the rates of common cancers following a breast cancer diagnosis. A Dutch study of 58,068 survivors of breast cancer has demonstrated an absolute excess risk of a second cancer (excluding breast cancer) of 13.6 per 10,000 women-years (95 % CI 9.7–17.6) when compared to the general population [8]. Of those patients followed up for a 10 year period the cumulative incidence of a second cancer was 5.4 % (95 % CI 5.1–5.7 %) [8]. The most prevalent tumors were of the uterus, lung, colon, ovaries and skin (melanoma), but tumors of the esophagus, stomach, rectum, kidney, bladder, soft tissue, non-hodgkin lymphoma and leukemia were also seen. Similarly in an analysis of the SEER database in the US a statistically significant increased incidence of breast cancer (standardized incidence ratio, SIR 1.55) followed by uterine cancer (SIR 1.36), ovarian cancer (SIR 1.27) and thyroid cancer (SIR 1.19) following a diagnosis of primary breast cancer [4].

This chapter will focus on treatment-associated malignancies. Interpretation of the data is complex because patients often receive multi-modality treatment each with effects on breast cancer outcome and ability to cause a second malignancy. Similarly, an individual's ability to benefit from any defined treatment is variable, depending on their risk of recurrence and this must be taken into account when considering management strategy. The ability of a treatment to induce carcinogenesis is related to treatment variables for example, dose given, dose intensity, and patient related clinic-pathological variables, such as age and a family history [9].

Cross-study comparisons are to be done with caution, as cohorts of women are often intrinsically different on a number of levels, such as ethnicity, treatment received and follow-up time.

When interpreting published data summarized in this chapter, it must be appreciated that treatment strategies have changed since data on second malignancies was first published and historic risks quoted may now be less due to refined treatment strategies. The most reliable data originates from randomized control trials, however since second malignancies are uncommon events, the numbers of patients affected in such prospective studies are very small, hence retrospective data from registries or case-control studies are often used. These types of study are more likely to be affected by bias.

In this chapter we review the risk of second cancers in breast cancer survivors, contributory factors and their interactions and suggest possible ways to enhance our ability to predict this risk. The main focus will be on treatment related factors, but we will also briefly discuss host related factors at the end of the chapter which will be discussed in more detail in Chap. 5.

## Treatment-Associated Cancers

When the three modalities of treatment are considered (radiotherapy, chemotherapy and hormone therapy) the increased risk of a second cancer varies with age and with time elapsed since treatment. In the general population, cancer risk increases with increasing age, but following therapy for breast cancer, the incidence of most second cancers has been shown to decrease over time. In the Dutch cohort study previously described, the breast cancer survivors under 50 years old had an increased risk of second cancers following radiotherapy with a hazard ratio (HR) of 1.04 (95 % CI 0.83–1.29), a reduced risk following chemotherapy with a HR of 0.79 (95 % CI 0.63–0.98) and reduced risk for endocrine therapy with a HR of 0.88 (95 % CI 0.64–1.22). In the cohort of patients over 50 years old, the HR was 1.00 for radiotherapy (95 % CI 0.91–1.10), 1.03 for chemotherapy (95 % CI 0.85–1.25) and 1.10 for endocrine therapy (95 % CI 1.01–1.21). A recent meta-analysis of 15 retrospective population based or hospital based cohort studies defined the SIR of a second cancer as 1.51 (95 % CI 1.35–1.70) for women younger than 50, and 1.11 (95 % CI 1.02–1.21) for women older than 50 [10]. The relative risk (RR) of a second cancer also increases over time, and was defined as 1.19 (95 % CI 1.06–1.33) in the first 10 years after diagnosis and 1.26 (95 % CI 1.05–1.52) thereafter [10].

The EPIC cohort study collected data on 10,000 breast cancer survivors over 11 years and found a 30 % increased risk (95 % CI 18–42) in the development of a second cancer (excluding contralateral breast cancer). Risks were increased for colorectal cancer (SIR 1.71, 95 % CI 1.43–2.00), lymphoma (SIR 1.80, 95 % CI 1.31–2.40), melanoma (SIR 2.12, 95 % CI 1.63–2.70), endometrial cancer (SIR 2.18, 1.75–2.70) and kidney cancer (SIR 2.40, 1.57–3.52) [11].

Although second primary malignancies are not common after a breast cancer diagnosis, a diagnosis of a subsequent cancer has been shown in one cohort to lead to a four-fold increased risk of death (HR 3.98; 95 % CI 3.77–4.20) in those affected and so is an important consideration [8]. An informed discussion when taking consent for treatment is thus of paramount importance.

## *Radiotherapy Induced Cancers*

The absolute benefit of adjuvant radiotherapy has been confirmed in the Early Breast Cancer Trialists Collaborative Group (EBCTCG) review of 10,801 women which showed that at least one breast cancer death is avoided by year 15 for every 4 recurrences avoided by year 10 with radiotherapy treatment, and the mortality reduction did not differ significantly in node positive or node negative disease [12]. When discussing curative radiotherapy, the small chance of secondary cancers has to be weighed against the significant benefit in terms of loco-regional and distant recurrence for majority of patients.

Much of the data on radiation induced tumorigenesis comes from data on atomic bomb survivors and historical use of low-dose radiotherapy to treat benign conditions. Sadamori et al. [13] showed that in the long-term follow-up of individuals exposed to atomic bomb fallout there was an increased risk of tumor development. Radiation induced tumorigenesis occurs at low doses and risk increases with dose; dose is affected by volume irradiated and technique used [14]. The latency of tumor detection is typically several years after exposure and can extend to decades [15, 16], and the younger the age at time of exposure, the higher the risk of tumorigenesis [17]. Concomitant treatment with chemotherapeutic or targeted therapies may also impact upon this risk by causing further damage to cellular DNA [18, 19]. The relative risk of a second cancer is also affected by host behaviors and genetic makeup [20]. SEER reviewed data from 328,691 women and identified an increased risk of contralateral breast cancer and other solid cancers namely lung, esophagus and soft tissue following radiotherapy treatment compared to those treated with surgery alone [21]. For those receiving radiotherapy and surviving beyond 5 years they found an 8 % (3–14 %) excess attributable risk of contralateral breast cancer and 10 % (5–14 %) of other solid cancers.

### Mechanisms of Radiation Damage

Ionizing radiation causes single and double strand DNA breaks to occur in the cell as well as DNA base damage and crosslinks. This damage may be repaired but if it is not, the cell will either undergo cell cycle arrest or cell death [22]. Aberrant cell cycle control, incorrect repair mechanisms or evasion of apoptosis induction can result in carcinogenesis in normal tissue in response to ionizing radiation. Germline mutations in p53 or BRCA1 and 2 could put individuals at higher risk of induction of second primary malignancy as the normal repair mechanisms are disrupted. The prevalence of these genetic mutations is quite low and Oeffinger et al. [23] suggested that radiation induced tumorigenesis is via DNA damage leading to other low penetrance genetic mutations, which may occur commonly across cancer patients. These low penetrance genes have been investigated and PRDM1, Glutathione S transferase and XRCC 3 as part of base excision repair have been shown to have an association with increased risk second primary cancers [24–26].

According to Broeks et al. radiotherapy may induce distinctive genomic aberrations and subsequent gene expression increasing risk of breast cancer through induction of a specific breast tumor molecular profile [27]. They compared 22 patients with breast cancer who had historically received thoracic irradiation for Hodgkin lymphoma to 20 breast cancer controls with no radiotherapy history. They found that the previously irradiated breast cancers tended to correlate more with a chromosomal instability gene profile, which is associated with basal cell subtype, higher grade and a poor clinical outcome, than the controls ($p=0.058$). Whilst this data is not related to breast cancer radiotherapy and represents a small study, it is an area that warrants further research as others have suggested that radiation induced breast cancers are of similar type to those seen in the general population [28].

Radiation induced cancers following curative radiotherapy for breast cancer include contralateral breast, lung and other less common cancers.

## Breast Cancer

Second breast cancer risk is increased in those who have had radiotherapy to the breast. When one considers the risk of contralateral breast cancer following breast radiotherapy one needs to consider the dose–response relationship, the age at exposure and the volume irradiated.

Hooning et al. [18] showed that contralateral breast cancers occur following radiation with a 1.5 fold overall increased risk. These cancers tend to be adenocarcinomas, but can also be sarcomas. Sarcomas of the breast usually occur 3–15 years after radiotherapy. Angiosarcomas are extremely rare accounting for <0.04 % breast neoplasms. However in a retrospective survey of nearly 200,000 women with breast cancer, those who had radiotherapy had a 16 fold increased lifetime risk [29]. The absolute risk is 0.5 % at 15 years.

The EBCTCG reviewed recurrence rates, breast cancer mortality and all-cause mortality in 42,000 patients who had had surgery alone or surgery and radiotherapy for early breast cancer [30]. They included all trials that had started recruiting by 1995, which led to a minimum follow up period of ten years. There was an excess of contralateral breast cancer incidence in those receiving radiotherapy, total cases 1451 (rate ratio 1.18, $2p=0.002$) calculated from the observed-expected rates divided by the variance. An excess of contralateral breast cancer occurs mainly in the 5–14 year period after follow up with the risk appearing to be most significant in those >50 years at time of treatment. This is contrary to other studies who found an increased risk in younger patients [21, 31]. The authors acknowledge that many of these patients were treated in the early seventies when radiotherapy techniques irradiated larger volumes of normal tissue than presently, thus giving a larger risk than more recently treated patients may have. Boice et al. found an increased rate of contralateral breast cancer occurring in those patients irradiated for EBC with 23 % of patients in the exposed cohort and 20 % of patients in the unexposed cohort developing second breast cancer, RR 1.19 (95 % CI 0.94–1.50). The risk increased with dose of radiation received 0.01–1.99 Gy RR 1.02, 2–3.99 Gy RR 1.07, >4 Gy RR 1.35. This risk at ten years was seen particularly in those exposed under 45 years of age (<45 RR 1.85 (95 % CI 1.15–2.97) and >45 RR 1.08 (95 % CI 0.74–1.57)). More recently, Berrington de Gonzalez et al. [21] showed that the RR of contralateral breast cancer in patients undergoing surgery and radiotherapy versus surgery alone was 1.09 (95 % CI 1.04–1.15). They demonstrated an increased risk at earlier age of exposure <40 years RR 1.30 (95 % CI 1.11–1.50), 40–49 years RR 1.08 (95 % CI 0.97–1.20), 50–59 years RR 0.98 (95 % CI 0.89–1.08) and >60 years RR 1.14 (95 % CI 1.04–1.26).

A review in 2004 of 64,782 women in the Thames Cancer Registry of which 33,763 received breast radiotherapy [32] showed that there was a significant increased risk of second breast, esophageal and lung cancers in breast cancer patients receiving radiotherapy. With regard to breast cancer there was an increased risk in both surgical and radiotherapy arms suggesting other underlying risk factors but there was an excess in the radiotherapy arm in the 5–10 years follow up group RR 1.34 (95 % CI 1.10–1.63) and the group followed for more than 15 years had a RR 1.26 (95 % CI 1.00–1.59).

Historically reduction of volume of tissue irradiated for Hodgkin lymphoma via involved field radiotherapy has been shown to reduce the dose to breast tissue [33]. This resulted in a 2–2.5 fold reduction in risk of radiation induced breast cancer [34, 35]. We can extrapolate that reduced volume of breast irradiated may reduce the dose to the contralateral breast and therefore the risk of breast cancer.

In high risk patients with node positive breast cancer, recent research has focused on the feasibility of regional nodal radiotherapy as an alternative to more extensive nodal surgery [36]. The resulting increased volume of tissue may increase risk of contralateral breast cancer or other cancers. This has not been shown in either of the two large recent randomized trials investigating regional nodal irradiation [37, 38], however longer follow up may be required.

## Lung Cancer

Darby et al. performed a prospective cohort analysis of 300,000 women with breast cancer of known laterality in SEER cancer registries between 1973 and 2001. They reviewed data for all-cause mortality focusing on cardiac mortality and lung cancer mortality [39]. In this study 37 % of women received breast radiotherapy. Among the un-irradiated cohort, lung cancer mortality ratio between ipsilateral versus contralateral lung cancer was 0.96 with no significant trend for increased incidence with time from diagnosis. However among women irradiated between 1973 and 1982 the lung cancer mortality ratio of ipsilateral versus contralateral lung cancer was 1.42. This mortality ratio increased with time since diagnosis. Those who had been diagnosed and irradiated 15 years or more prior to lung cancer diagnosis had a mortality ratio of ipsilateral versus contralateral lung cancer of 2.71 (57 vs 23 lung cancer deaths). In the study there was insufficient data on women irradiated after 1982 to review the ratio of lung cancer mortality as not enough time had elapsed [39].

In a single institution review in 2007 of 16,705 patients treated for EBC, 13,472 received radiotherapy. In total 709 s primary malignancies occurred. The incidence was 596 (4.4 %) in the radiotherapy group and 113 (3.5 %) in the non-radiotherapy group, with a significant increase in sarcoma and lung cancer [40].

When considering the risk of lung cancer one needs to consider the dose of radiotherapy received to the lung, the age of the patient at exposure and the volume irradiated. Grantzau et al. [41] conducted a study using the Danish Cancer Registry to identify 23,627 women who had received radiotherapy for breast cancer and identified those who developed second lung cancers. The 151 cases were matched to control patients who did not develop lung cancer. The mean dose of radiotherapy at the lung cancer site was 8.7 Gy (0.04–52.2 Gy) for the cases and 5.6 Gy (0.01–52.3 Gy) for the controls. Seventy percent of the lung cancers occurred after 5 years following treatment and 40 % at over 10 years, with significantly more smokers in the lung cancer group. When adjusted for this and adjuvant systemic therapy, the risk of lung cancer at 5 years was 3 fold for doses greater than 15 Gy and at ten years the risk was 6 fold for doses greater than 25 Gy OR 6.27 (95 % CI 1.1–34.8 $p<0.0001$). The excess RR per Gy at 5 years or more was 8.5 % (95 % CI 3.1–23.3 % $p<0.005$). Considering ever smokers alone the excess RR per Gy was 17.5 % (95 % CI 4.5–54 %). The excess risk in never smokers was difficult to calculate as numbers were so small but did not vary appreciably from baseline.

Roychouduri et al. in their 2004 [32] review of 64,000 women found an increased incidence of lung cancer in patients receiving radiotherapy to the breast. The risk was not elevated in the first 5 years after treatment but at 10–14 years the RR was 1.62 (95 % CI 1.05–2.54) and following 15 years the RR was 1.49 (95 % CI 1.05–2.14). They did not have data available on smoking status of patients in this study.

Kaufman et al. [42] also reviewed the risk of lung cancer after breast radiotherapy in a nested case control cohort. In their study 119 women with breast cancer and previous radiotherapy who developed lung cancer were matched to controls with no lung cancer. They found no increased risk in women who had never smoked for radiotherapy to the breast in general, but there was an increased risk of ipsilateral lung cancer OR 1.9 (95 % CI 1.1–3.4) versus contralateral OR 0.6 (95 % CI 0.3–1.3). They found excess risks in unirradiated ever smokers who had not received radiation therapy with an increase OR ipsilateral lung cancer of 10.3 (95 % CI 2.9–36.4) and contralateral lung cancer of 4.9 (95 % CI 1.7–14.0). This was multiplied in ever smokers who had breast radiotherapy OR ipsilateral 37.6 (95 % CI 10.2–139.0) contralateral 10.5 (95 % CI 2.9–37.8).

When considering the volume of lung tissue irradiated several studies [19, 39, 41, 42] suggest that the increased incidence of lung cancer was greater in those patients who received radiotherapy in the era of the 1970–1980s. They comment that during this era CT planning was not routinely used and restrictions on maximal depth of lung in radiation field were less rigorous, moreover frequently nodal regions were irradiated routinely increasing total dose of lung irradiated. Rates of lung cancer from more modern techniques are not yet established [18]; however we must be mindful of the increased volumes now exposed to low doses of radiation with techniques such as IMRT, VMAT and tomotherapy [43].

## Thyroid Cancer

The thyroid gland is not usually irradiated in breast-only radiotherapy but in the modern era we are increasingly irradiating nodal regions as an alternative to surgery. The thyroid gland is one of the most radiation sensitive tissues in the body and Ron et al. [44] showed that doses as low as 100 mGy can cause excess risk.

There is a linear exponential relationship between radiation dose and thyroid cancer with the peak risk occurring between doses of 15–20 Gy and reduced risk in doses over 30 Gy [45]. This is likely due to cell killing at higher doses. The Thames cancer registry study [32] did not identify any excess of thyroid cancers in patients who were irradiated for EBC. This may be due to the dose used for nodal regional radiotherapy being in the order of 40–50 Gy.

## Esophageal Cancer

The EBCTCG review of 42,000 patients who had surgery versus surgery and radiotherapy for EBC found an increased risk of esophageal cancer (150 cases; rate ratio 2.06, $2p=0.05$) and esophageal cancer mortality (rate ratio 2.40, $2p=0.0004$) in the radiotherapy arm but further analysis of this was difficult due to small numbers [30]. The Thames Cancer Registry study [32] revealed an increased risk of esophageal cancer at 15 years following diagnosis in those receiving radiotherapy for breast cancer, RR 2.19 % (95 % CI 1.10–4.62). A study in 2012 [46] reviewed the risk of esophageal cancer in patients treated with breast radiotherapy using international cancer registries. This study calculated the radiation dose received to different levels of the esophagus using a variety of radiotherapy techniques. Increased doses of radiation to the esophagus were seen in those patients receiving supraclavicular fossa and internal mammary chain radiotherapy. They identified 167 cases and 285 matched controls. Esophageal cancer risk increased with increasing dose to the esophagus with little evidence of increased risk at doses below 20 Gy. They estimated that 30 % of second esophageal cancers in their study could be attributed to radiotherapy overall but in those women receiving over 20 Gy (71 cases) to the esophagus 72 % could be attributed. Subgroup analysis revealed no effect of age at breast cancer radiotherapy. The overall risk is low; among 1,000 women aged 60 at breast cancer diagnosis receiving an esophageal radiation dose of 30 Gy an excess of 5 esophageal cancers due to radiotherapy might be expected over a 25-year period [46].

### Skin Cancer

We could find no published data on the incidence of non-melanoma skin cancer following breast radiotherapy, and Roychoudhuri et al. found no significant increased risk of malignant melanoma after breast cancer radiotherapy [32].

### Hematological Malignancies

The risk of induction of hematological malignancies after low dose radiotherapy for benign conditions has been known for some time [47]. Adjuvant treatment with breast radiotherapy is known to increase the subsequent risk of myelodysplastic syndrome (MDS) and acute myeloid leukemia (AML), although the absolute numbers are small. It has been reported that patients treated with radiotherapy alone for ductal carcinoma in situ are at a slightly increased risk of subsequent AML [48]. The risk increases with increasing field size and increasing doses administered. For example, Le Deley showed in their study of 182 patients with subsequent AML following breast cancer treatment in a univariate analysis that patients who were treated with radiotherapy to the breast only had a 2.39 increased risk (95 % CI 0.84–6.77) whereas for patients who had had regional radiotherapy, the risk was multiplied by 5.17 (95 % CI 1.98–13.5) [49]. The same group also showed that an increase in 1 Gy was associated with an increased risk of 1.14 (95 % CI 1.04–1.25) for development of subsequent AML.

Kaplan et al. have published data from 5,790 patients treated for breast cancer and found that there was an increased risk in patients treated with radiation alone for breast cancer (RR 3.32 95 % CI 1.42–6.45), and that this risk was higher for patients treated with radiation and chemotherapy (6.32 95 % CI 3.03–11.45) [50]. Smith et al. showed in their review of six NSABP adjuvant breast cancer studies that the relative risk of developing MDS/AML with these chemotherapy agents when radiotherapy was also given was 2.38 (95 % CI 1.29–4.40; $p=0.006$) [51]. Using the SEER database, Calip et al. reported the HR for chemotherapy alone to be 1.38 (95 % CI 0.98–1.93) and chemotherapy and radiation to be 1.77 (95 % CI 1.25–2.51) [52]. Those who received radiotherapy and surgery alone had no increased risk of AML/MDS.

## *Systemic Therapy Induced Cancers*

Systemic therapy following a diagnosis of breast cancer may include chemotherapy, endocrine therapy and biological therapy. This section will focus on chemotherapy and endocrine therapy as data suggests these two modalities contribute the most to the development of second cancers.

## Chemotherapy

The decision as to whether to offer adjuvant (or neoadjuvant) cytotoxic chemotherapy to a woman with early breast cancer is determined by her individual risk of disease relapse and co-morbidity. Breast cancer mortality is significantly reduced at 10-years with the addition of anthracycline-containing chemotherapy with a RR of 0.79 (95 % CI 0.72–0.85) [53]. Several studies have shown that when compared to the general population, breast cancer survivors who have been treated with chemotherapy do not have subsequent increased frequency of second malignancies [54–59]. For example, a review of 797 patients treated at MD Anderson Hospital between 1974 and 1982 in clinical trials where adjuvant chemotherapy had been administered, were compared to 186 controls who had not received chemotherapy, and didn't show any increased incidence of second cancers [57]. Reasons for a possible reduced risk of subsequent second cancers following chemotherapy are likely multifactorial; for example in a pre-menopausal patient the resulting ovarian function disruption may have a beneficial effect in reducing future incidence of certain cancers.

The second primary malignancy with the strongest evidence of being related to previous chemotherapy in the setting of EBC is leukemia. Between 10 and 30 % of all cases of AML are secondary to therapy, and in the GIMEMA archive of 2,964 patients more than half of the cases were following a diagnosis of breast cancer or lymphoma [60]. Large groups of patients previously treated with systemic chemotherapy have been studied from groups including the NSABP, Eastern Co-operative Oncology Group, University of Texas, MD Anderson Cancer Center, International Collaborative Cancer Group, CALGB, French Adjuvant Study Group, and data published on more modern chemotherapy regimens and their association with hematological malignancies [51, 61–67]. The cumulative incidence of AML following breast cancer chemotherapy is less than 1 % in most studies of modern therapy. The MD Anderson Cancer Center experience also showed an increased risk of AML when the FAC (fluorouracil, doxorubicin and cyclophosphamide) regime was used with a 10 year estimated leukemia rate of 1.5 % (95 % CI 0.7–2.9 %) [62]. The majority of patients in this study had also received radiotherapy. More recently, in the 2012 EBCTCG review of 14,250 women given poly-chemotherapy in the context of randomized trials there was a non-significant excess mortality of 0.2 % from leukemias, lymphomas and cardiovascular disease reported with an average of 6 years follow up [53].

Treatment related factors influencing subsequent leukemia risk include drug regimen, drug dose and dose intensity. Alkylating agents such as cyclophosphamide, and topoisomerase II inhibitors such as anthracyclines, are classes of drug most strongly associated with the subsequent development of MDS and AML [68]. Curtis et al. reported a doubling of risk of AML in a case control study of women treated with 6 months of cyclophosphamide, methotrexate and 5-fluourouracil (CMF) [69]. Similarly Haas et al. reported a statistically significant RR of 2.7 (95 % CI 1.2–6.3) in a historic study of 93 women who developed leukemia matched to 185 controls [70]. However, other studies have not shown such associations with cyclophosphamide [56, 61].

The evidence for second malignancy with anthracyclines/anthracycline combinations is more compelling. Crump et al. reported a retrospective study of 1,545 women treated in National Canadian breast cancer trials where they compared the risk of developing MDS/AML following adjuvant CMF or anthracycline containing regimens. They found a slightly increased risk of MDS/AML in patients who had received regimens containing anthracyclines [71]. When compared at a median follow up of 8 years, the conditional probability of developing AML following anthracycline-based chemotherapy was 1.3–1.7 % (95 % CI 0.5–3.6 % for CEF and 0–4.7 % for AC) and 0.4 % (95 % CI 0–1.3 %) for CMF chemotherapy. A French case–control study [49] compared 182 patients who developed AML after breast cancer treatment between 1985 and 2001 alongside 534 matched controls. The risk of leukemia was markedly increased after chemotherapy that included a topoisomerase-II inhibitor ($P < .0001$), and was higher after mitoxantrone than after anthracyclines (RR 15.6, 95 % CI 7.1–34.2; RR 2.7, 95 % CI 1.7–4.5 respectively) [49]. The NSABP published their outcome data with respects to MDS and leukemia following 4 cycles of anthracycline based chemotherapy (doxorubicin 60 $mg/m^2$, cyclophosphamide 600 $mg/m^2$) and reported that at 8 years follow-up the risk was 0.3 % [51, 72].

Increasing chemotherapy dose has also been shown to increase the risk of hematological malignancy. In a Curtis et al. case control study, a median dose of 7,350 mg of cyclophosphamide led to a RR of 1.5 (95 % CI 0.3–8.9); when this rose to over 30,000 mg the RR of AML/MDS increased to 9.4 (95 % CI 0.9–103) [69]. Patients given standard doses of epirubicin ($\leq$720 $mg/m^2$) or cyclophosphamide ($\leq$6,300 $mg/m^2$) had an 8-year cumulative probability of developing AML/MDS of 0.37 % (95 % CI, 0.13–0.61 %) compared with 4.97 % (95 % CI 2.06–7.87 %) for patients given higher doses. The NSABP study found no increased risk with increasing doses of doxorubicin (60, 75, 90 $mg/m^2$) [66]. The risk of subsequent AML was the same when the anthracyclines doxorubicin and epirubicin were considered separately.

A review of 19 randomized studies involving 9,796 women by Praga et al. showed that subsequent risk of MDS/AML developing after anthracycline based chemotherapy increases with increasing cumulative dose of anthracycline given [72]. Chemotherapy dose intensity has also been shown to impact on future leukemia risk. Smith et al. assessed regimens containing doxorubicin and cyclophosphamide in six adjuvant studies run by the NSABP (B-15, B-16, B-18, B-22, B-23 and B-25) involving 8,563 women [51]. They found that 43 patients treated in these studies subsequently developed MDS or AML. The study found that at standard doses of doxorubicin-cyclophosphamide the incidence of AML/MDS was 0.32 cases per 1,000 years (95 % CI 0.16–0.57 %), but in those patients treated with intense cyclophosphamide (2 or 4 cycles of cyclophosphamide at 2,300 $mg/m^2$ requiring G-CSF support), the risk of hematological malignancy was substantially increased, to a relative risk of 6.16 ($p < 0.0001$) and an incidence rate of 1.75 cases per 1,000 patients years (95 % CI 1.04–2.77). Interestingly, even when the data was censored at the time of relapse or development of another second primary cancer (for which more treatment might have been given) the increased risk in MDS or AML remained similar.

Following breast cancer chemotherapy at least four other risk factors have been reported to affect risk of MDS/AML development: patient age at diagnosis, delivery of adjuvant radiotherapy, inherited predisposition and concomitant use of G-CSF.

The MDS/AML incidence rate is known to rise with age in a population. In Kaplan's study of 306,691 women treated for breast cancer from 18 SEER registries, survivors aged between 20 and 49 had the highest relative risk of subsequent MDS/AML [48]. When patients aged 20–49 were compared to those aged 65–74, RRs were 10.6 (95 % CI 8.57–12.93) and 2.94 (95 % CI 2.45–3.50) respectively. However, it is likely that older patients may not have received any chemotherapy, as the SEER database does not collect this information. In this study a higher risk of MDS compared to AML was seen across all age groups with a rate ratio of 2.75 (95 % CI 2.51–3.00). Conversely, Smith et al. found that there was a greater incidence of MDS/AML in women over 50 years old treated in the NSABP studies, with a RR of 2.37 (95 % CI 1.26–4.44; $p=0.08$) when compared to younger women [51]. Similarly the Dutch study of breast cancer survivors found that chemotherapy was associated with increased risk of AML in patients over 50 years old at a median follow up of 10 years with a HR of 3.18 (95 % CI 1.39–7.28), compared to patients under 50 years old who had a HR of 1.78 (95 % CI 0.55–5.74) [8].

Several polymorphisms associated with genes that control the enzymes responsible for drug metabolism have been identified as increasing predisposition to the development of MDS/AML if exposed to a mutagen. Examples include the NQ01-187Ser single nucleotide polymorphism which has been shown by one group to lead to a 2.09 (95 % CI 1.08–4.03) fold increased risk [73]. Therapy-related AML is generally associated with adverse cytogenetics and has a poorer outcome [68, 74]. Leukemias related to topoisomerase inhibitors tend to have translocations involving chromosome 11q23 or 9, 19 or 4 whereas those associated with alkylating agents typically have deletions of chromosome 13 or a complete or partial loss of chromosome 5 or 7 [60][75]. In addition, leukemias following alkylating agents usually occur after around 5–7 years and are preceded by MDS, as opposed to a shorter latency following topoisomerase II inhibitors [60]. Data suggests that the majority of cases of MDS/AML occur in the first 2 years following treatment and that 84 % of cases are diagnosed by 5 years [48].

## Endocrine Therapy

The majority of breast cancers are hormone receptor positive and adjuvant endocrine therapy is offered as a risk reduction strategy towards the development of recurrent breast cancer, a new breast cancer and metastatic disease [76]. Breast cancer mortality is significantly reduced by about 40 % with the addition of endocrine therapy in this setting, with aromatase inhibitors leading to the greatest proportional reductions [76]. Tamoxifen increases the risk of developing endometrial hyperplasia, polyps, carcinomas and sarcoma [76–79]. Aromatase inhibitors, by contrast, confer no increased risk of subsequent gynecological malignancies and may reverse tamoxifen associated gynecological abnormalities [80, 81]. When compared to women who have received no endocrine therapy, women on aromatase inhibitors have been shown to have a non-statistically significant reduced incidence of endometrial cancer [82].

A retrospective review of 45,575 survivors of breast cancer in the Osaka Cancer Registry in Japan showed that when endocrine therapy was considered, the only cancer that patients were subsequently at increased risk of was uterine cancer [83]. Other retrospective studies showed that the risk of endometrial and cervical cancer was associated with endocrine therapy in breast cancer patients and that the SIR was 1.6 (95 % CI 1.34–1.89) [19]. In 2015 the EBCTCG [84] reviewed 31,920 women from studies and assessed the RR of subsequent endometrial cancer following adjuvant aromatase inhibitor or tamoxifen and found the 10 year incidence to be 0.4 % versus 1.2 % respectively (absolute different 0.8 %, 95 % CI 0.6–1.0; $p<0.0001$) including 5 versus 9 deaths from endometrial cancer [76]. They found a proportional decrease in endometrial cancer incidence with a RR of 0.33 (95 % CI 0.21–0.51) with aromatase inhibitors and that this was independent of age and persisted for years after treatment finished.

There are factors that affect the subsequent likelihood of developing endometrial cancer following Tamoxifen use. The first of these relates to duration of use. Sequencing studies investigating 2–3 years of Tamoxifen followed/preceded by 2–3 years of an aromatase inhibitor showed a non-significant increase incidence of endometrial cancer although they did show increased numbers of patients with endometrial abnormalities in patients on Tamoxifen [85, 86]. Recently published studies have demonstrated improvements with respects to breast cancer outcome with extended adjuvant Tamoxifen for 10 years. The ATLAS trial showed that the risk of developing endometrial cancer was increased following adjuvant Tamoxifen use for 10 years compared to 5 years with incidence of 3.1 % versus 1.6 % respectively [87]. Similarly, the aTTOM study also showed an increased cumulative incidence of endometrial cancer with an increased risk of endometrial cancer (rate ratio 2.20, 95 % CI 1.31–2.34) and deaths from endometrial cancer (rate ratio 1.83, 95 % CI 1.09–3.09) [88].

Another factor is age, with post-menopausal patients being at the highest risk of second cancers overall. Gray et al. in the aTTom trial showed that there was no significant increased risk of endometrial cancer in pre-menopausal women following 10 years of Tamoxifen treatment [88]. In the 2015 EBCTCG study the absolute excess endometrial cancer seen with 5 years of Tamoxifen was 0.7 % (95 % CI 0.5–0.9) at ages 55–69 and 1.4 % (95 % CI 0.5–2.4) at older ages [76].

The molecular mechanisms of Tamoxifen induced endometrial cancer are complex, involving many pathways that have been described but are not fully understood [89]. Similar to treatment induced MDS/AML, data suggests that Tamoxifen induced endometrial adenocarcinoma has a worse outcome than de-novo endometrial adenocarcinoma [77, 87, 90]. However, most are low-grade tumors, which can be treated with surgery alone [91, 92]. A SEER analysis of 289,933 breast cancer survivors showed increased risk of endometrial cancer irrespective of ER/PR status, indicating that common etiological factors of both cancers may exist [93].

Whilst it is important that women diagnosed with breast cancer are informed of the slightly increased risk of endometrial cancer induced by adjuvant Tamoxifen for five or ten years, it must be highlighted that in all but very low risk women this risk is likely to be offset by the relative risk reduction in breast cancer recurrence by Tamoxifen. The greatest risk, albeit small, lies with postmenopausal women who are generally offered aromatase inhibitors.

## Targeted Therapies

There is no published data showing increased risk of second malignancies with targeted agents such as monoclonal antibodies or small molecules routinely used in the treatment of breast cancer but long-term data on these agents is not yet available.

## Granulocyte Colony Stimulating Factor (G-CSF)

G-CSF is used to stimulate the proliferation and differentiation of white blood cells following chemotherapy in order to maintain dose intensity and reduce risk of life threatening neutropenic sepsis. It has been postulated that co-administration of G-CSF during adjuvant chemotherapy could allow myeloid cells with abnormal chromosomes to survive and hence increase the subsequent risk of developing MDS/AML [94]. Historical studies have shown mixed results with respects to whether there is an increased risk or not, but a meta-analysis by Lyman in 2010 looking at G-CSF use in seven different tumor types (including breast cancer) showed there was an increased risk of MDS/AML with its use with a RR of 1.92 (95 % CI, 1.19–3.07; $p=0.007$) [95]. However, absolute increased cases of leukemia were small and it must be noted that all-cause mortality was lower with G-CSF use due to reduced deaths from neutropenic sepsis. More recently Calip et al. have shown that when adjusted for type of chemotherapy used there was a non-significant increased risk of AML in breast cancer patients treated with G-CSF in the adjuvant setting [52]. The risk was only observed with filgrastim use HR 1.47 (95 % CI 1.05–2.06). Pegfilgrastim was not associated with increased risk. The risk with filgrastim was only seen in anthracycline containing regimens with an increased risk with more than 6 doses of G-CSF leading to a HR of 2.70 (95 % CI 1.33–2.58). The NSABP group [51] also studied risk of MDS or AML in patients who had received more than 242 mcg/kg of GCSF. They found that when patients who had subsequently developed a relapse of their breast cancer, or developed a second cancer were excluded the increased risk of MDS/AML was not statistically significant [51].

In the future it is hoped that the use of prognostic and predictive tools of chemotherapy benefit, such as Oncotype Dx and IHC4, will personalize chemotherapy recommendations, so that only women most likely to significantly benefit from adjuvant chemotherapy are exposed to these risks of second malignancies.

## Host Related Factors

Factors contributing to an individual's risk of second primary neoplasms include host environment and genetic factors. The second cancer sites for which increased risks are observed following a diagnosis of a primary breast cancer often share common etiological factors involving either lifestyle factors (such as obesity and reproductive factors), or genetic susceptibility (such as BRCA 1 or 2 mutations) [96, 97].

### *Host Environment*

Lifestyle factors can significantly affect the chance of developing a second primary malignancy and will be discussed in Chapter x. Here we only consider three examples of the interaction of therapy and lifestyle factors [98].

Kaufman et al. 2008 reviewed the risk of breast radiotherapy induced lung cancer in smokers and non-smokers. They found irradiated never smokers had no significant increased risk of second lung cancer. Previous smokers and current smokers had increased risk further increased by having radiotherapy. For smokers not receiving radiotherapy the OR was 5.9 (95 % CI 2.7–12.8) versus the OR for irradiated smokers, which was 18.9 (95 % CI 7.9–45.4). This multiplicative risk has been replicated in subsequent research [41].

In a study by Morton et al. examining the risk of secondary esophageal cancer after breast radiotherapy the authors assessed whether alcohol and smoking status increased risk after breast radiotherapy as part of subgroup analysis. The risk of developing esophageal cancer was increased in patients who were heavy smokers OR 2.4 (95 % CI 1.1–5.7) and in moderate to heavy drinkers OR 6.9 (95 % CI 1.1–8.5). In patients irradiated with a dose to esophagus >20 Gy the ORs were 2.9 (95 % CI 1.4–6.4) for light smokers (<one pack per day) versus 16.3 (95 % CI 2.2–340) for heavy smokers; 2.7 (95 % CI 0.5–21) in light or non-drinkers versus 4.2 (95 % CI 1.4–13) in moderate to heavy drinkers.

Swerdlow et al. investigated the features that differed between 813 patients who developed endometrial cancer following Tamoxifen use and compared them to 1,067 controls. One factor affecting the risk of endometrial cancer development following Tamoxifen was body weight, with higher body weight significantly increasing the risk in post-menopausal women [99]. The same study also showed an increased risk in those patients who had had pelvic radiotherapy 5 years earlier (OR 11.7, 95 % CI 1.5–548.2) [82].

### *Germline Mutations*

Mutations in the BRCA1 and 2 genes result in increased risk of breast cancer and ovarian cancer. Mutations in these genes account for 0.25 % of all cancers and 3 % of breast cancers [100]. Mutations in the BRCA gene result in reduced repair of

DNA damage; therefore theoretically radiation induced DNA damage may increase the risk of second malignancy in these patients. However, Bernstein et al. in their 2013 study found that while prior radiotherapy and BRCA mutation both resulted in increased risk of contralateral breast cancer there was no significant multiplicative risk [101]. This is reassuring but in view of the increased lifetime risk of breast cancer in BRCA carriers bilateral mastectomy and reconstruction are often discussed in an attempt to reduce their future cancer risk.

Li-Fraumeni syndrome is a rare autosomal dominant inherited disorder of germline mutations in the tumor suppressor gene p53. Mutations in this gene result in increased risk of early onset malignancies including sarcomas, premenopausal breast cancer, brain tumors, leukemias and other cancers [102]. One study of 200 patients with Li-Fraumeni family history found a cumulative probability of second cancer of 57 % at 30 years post primary malignancy [103]. The same researchers found that ionizing radiation played a role in sensitivity of patients in development of subsequent malignancies.

Lynch syndrome is an autosomal dominant collection of mutations in DNA mismatch repair including mutations in MLH1, MSH2, MSH6 and PMS1. This results in increased risk of colon cancers but also stomach, hepatobiliary, endometrial, breast, ovary and prostate cancers [104]. Morioka et al. [105] studied mice with mutations in MLH1 and exposed them to radiation and inflammatory colitis to see if this affected risk of developing colonic tumors. The results showed that the number of colonic tumors was increased if inflammation and radiation effects were present in the colon. This was not shown for breast cancer. More recently CHEK2*1100delC heterozygosity has been associated with increased risks of a second breast cancer in breast cancer survivors [106].

Identifying carriers of germline mutations via family history guides treatment decisions and future surveillance for patients and families. Further research into the effect of treatment such as radiotherapy on second malignancy risk is needed in these rare subgroups of patients.

## Screening and Predicting Risk of Second Primary Cancers

Prediction models are widely used in medicine to advise clinicians on merits of treatment and also to predict absolute risk of subsequent medical conditions. We should be able to develop prediction models to identify patients at particular risk of second primary neoplasms and suggest increased surveillance. However, very few of these models exist and virtually none have been externally validated [23]. Oeffinger and colleagues from the Childhood Cancer Survival Study (CCSS) group along with van Leeuwen and colleagues from the Dutch long-term effects (LATER) cohort are developing a web-based calculator to predict absolute risk of second primary breast cancer that integrates treatment related and traditional risk factors [23]. Donovan et al. used the BIER VII model to review the doses of radiotherapy received at distant organ sites using more complex modern radiotherapy techniques versus standard radiotherapy for breast cancer using phantom model. This showed no theoretical increased risk with standard radiotherapy planning constraints [107]. Further prediction models are needed and should facilitate decision making for medical professionals and patients. Current American Cancer Society/American Society of Clinical Oncology Breast Cancer Survivorship Care Guidelines advise that primary care physicians should screen for cancers as they would in patients in the general population and provide an annual gynecological assessment for post-menopausal women on selective estrogen receptor modulator therapy [108]. Most follow-up guidelines suggest annual mammography of residual breast tissue following a diagnosis of breast cancer and the consenting process and survivorship care plans should document risk of future cancers where appropriate. It is not currently clear if screening programs for treatment induced malignancies following breast cancer improve outcomes [109].

## Conclusion

Although the risk of a second malignancy following a diagnosis of breast cancer is important to consider, the absolute risk remains extremely low. It is likely that with improved treatment the risks may be lower than quoted in historical series. After a primary breast cancer, the risk of a second breast cancer unrelated to treatment is more likely than any treatment induced cancer. The benefit from appropriately selected and delivered treatment is likely to outweigh treatment-induced malignancy in the majority of patients. Of the treatment associated malignancies the most important to be aware of are MDS and leukemias following chemotherapy, uterine cancers following endocrine therapy with Tamoxifen and breast and lung cancers following radiotherapy. Follow up appointments must be used as an opportunity to encourage change to adverse lifestyle behaviors which can modify risk of treatment related and unrelated cancers. Hopefully future prediction models and improved understanding of factors associated with development of second cancers will allow us to predict those at increased risk and modify their treatment to provide individualized therapy.

## References

1. Howlader N, Noone AM, Krapcho M, Garshell J, Neyman N, Altekruse SF, Kosary CL, Yu M, Ruhl J, Tatalovich Z, Cho H, Mariotto A, Lewis DR, Chen HS, Feuer EJ, Cronin KA, editors. SEER cancer statistics review, 1975–2010. Bethesda: National Cancer Institute. http://seer.cancer.gov/csr/1975_2010/. Based on November 2012 SEER data submission, posted to the SEER web site; 2013.
2. Chen Y, et al. Epidemiology of contralateral breast cancer. Cancer Epidemiol Biomarkers Prev. 1999;8(10):855–61.
3. Heron DE, et al. Bilateral breast carcinoma: risk factors and outcomes for patients with synchronous and metachronous disease. Cancer. 2000;88(12):2739–50.

4. Hayat MJ, et al. Cancer statistics, trends, and multiple primary cancer analyses from the Surveillance, Epidemiology, and End Results (SEER) Program. Oncologist. 2007;12(1):20–37.
5. Hankey BF, et al. A retrospective cohort analysis of second breast cancer risk for primary breast cancer patients with an assessment of the effect of radiation therapy. J Natl Cancer Inst. 1983;70(5):797–804.
6. Nichols HB, et al. Declining incidence of contralateral breast cancer in the United States from 1975 to 2006. J Clin Oncol. 2011;29(12):1564–9.
7. Rasmussen CB, et al. Incidence of metachronous contralateral breast cancer in Denmark 1978–2009. Int J Epidemiol. 2014;43(6):1855–64.
8. Schaapveld M, et al. Risk of new primary nonbreast cancers after breast cancer treatment: a Dutch population-based study. J Clin Oncol. 2008;26(8):1239–46.
9. Shankar A, et al. Contralateral breast cancer: a clinico-pathological study of second primaries in opposite breasts after treatment of breast malignancy. Asian Pac J Cancer Prev. 2015;16(3):1207–11.
10. Molina-Montes E, et al. Risk of second cancers cancer after a first primary breast cancer: a systematic review and meta-analysis. Gynecol Oncol. 2015;136(1):158–71.
11. Ricceri F, et al. Risk of second primary malignancies in women with breast cancer: results from the European prospective investigation into cancer and nutrition (EPIC). Int J Cancer. 2015;137(4):940–8.
12. Early Breast Cancer Trialists' Collaborative Group, et al. Effect of radiotherapy after breast-conserving surgery on 10-year recurrence and 15-year breast cancer death: meta-analysis of individual patient data for 10,801 women in 17 randomised trials. Lancet. 2011;378(9804):1707–16.
13. Sadamori N, et al. Incidence of intracranial meningiomas in Nagasaki atomic-bomb survivors. Int J Cancer. 1996;67(3):318–22.
14. Braunstein S, Nakamura JL. Radiotherapy-induced malignancies: review of clinical features, pathobiology, and evolving approaches for mitigating risk. Front Oncol. 2013;3:73.
15. Ron E, Modan B, Boice Jr JD. Mortality after radiotherapy for ringworm of the scalp. Am J Epidemiol. 1988;127(4):713–25.
16. Ron E, et al. Tumors of the brain and nervous system after radiotherapy in childhood. N Engl J Med. 1988;319(16):1033–9.
17. Watt TC, et al. Radiation-related risk of basal cell carcinoma: a report from the Childhood Cancer Survivor Study. J Natl Cancer Inst. 2012;104(16):1240–50.
18. Hooning MJ, et al. Roles of radiotherapy and chemotherapy in the development of contralateral breast cancer. J Clin Oncol. 2008;26(34):5561–8.
19. Kirova YM, et al. Second malignancies after breast cancer: the impact of different treatment modalities. Br J Cancer. 2008;98(5):870–4.
20. Kleinerman RA. Radiation-sensitive genetically susceptible pediatric sub-populations. Pediatr Radiol. 2009;39 Suppl 1:S27–31.
21. Berrington de Gonzalez A, et al. Second solid cancers after radiotherapy for breast cancer in SEER cancer registries. Br J Cancer. 2010;102(1):220–6.
22. Tannock I. The basic science of oncology. 4th ed. New York: McGraw-Hill, Medical Pub. Division; 2005. Chapter 14.
23. Oeffinger KC, et al. Solid tumor second primary neoplasms: who is at risk, what can we do? Semin Oncol. 2013;40(6):676–89.
24. Best T, et al. Variants at 6q21 implicate PRDM1 in the etiology of therapy-induced second malignancies after Hodgkin's lymphoma. Nat Med. 2011;17(8):941–3.
25. Au WW, Salama SA, Sierra-Torres CH. Functional characterization of polymorphisms in DNA repair genes using cytogenetic challenge assays. Environ Health Perspect. 2003;111(15):1843–50.
26. Mertens AC, et al. XRCC1 and glutathione-S-transferase gene polymorphisms and susceptibility to radiotherapy-related malignancies in survivors of Hodgkin disease. Cancer. 2004;101(6):1463–72.

27. Broeks A, et al. Radiation-associated breast tumors display a distinct gene expression profile. Int J Radiat Oncol Biol Phys. 2010;76(2):540–7.
28. Henderson TO, et al. Systematic review: surveillance for breast cancer in women treated with chest radiation for childhood, adolescent, or young adult cancer. Ann Intern Med. 2010;152(7):444–55; W144–54.
29. Henderson TO, et al. Secondary sarcomas in childhood cancer survivors: a report from the Childhood Cancer Survivor Study. J Natl Cancer Inst. 2007;99(4):300–8.
30. Yap J, et al. Sarcoma as a second malignancy after treatment for breast cancer. Int J Radiat Oncol Biol Phys. 2002;52(5):1231–7.
31. Boice Jr JD, et al. Cancer in the contralateral breast after radiotherapy for breast cancer. N Engl J Med. 1992;326(12):781–5.
32. Roychoudhuri R, et al. Radiation-induced malignancies following radiotherapy for breast cancer. Br J Cancer. 2004;91(5):868–72.
33. Koh ES, et al. A comparison of mantle versus involved-field radiotherapy for Hodgkin's lymphoma: reduction in normal tissue dose and second cancer risk. Radiat Oncol. 2007;2:13.
34. De Bruin ML, et al. Breast cancer risk in female survivors of Hodgkin's lymphoma: lower risk after smaller radiation volumes. J Clin Oncol. 2009;27(26):4239–46.
35. Swerdlow AJ, et al. Breast cancer risk after supradiaphragmatic radiotherapy for Hodgkin's lymphoma in England and Wales: a National Cohort Study. J Clin Oncol. 2012;30(22):2745–52.
36. Donker M, et al. Radiotherapy or surgery of the axilla after a positive sentinel node in breast cancer (EORTC 10981–22023 AMAROS): a randomised, multicentre, open-label, phase 3 non-inferiority trial. Lancet Oncol. 2014;15(12):1303–10.
37. Poortmans PM, et al. Internal mammary and medial supraclavicular irradiation in breast cancer. N Engl J Med. 2015;373(4):317–27.
38. Whelan TJ, et al. Regional nodal irradiation in early-stage breast cancer. N Engl J Med. 2015;373(4):307–16.
39. Darby SC, et al. Long-term mortality from heart disease and lung cancer after radiotherapy for early breast cancer: prospective cohort study of about 300,000 women in US SEER cancer registries. Lancet Oncol. 2005;6(8):557–65.
40. Kirova YM, et al. Risk of second malignancies after adjuvant radiotherapy for breast cancer: a large-scale, single-institution review. Int J Radiat Oncol Biol Phys. 2007;68(2):359–63.
41. Grantzau T, et al. Risk of second primary lung cancer in women after radiotherapy for breast cancer. Radiother Oncol. 2014;111(3):366–73.
42. Kaufman EL, et al. Effect of breast cancer radiotherapy and cigarette smoking on risk of second primary lung cancer. J Clin Oncol. 2008;26(3):392–8.
43. Kim DW, et al. Risk of secondary cancers from scattered radiation during intensity-modulated radiotherapies for hepatocellular carcinoma. Radiat Oncol. 2014;9:109.
44. Ron E, et al. Thyroid cancer after exposure to external radiation: a pooled analysis of seven studies. Radiat Res. 1995;141(3):259–77.
45. Sigurdson AJ, et al. Primary thyroid cancer after a first tumour in childhood (the Childhood Cancer Survivor Study): a nested case–control study. Lancet. 2005;365(9476):2014–23.
46. Morton LM, et al. Risk of treatment-related esophageal cancer among breast cancer survivors. Ann Oncol. 2012;23(12):3081–91.
47. Michels SD, et al. Therapy-related acute myeloid leukemia and myelodysplastic syndrome: a clinical and morphologic study of 65 cases. Blood. 1985;65(6):1364–72.
48. Kaplan HG, et al. Age related risk of myelodysplastic syndrome and acute myeloid leukemia among breast cancer survivors. Breast Cancer Res Treat. 2013;142(3):629–36.
49. Le Deley MC, et al. Anthracyclines, mitoxantrone, radiotherapy, and granulocyte colony-stimulating factor: risk factors for leukemia and myelodysplastic syndrome after breast cancer. J Clin Oncol. 2007;25(3):292–300.
50. Kaplan HG, Malmgren JA, Atwood MK. Increased incidence of myelodysplastic syndrome and acute myeloid leukemia following breast cancer treatment with radiation alone or combined with chemotherapy: a registry cohort analysis 1990–2005. BMC Cancer. 2011;11:260.

51. Smith RE, et al. Acute myeloid leukemia and myelodysplastic syndrome after doxorubicin-cyclophosphamide adjuvant therapy for operable breast cancer: the National Surgical Adjuvant Breast and Bowel Project Experience. J Clin Oncol. 2003;21(7):1195–204.
52. Calip GS, et al. Myelodysplastic syndrome and acute myeloid leukemia following adjuvant chemotherapy with and without granulocyte colony-stimulating factors for breast cancer. Breast Cancer Res Treat. 2015;154(1):133–43.
53. Early Breast Cancer Trialists' Collaborative Group, et al. Comparisons between different polychemotherapy regimens for early breast cancer: meta-analyses of long-term outcome among 100,000 women in 123 randomised trials. Lancet. 2012;379(9814):432–44.
54. Holdener EE, et al. Second malignant neoplasms in operable carcinoma of the breast. Recent Results Cancer Res. 1984;96:188–96.
55. Arriagada R, Rutqvist LE. Adjuvant chemotherapy in early breast cancer and incidence of new primary malignancies. Lancet. 1991;338(8766):535–8.
56. Valagussa P, et al. Second malignancies following CMF-based adjuvant chemotherapy in resectable breast cancer. Ann Oncol. 1994;5(9):803–8.
57. Herring MK, et al. Second neoplasms after adjuvant chemotherapy for operable breast cancer. Am J Clin Oncol. 1986;9(3):269–75.
58. Rubagotti A, et al. Risk of new primaries after chemotherapy and/or tamoxifen treatment for early breast cancer. Ann Oncol. 1996;7(3):239–44.
59. Yi M, et al. Other primary malignancies in breast cancer patients treated with breast conserving surgery and radiation therapy. Ann Surg Oncol. 2013;20(5):1514–21.
60. Leone G, et al. The incidence of secondary leukemias. Haematologica. 1999;84(10):937–45.
61. Tallman MS, et al. Leukemogenic potential of adjuvant chemotherapy for early-stage breast cancer: the Eastern Cooperative Oncology Group experience. J Clin Oncol. 1995;13(7): 1557–63.
62. Diamandidou E, et al. Treatment-related leukemia in breast cancer patients treated with fluorouracil-doxorubicin-cyclophosphamide combination adjuvant chemotherapy: the University of Texas M.D. Anderson Cancer Center experience. J Clin Oncol. 1996;14(10):2722–30.
63. Wils JA, et al. Epirubicin plus tamoxifen versus tamoxifen alone in node-positive postmenopausal patients with breast cancer: a randomized trial of the International Collaborative Cancer Group. J Clin Oncol. 1999;17(7):1988–98.
64. Fumoleau P, et al. Randomized trial comparing six versus three cycles of epirubicin-based adjuvant chemotherapy in premenopausal, node-positive breast cancer patients: 10-year follow-up results of the French Adjuvant Study Group 01 trial. J Clin Oncol. 2003;21(2):298–305.
65. Levine MN, et al. Randomized trial of intensive cyclophosphamide, epirubicin, and fluorouracil chemotherapy compared with cyclophosphamide, methotrexate, and fluorouracil in premenopausal women with node-positive breast cancer. National Cancer Institute of Canada Clinical Trials Group. J Clin Oncol. 1998;16(8):2651–8.
66. Henderson IC, et al. Improved outcomes from adding sequential Paclitaxel but not from escalating Doxorubicin dose in an adjuvant chemotherapy regimen for patients with node-positive primary breast cancer. J Clin Oncol. 2003;21(6):976–83.
67. Citron ML, et al. Randomized trial of dose-dense versus conventionally scheduled and sequential versus concurrent combination chemotherapy as postoperative adjuvant treatment of node-positive primary breast cancer: first report of Intergroup Trial C9741/Cancer and Leukemia Group B Trial 9741. J Clin Oncol. 2003;21(8):1431–9.
68. Godley LA, Larson RA. Therapy-related myeloid leukemia. Semin Oncol. 2008;35(4):418–29.
69. Curtis RE, et al. Risk of leukemia after chemotherapy and radiation treatment for breast cancer. N Engl J Med. 1992;326(26):1745–51.
70. Haas JF, et al. Risk of leukaemia in ovarian tumour and breast cancer patients following treatment by cyclophosphamide. Br J Cancer. 1987;55(2):213–8.
71. Crump M, et al. Risk of acute leukemia following epirubicin-based adjuvant chemotherapy: a report from the National Cancer Institute of Canada Clinical Trials Group. J Clin Oncol. 2003;21(16):3066–71.

72. Praga C, et al. Risk of acute myeloid leukemia and myelodysplastic syndrome in trials of adjuvant epirubicin for early breast cancer: correlation with doses of epirubicin and cyclophosphamide. J Clin Oncol. 2005;23(18):4179–91.
73. Bolufer P, et al. Profile of polymorphisms of drug-metabolising enzymes and the risk of therapy-related leukaemia. Br J Haematol. 2007;136(4):590–6.
74. Larson RA. Etiology and management of therapy-related myeloid leukemia. Hematology Am Soc Hematol Educ Program. 2007:453–9.
75. Ahuja HG, Felix CA, Aplan PD. Potential role for DNA topoisomerase II poisons in the generation of t(11;20)(p15;q11) translocations. Genes Chromosomes Cancer. 2000;29(2):96–105.
76. Early Breast Cancer Trialists' Collaborative Group, et al. Aromatase inhibitors versus tamoxifen in early breast cancer: patient-level meta-analysis of the randomised trials. Lancet. 2015;386(10001):1341–52.
77. Jones ME, et al. Endometrial cancer survival after breast cancer in relation to tamoxifen treatment: pooled results from three countries. Breast Cancer Res. 2012;14(3):R91.
78. van Leeuwen FE, et al. Risk of endometrial cancer after tamoxifen treatment of breast cancer. Lancet. 1994;343(8895):448–52.
79. Bernstein L, et al. Tamoxifen therapy for breast cancer and endometrial cancer risk. J Natl Cancer Inst. 1999;91(19):1654–62.
80. Morales L, et al. Endometrial safety of third generation aromatase inhibitors versus tamoxifen in breast cancer patients. Int J Gynecol Cancer. 2006;16 Suppl 2:515–7.
81. Morales L, et al. Third generation aromatase inhibitors may prevent endometrial growth and reverse tamoxifen-induced uterine changes in postmenopausal breast cancer patients. Ann Oncol. 2005;16(1):70–4.
82. Chlebowski RT, et al. Aromatase inhibitors, tamoxifen, and endometrial cancer in breast cancer survivors. Cancer. 2015;121(13):2147–55.
83. Kamigaki Y, Kawakami K. Risk of second cancer after initial treatment of breast cancer: an Osaka Cancer Registry Database study. Oncol Lett. 2011;2(5):963–73.
84. Early Breast Cancer Trialists' Collaborative Group, et al. Relevance of breast cancer hormone receptors and other factors to the efficacy of adjuvant tamoxifen: patient-level meta-analysis of randomised trials. Lancet. 2011;378(9793):771–84.
85. Bertelli G, et al. Long-term endometrial effects in postmenopausal women with early breast cancer participating in the Intergroup Exemestane Study (IES) – a randomised controlled trial of exemestane versus continued tamoxifen after 2–3 years tamoxifen. Ann Oncol. 2010;21(3):498–505.
86. Kieback DG, et al. Endometrial effects of exemestane compared to tamoxifen within the Tamoxifen Exemestane Adjuvant Multicenter (TEAM) trial: results of a prospective gynecological ultrasound substudy. Gynecol Oncol. 2010;119(3):500–5.
87. Davies C, et al. Long-term effects of continuing adjuvant tamoxifen to 10 years versus stopping at 5 years after diagnosis of oestrogen receptor-positive breast cancer: ATLAS, a randomised trial. Lancet. 2013;381(9869):805–16.
88. Gray RG, et al. aTTom: Long-term effects of continuing adjuvant tamoxifen to 10 years versus stopping at 5 years in 6,953 women with early breast cancer. J Clin Oncol. 2013;31(suppl):abstr 5.
89. Hu R, Hilakivi-Clarke L, Clarke R. Molecular mechanisms of tamoxifen-associated endometrial cancer (Review). Oncol Lett. 2015;9(4):1495–501.
90. Wilder JL, et al. Tamoxifen-associated malignant endometrial tumors: pathologic features and expression of hormone receptors estrogen-alpha, estrogen-beta and progesterone; a case controlled study. Gynecol Oncol. 2004;92(2):553–8.
91. Bergman L, et al. Risk and prognosis of endometrial cancer after tamoxifen for breast cancer. Comprehensive Cancer Centres' ALERT Group. Assessment of Liver and Endometrial cancer Risk following Tamoxifen. Lancet. 2000;356(9233):881–7.
92. Fisher B, et al. Endometrial cancer in tamoxifen-treated breast cancer patients: findings from the National Surgical Adjuvant Breast and Bowel Project (NSABP) B-14. J Natl Cancer Inst. 1994;86(7):527–37.

93. Liu J, et al. Elevated risks of subsequent endometrial cancer development among breast cancer survivors with different hormone receptor status: a SEER analysis. Breast Cancer Res Treat. 2015;150(2):439–45.
94. Kaushansky K. Lineage-specific hematopoietic growth factors. N Engl J Med. 2006;354(19): 2034–45.
95. Lyman GH, et al. Acute myeloid leukemia or myelodysplastic syndrome in randomized controlled clinical trials of cancer chemotherapy with granulocyte colony-stimulating factor: a systematic review. J Clin Oncol. 2010;28(17):2914–24.
96. Wang J, et al. Associations of body mass index with cancer incidence among populations, genders, and menopausal status: a systematic review and meta-analysis. Cancer Epidemiol. 2016;42:1–8.
97. Couch FJ, Nathanson KL, Offit K. Two decades after BRCA: setting paradigms in personalized cancer care and prevention. Science. 2014;343(6178):1466–70.
98. Jegu J, et al. The effect of patient characteristics on second primary cancer risk in France. BMC Cancer. 2014;14:94.
99. Swerdlow AJ, Jones ME; G. British Tamoxifen Second Cancer Study, Tamoxifen treatment for breast cancer and risk of endometrial cancer: a case-control study. J Natl Cancer Inst. 2005;97(5):375–84.
100. Petrucelli N, Daly MB, Feldman GL. Hereditary breast and ovarian cancer due to mutations in BRCA1 and BRCA2. Genet Med. 2010;12(5):245–59.
101. Bernstein JL, et al. Contralateral breast cancer after radiotherapy among BRCA1 and BRCA2 mutation carriers: a WECARE study report. Eur J Cancer. 2013;49(14):2979–85.
102. Li FP, et al. A cancer family syndrome in twenty-four kindreds. Cancer Res. 1988;48(18):5358–62.
103. Hisada M, et al. Multiple primary cancers in families with Li-Fraumeni syndrome. J Natl Cancer Inst. 1998;90(8):606–11.
104. Win AK, et al. Risks of primary extracolonic cancers following colorectal cancer in lynch syndrome. J Natl Cancer Inst. 2012;104(18):1363–72.
105. Morioka T, et al. Ionizing radiation, inflammation, and their interactions in colon carcinogenesis in Mlh1-deficient mice. Cancer Sci. 2015;106(3):217–26.
106. Weischer M, et al. CHEK2*1100delC heterozygosity in women with breast cancer associated with early death, breast cancer-specific death, and increased risk of a second breast cancer. J Clin Oncol. 2012;30(35):4308–16.
107. Donovan EM, et al. Second cancer incidence risk estimates using BEIR VII models for standard and complex external beam radiotherapy for early breast cancer. Med Phys. 2012;39(10):5814–24.
108. Runowicz CD, et al. American Cancer Society/American Society of Clinical Oncology Breast Cancer Survivorship Care Guideline. CA Cancer J Clin. 2016;66(1):43–73.
109. Corkum M, et al. Screening for new primary cancers in cancer survivors compared to non-cancer controls: a systematic review and meta-analysis. J Cancer Surviv. 2013;7(3):455–63.

# Chapter 18
# The Effects of Breast Cancer Treatments on Cognition

**Helena Harder and Valerie Jenkins**

**Abstract** There is growing concern among patients with early-stage breast cancer about self-perceived or objective cognitive changes following their diagnosis and treatment. Symptoms include difficulties with multi-tasking, short-term memory, attention and concentration and word-finding, which may have a detrimental effect on quality of life. The severity of symptoms varies widely, when assessed objectively, the problems are generally subtle. Early clinical observational studies accumulated evidence that suggested cognitive problems could be attributed to the direct neurotoxic effects of chemotherapy. However, observations of cognitive deficits before the start of any treatment question the singular role of chemotherapy. Additionally, results from studies examining the effect of endocrine therapies on cognitive function are mixed.

Recent neuroimaging techniques have reported structural and functional neural changes associated with breast cancer treatments. Also, translational research has accumulated evidence for the role of immune dysregulation and neurotoxicity from (pro-) inflammatory cytokines. It is clear that cognitive changes associated with breast cancer and its treatment are still far from being fully understood. Other contributing factors such as surgery, radiotherapy, the psychological burden of having cancer treatment, and treatment-related side effects, in particular fatigue may all play a role. Research into pharmacological and non-pharmacological interventions for cognitive impairment is in preliminary stages. Cognitive impairment following breast cancer diagnosis and treatment remains an important priority in breast cancer survivorship. Further investigations are needed to better understand symptoms and processes involved to enable the development of appropriate support for patients and survivors.

**Keywords** Breast cancer • Cognition • Memory • Chemotherapy • Endocrine therapy • Neuroimaging • Cytokines • Neurocognitive interventions

---

H. Harder, PhD, MSc, BSc (✉) • V. Jenkins, DPhil, BSc
Sussex Health Outcomes Research & Education in Cancer (SHORE-C), Brighton & Sussex Medical School, University of Sussex, Brighton, East Sussex, UK
e-mail: h.harder@sussex.ac.uk; val@sussex.ac.uk


A. Ring, M. Parton (eds.), *Breast Cancer Survivorship*,
DOI 10.1007/978-3-319-41858-2_18

## Introduction

Women receiving chemotherapy and endocrine therapy for early-stage breast cancer may experience problems with their memory and attention, which can be distressing and interfere with quality of life. Changes primarily include difficulties with concentration/focus, word finding, planning/multi-tasking, and forgetfulness or difficulty with recall of names or numbers. These problems are reported after diagnosis, during treatment or sometimes years later. While most breast cancer patients experience minor difficulties that tend to resolve over time, a subgroup report more severe and longer lasting impairments. This can be of great concern and may have a negative impact for some individuals on their day-to-day activities and quality of life, such as social functioning, family-life, professional reintegration and leisure activities.

Cognitive changes following cancer treatments often are referred to as 'chemobrain' or 'chemofog', although most breast cancer patients receive multi-modality treatment, and evidence for a direct link between the neurotoxic effects of chemotherapy and the symptoms is debatable. A better descriptor of the problem is the term 'cancer-related cognitive impairment' (CRCI) [1]. Whatever the underpinning causal factors, the phenomenon continues to cause problems for patients and impact negatively on their quality of life. In this chapter, we summarize the evidence for CRCI in breast cancer patients including its nature, incidence, risk factors and possible underlying mechanisms, focusing on the contributions of chemotherapy and endocrine therapy.

## Chemotherapy and Cognition

### *Evidence from Cross-Sectional Studies*

Observations of cognitive changes in cancer patients were first reported more than three decades ago [2]. Initial research with breast cancer patients incorporated cross-sectional designs with relatively small sample sizes. These studies provided only a 'snap shot' of potential cognitive impairment found post-chemotherapy without evidence for changes in relation to pre-treatment cognitive status. Data showed that during formal neuropsychological evaluation, breast cancer patients treated with chemotherapy performed significantly worse than those not receiving chemotherapy or healthy controls or when compared to normative test data [3–5]. Changes were observed in the following cognitive domains: attention, processing speed, executive function, working memory, short-term memory, and motor function. Greater cognitive impairment was usually reported in studies comparing chemotherapy groups with healthy control groups or normative data. Incidence rates of impairment varied widely from 16 to 75 % in patients with breast cancer undergoing chemotherapy compared with 4–11 % in healthy controls [6, 7].

Several meta-analyses have examined the nature and severity of cognitive impairment in women with breast cancer [8–10]. A recent meta-analysis by Ono et al. [11] found evidence for subtle cognitive decline following treatment. They reported a small significant grand mean effect size (−0.12) for cross-sectional studies with a comparison group that consisted of healthy individuals or breast cancer patients not receiving chemotherapy (e.g. local therapy only). However, the level of impairment in those treated with chemotherapy was not significantly different to chemotherapy naïve patients. In addition, level of education (but not time since treatment or age) was found to significantly moderate the magnitude of cognitive impairment. The authors concluded that subtle cognitive changes were common among breast cancer patients regardless of a history of chemotherapy or different treatment regimens.

## *Evidence from Prospective Longitudinal Studies*

Over the past decade, prospective longitudinal research studies have been conducted to examine cognitive changes developing pre- and post-chemotherapy, and throughout the treatment pathway. Some prospective neuropsychological studies have found evidence for an association between chemotherapy exposure and cognitive function by demonstrating a significant progressive decline over time (i.e. over the course of chemotherapy treatment) relative to a matched healthy control group or published normative data [12, 13]. Incidence rates of cognitive decline after chemotherapy generally varied widely between 20 and 60 % [8]. Other factors such as fatigue, depression, anxiety or stress may also influence cognitive outcomes and perhaps contribute to CRCI [14, 15]. However these are not consistent findings and several prospective studies have not found evidence for cognitive changes associated with chemotherapy at different time points following treatment; at 4–6 weeks [16], 6 months [17], and 18 months after completion of chemotherapy [18].

Inclusion of pre-treatment assessments in prospective research has also revealed an unanticipated result; it has been found that 20–30 % of breast cancer patients had lower than expected cognitive performance prior to receiving chemotherapy in comparison to reference data of healthy controls [19]. Until now, no clear explanation has been found for decreased function prior to chemotherapy. Surgery (e.g. a general anesthetic), comorbidities [20], stress-related factors or fatigue may play a role [21, 22]. However, the effect of surgery may be minimal as poor performances have been recorded in patients prior to receiving neoadjuvant chemotherapy. Hermelink et al. [23] assessed cognitive performance in 101 patients before and towards completion of neoadjuvant chemotherapy (epirubicin, cyclophosphamide and paclitaxel). Cognitive deficits, in particular on tests measuring divided attention, concentration and executive function were observed in 31 % before the start of treatment compared to normative data.

These observations emphasize the importance of taking into account baseline assessments before an assumption of causality can be made between chemotherapy exposure and cognitive decline.

## *Research into Late Cognitive Effects*

If cognitive effects are detected in women who are receiving chemotherapy, a key question is whether these changes persist over time. Most prospective studies have followed patients for 1 or 2 years post-chemotherapy and it appears that the natural course is for cognitive changes to improve in many patients. Zheng and colleagues [24] investigated cognitive function from 18 to 36 months after diagnosis in 1059 breast cancer patients. They reported that short term memory, attention, executive function and delayed memory significantly improved over time. A recent meta-analysis provides further evidence that cognitive performance in breast cancer patients treated with chemotherapy improves marginally over time [11].

Few studies have investigated the long-term and late effects of chemotherapy. One, in older breast cancer patients (>65 years; n=30) who remained disease-free for more than a decade, reported that long-term cancer survivors scored significantly lower compared to matched healthy controls in executive functioning, working memory, and divided attention [25]. A larger case-cohort study (n=196) confirmed potential late effects when comparing cognitive functioning in breast cancer patients who were treated with CMF chemotherapy (cyclophosphamide, methotrexate, 5-fluorouracil) on average 20 years previously with that of a population-based sample of women never diagnosed with cancer (n=1509). The breast cancer patients were more likely to have lower performance on memory, information processing speed and psychomotor speed compared healthy controls [26].

In contrast, a recent large nationwide cohort of recurrence-free breast cancer patients (n=1889) 7–9 years after primary treatment revealed no differences in long-term cognitive function between women who had or who had not received systemic therapies [27]. Cognition was assessed using a self-report measure, the Cognitive Failures Questionnaire [28] and not by objective neuropsychological testing, which may explain the different outcome. In addition, results showed that the observed proportion of patients with significant subjective cognitive complaints was comparable to healthy controls.

It remains uncertain whether or not there is a link between the discrepancies found in objective cognitive testing and subjective/perceived cognitive impairment, which is measured with self-report questionnaires and/or interviews. A review showed that most studies fail to find an association between objective and subjective cognitive function [29]. However, qualitative studies with in-depth face-to-face interviews frequently report a detrimental effect of cognitive changes on personal and professional life [30–32]. Boykoff et al. [30] interviewed 74 breast cancer survivors. The majority (70 %) considered cognitive impairment to be the most problematic side-effect of treatment. Several indicated that the cognitive changes had reduced their independence (e.g. they needed help with finances) or affected them professionally (e.g. they were unable to complete education or keep a job). Von Ah et al. [31] interviewed 22 breast cancer survivors who were at least 1 year post-treatment. They primarily expressed concerns in short and long-term memory, processing speed, concentration, language and executive functioning. All found these impairments frustrating, and some reported a negative impact on self-confidence and social relationships. Those who were employed reported working harder to perform tasks and used compensatory strategies to complete work tasks. Player et al. [32] conducted a qualitative study with 9 women who were at different stages of their breast cancer treatment. A key concern was the impact the cognitive changes had on their employment or work-related abilities. Some had to rely on family and friends to complete routine daily tasks. Others were unable to drive or complete domestic tasks or were no longer able to coordinate running their household and experienced a loss of independence. These qualitative studies show that perceived cognitive changes may have broad implications for the well-being of patients, however experiences are highly variable and individual.

## *Neuroimaging and Translational Research*

Ongoing developments in research techniques, in particular neuroimaging and translational research have led to greater insight into the association between chemotherapy and cognition and a better understanding of the underlying processes [33–36].

Neuroimaging techniques, including (functional) magnetic resonance imaging (MRI, fMRI) and positron emission tomography (PET) have been applied to investigate the neural substrate of potential cognitive changes. These methods are capable of detecting alterations in gray matter (GM) and white matter (WM) tissue in the brain or differences in brain functioning (fMRI, PET). Results have shown that chemotherapy is associated with structural changes (decrease in GM volume) and functional changes (in patterns of activation and resting state metabolism), particularly in the frontal regions that are involved in executive function and memory [37, 38]. Abnormal microstructural properties in WM regions involved in cognition have also been demonstrated [39]. In some studies, changes were associated with cognitive dysfunction or self-reported cognitive complaints [40–42]. Additionally, there is evidence that structural changes can be detected long after completion of chemotherapy. Long-term effects of chemotherapy in brain function were examined in 184 chemotherapy-exposed breast cancer patients more than 20 years after systemic chemotherapy [38]. Smaller total brain and global GM volumes were found compared to healthy controls.

Recent research that combined structural and functional MRI, neuropsychological assessment, and patient-reported outcomes reported lower cognitive performance, prefrontal hyperactivation and lower WM integrity in breast cancer patients prior to the start of adjuvant treatment compared to healthy controls [43]. The results suggested that fatigue might be an important contributing factor in cognitive changes because symptoms of fatigue were associated with observed abnormalities.

Growing evidence from translational research suggests that cytokines may also be involved in CRCI [36, 44]. Multiple clinical studies have demonstrated that administration of chemotherapy causes increases in cytokine levels, such as interleukin (IL)-1ß, IL-6, IL-8, IL-10, monocyte chemoattractant protein-1 (MCP-1), vascular endothelial growth factor (VEGF) and tumor necrosis factor (TNF)-$\alpha$ [41, 45]. These changes were more prominent in patients who experienced cognitive dysfunctions [41, 44, 46, 47]. However, there is still limited evidence for an association between the severity of the impairment and dysregulation in cytokines. In addition, the influence of certain disease characteristics such as estrogen receptor (ER) status and tumor size remains unclear [48]. Ongoing research in this area may facilitate identification of those at risk of cognitive impairment and the planning of interventions.

## Endocrine Therapy and Cognition

### *Estrogen and Cognitive Function*

The suggestion that endocrine therapy may affect cognition stems from the observation that estrogen receptors, ERα and ERß, are found in the prefrontal cortex, hippocampus and related cortical areas and the amygdala [49]. These are areas in the brain involved in cognitive performance, although the exact role of estrogen within the memory system is more complex [50].

Evidence that endocrine therapy may interfere with cognition is difficult to assess in women treated for breast cancer due to other influencing factors such as the effects of surgery, chemotherapy and radiotherapy regimens. Also, there are different types of endocrine treatments and the degree to which they impact on an individual may depend on age (pre- or post-menopause), previous use of hormone replacement therapy and the severity of side effects (e.g. lack of sleep due to night sweats causing fatigue and/or poor concentration). All these factors need to be considered when interpreting the data presented in research articles implicating endocrine therapy as detrimental to cognitive performance.

Endocrine therapies can be categorized into two groups, the selective estrogen receptor modulators (SERMs) and the aromatase inhibitors (AIs). The SERM tamoxifen, is a mixed agonist/antagonist, it binds to the estrogen receptors ERα and ERß amongst others, but there is conflicting evidence as to whether it acts as an agonist or an antagonist in the brain. The enzyme aromatase converts adrenal androgens to estrogens, and aromatase inhibitors are widely used in postmenopausal women with estrogen receptor positive breast cancer. Aromatase is found in numerous sites in the brain, particularly the hippocampus and the cortex [51]. However, the biochemical changes occurring as a result of the introduction of AIs drugs and the subsequent consequences for cognition are less well known. In order to get a clearer picture of the effect of these therapies it is useful to focus on studies where the drugs are used in women who did not receive prior chemotherapy and in breast cancer prevention in order to minimize the impact of confounding factors.

### *Evidence from Cross-Sectional and Observational Studies*

A cross-sectional study of elderly nursing home patients showed a reduced risk of Alzheimer's disease, improved activities of daily living, and improved decision making in women treated with tamoxifen [52]. This result implies that tamoxifen may have a favorable effect on the aging brain, a finding supported by Ernst and colleagues [53] who examined the impact of tamoxifen and estrogen on brain metabolism in 43 elderly women (65–80 years) compared with 33 matched controls. These data showed that tamoxifen had a similar effect to estrogen, albeit in small numbers of individuals. However, observational studies have provided mixed evidence concerning the effects of tamoxifen on cognition. For example, a study with early-stage breast cancer patients found that anastrozole compared to tamoxifen led to significant impairments in verbal and visual learning and memory [54]. However, other research has shown a deterioration in verbal abilities (verbal memory and fluency) in women following breast cancer treatment with tamoxifen compared to those who had surgery with or without radiotherapy or healthy controls [55].

## *Evidence from Randomized Controlled Trials*

Many international randomized clinical trials examining endocrine therapies have fortunately supported sub-protocols to examine cognition, for example the ATAC (anastrozole, tamoxifen alone or combined) and TEAM (tamoxifen and exemestane) trials, BIG 1–98 (letrozole and/or tamoxifen), NSABP Breast Cancer Prevention Trial (tamoxifen versus placebo) and the IBIS II study (double blind placebo controlled trial of anastrozole).

In a sub-study of the ATAC trial, cognition was examined in 100 chemotherapy naïve women who had been on the trial for a median of 36 months. Results showed a significantly poorer performance on tasks of verbal memory and processing speed in breast cancer patients compared with age matched controls but numbers were too small to conduct any between-group analyses to determine whether tamoxifen or anastrozole or the combination of drugs was implicated. Also there was no pretreatment baseline assessment to establish whether or not the effect was due to endocrine therapy per se [56].

The effect of tamoxifen on perceived cognitive function relative to placebo was assessed in the NSABP Breast Cancer Prevention Trial of 13,388 women [57]. Patients completed a quality of life symptom checklist that included aspects of cognition such as ease of concentration, and forgetfulness. At 1 year patients receiving tamoxifen had worse quality of life but no difference in self-reported cognitive function.

In the TEAM sub-study, cognition was assessed prior to starting and after 1 year of endocrine treatment in 80 patients on tamoxifen and 99 on exemestane [58]. Their results were compared to those of 120 healthy controls. After adjusting for baseline performance, patients on tamoxifen (but not those on exemestane) performed significantly worse than the controls on tasks of verbal memory and executive functioning. However, there were no significant differences regarding cognitive testing between the two therapies.

In the BIG 1–98 trial, change in cognitive function was assessed after cessation of treatment in 100 postmenopausal breast cancer patients who had received 5 years of adjuvant tamoxifen or letrozole alone or in sequence. Patients were assessed with a computerized battery of tests in the final year of treatment and 1 year later [59]. There was a moderate improvement in the composite cognitive score 1 year after cessation of treatment. Weaknesses of the study included small sample sizes (insufficient to compare differences between the groups), and lack of a control group and baseline assessment.

The randomized double blind placebo controlled prevention trial IBIS II explored the effects of anastrozole on cognition in a subset of 200 women over 2 years. No significant differences between the groups were found for any of the cognitive tasks [60]. By 6 months, 13 women in both groups reported changes to their memory and this decreased to five women in the placebo group and three women in the anastrozole group by the 24-month assessment. The strength of this study was its design, a double blind placebo controlled trial allowed a true evaluation of the effect of the drug on cognition.

The variability of results from the studies cited shows how difficult it is to tease out the effect of any endocrine therapy on cognition, especially when confounded with other factors associated with breast cancer treatments. In terms of patient care, there is insufficient evidence to select one endocrine therapy over another based on purported cognitive impact.

## Interventions for Management of Cognitive Changes

For most breast cancer patients the effects of cancer and its treatment on cognition are transient but for a subgroup symptoms may persist. If cognitive impairment is detected or reported by women after treatment, strategies to help them cope with these cognitive changes may be useful. There are broadly two approaches to manage cognitive changes after cancer treatment: pharmacological and nonpharmacological interventions. However, only a limited number of studies have been conducted in breast cancer patients and many of these are limited by methodological concerns [61].

Pharmacological interventions are usually targeted at the mechanism underlying CRCI or may be selected based on their known property to enhance cognitive function in other cognitively impaired populations [62]. The effectiveness of pharmacologic agents to reduce or prevent cognitive changes after breast cancer treatment is not well established. A review of prospective randomized controlled trials (RCTs) in breast cancer patients during or after chemotherapy or multimodal therapy (including chemotherapy) identified 6 pharmacological intervention RCTs with psycho or neurostimulants (i.e. methylphenidate, d-methylphenidate and modafinil), erythropoietin stimulating agents (i.e. epoetin alfa) or gingko biloba [61]. Outcomes were negative or inconclusive: there was no statistically significant difference in cognitive measures (evaluated within individual cognitive domains) in any of these studies. In addition, there are some safety concerns as adverse effects associated with the intervention or placebo were reported in the majority of the studies.

Nonpharmacological interventions may provide more effective alternatives for targeting functional impairments in cancer survivors. One of the most frequently employed nonpharmacological approaches is cognitive rehabilitation or cognitive training which is designed to help the patient learn and apply adaptive strategies to reduce or manage cognitive impairment. This usually involves an intervention focused on retraining (e.g. repeated and structured practice of tasks), acquisition of compensatory strategies or psychoeducation. Thus far there have been a limited number of studies in patients with breast cancer [63–67]. The majority of these studies demonstrated modest improvement in objective cognitive performance, perceived cognitive ability and quality of life. However, the efficacy of cognitive training depends highly on the intensity of treatment over an extended period of time and most studies lack a long-term evaluation. A recent study showed that web-based cognitive rehabilitation may be a promising intervention that can be applied for longer at low costs [68]. A RCT in 157 breast cancer patients (4.5 years post-diagnosis) who followed an intensive 6-weeks training program noted modest improvements on working memory and verbal learning up to 5-month after completion of the intervention.

Another approach is electroencephalography biofeedback or neurofeedback which addresses the underlying cause of cognitive problems rather than treating symptoms. It involves real-time display of brain electrical activity provided to the individual as visual or auditory information which may enable the individual to modify that brainwave activity. Neurofeedback was investigated in a small study by Alvarez et al. [69] with 23 breast cancer survivors 6–60 months post-chemotherapy. Improvements were noted in perceived cognitive function, but unfortunately objective cognitive performance was not assessed.

Recent research shows that exercise and mind-body interventions may be useful for improving cognitive function [70, 71]. In a randomized pilot study, mindfulness-based stress reduction (MBSR) was compared to psychoeducation and support [70]. Participants in the MBSR-arm reported a greater improvement in perceived cognitive impairment immediately after the 8-week intervention and 6 months later and showed greater accuracy on an attention test at both time points compared to the control arm. However, this small RCT targeted cancer-related fatigue as it included breast (and colorectal) cancer survivors (n=71) with moderate to severe fatigue.

A larger RCT (n=200) in early-stage breast cancer survivors showed that yoga may have the potential to effectively reduce cognitive complaints [71]. Participants (all post-treatment) were randomized to a 12-week Hatha yoga intervention (twice-weekly) or a wait-list control group. Three months after the intervention yoga participants reported fewer (23 % lower) cognitive problems compared to the wait-list controls, and group differences remained after adjusting for distress, fatigue and sleep quality. Within the yoga group, those who practiced more frequently noted significantly fewer cognitive complaints.

In conclusion, current evidence favors nonpharmacological management of cognitive changes associated with breast cancer treatment, but the durability of long-term effects remains uncertain. Further more rigorous RCTs with sufficient sample sizes and both objective and self-report measures of cognitive function are necessary.

## Conclusions

Research into breast cancer and cognition has grown over the past decades and has taken a multidisciplinary approach. At present the relationship between breast cancer treatment and cognition remains unclear despite the improvement in study design and methods. Controversy about the extent and the underlying mechanisms still exists, although it is recognized that CRCI is likely to be multifactorial. A combination of individual characteristics, genetic or biological factors are all likely to play a role in the predisposition to cognitive changes.

In response to the methodological limitations of current research, an international group of investigators has proposed common criteria for defining CRCI to increase homogeneity of study methods and to facilitate comparisons across studies [72]. This includes recommendations for study design and neuropsychological assessment (e.g. cognitive tests, analytical methods). Implementing these recommendations in future clinical trials could be a first step to gaining further insight into cognitive changes after a diagnosis of breast cancer. More large prospective studies in breast cancer patients and into effective and safe interventions are encouraged. Future evaluations should include patients exposed to targeted treatment, and investigation of the influence of comorbidities and aging. This may help to improve the understanding of the processes involved in CRCI, and contribute to informed decisions about treatment to maintain quality of life among breast cancer patients.

## References

1. Janelsins MC, Kesler SR, Ahles TA, et al. Prevalence, mechanisms, and management of cancer-related cognitive impairment. Int Rev Psychiatry. 2014;26:102–13.
2. Oxman TE, Silberfarb PM. Serial cognitive testing in cancer patients receiving chemotherapy. Am J Psychiatry. 1980;137:1263–5.
3. Wieneke MH, Dienst E. Neuropsychological assessment of cognitive functioning following chemotherapy for breast cancer. Psycho Oncol. 1995;4:61–6.
4. Van Dam FS, Schagen SB, Mueller MJ, et al. Impairment of cognitive function in women receiving adjuvant treatment for high-risk breast cancer: high-dose versus standard-dose chemotherapy. J Natl Cancer Inst. 1998;90:210–8.
5. Ahles TA, Saykin AJ, Furstenberg CT, et al. Neuropsychologic impact of standard-dose systemic chemotherapy in long-term survivors of breast cancer and lymphoma. J Clin Oncol. 2002;20:485–93.
6. Janelsins MC, Kohli S, Mohile SG, et al. An update on cancer- and chemotherapy-related cognitive dysfunction: current status. Semin Oncol. 2011;38:431–8.
7. Ahles TA. Brain vulnerability to chemotherapy toxicities. Psycho Oncol. 2012;21:1141–8.
8. Falleti MG, Sanfilippo A, Maruff P, et al. The nature and severity of cognitive impairment associated with adjuvant chemotherapy in women with breast cancer: a meta-analysis of the current literature. Brain Cogn. 2005;59:60–70.
9. Stewart A, Bielajew C, Collins B, et al. A meta-analysis of the neuropsychological effects of adjuvant chemotherapy treatment in women treated for breast cancer. Clin Neuropsychol. 2006;20:76–89.
10. Jim HS, Phillips KM, Chait S, et al. Meta-analysis of cognitive functioning in breast cancer survivors previously treated with standard-dose chemotherapy. J Clin Oncol. 2012;30:3578–87.
11. Ono M, Ogilvie JM, Wilson JS, et al. A meta-analysis of cognitive impairment and decline associated with adjuvant chemotherapy in women with breast cancer. Front Oncol. 2015;5:59. doi:10.3389/fonc.2015.00059.
12. Wefel JS, Lenzi R, Theriault RL, et al. The cognitive sequelae of standard-dose adjuvant chemotherapy in women with breast carcinoma: results of a prospective, randomized, longitudinal trial. Cancer. 2004;100:2292–9.

13. Collins B, Mackenzie J, Tasca GA, et al. Cognitive effects of chemotherapy in breast cancer patients: a dose–response study. Psycho Oncol. 2013;22:1517–27.
14. Ahles TA, Saykin AJ. Breast cancer chemotherapy-related cognitive dysfunction. Clin Breast Cancer. 2002;3:S84–90.
15. Vearncombe KJ, Rolfe M, Wright M, et al. Predictors of cognitive decline after chemotherapy in breast cancer patients. J Int Neuropsychol Soc. 2009;15:951–62.
16. Mehlsen M, Pedersen AD, Jensen AB, et al. No indications of cognitive side-effects in a prospective study of breast cancer patients receiving adjuvant chemotherapy. Psycho Oncol. 2009; 18:248–57.
17. Debess J, Riis JØ, Engebjerg MC, et al. Cognitive function after adjuvant treatment for early breast cancer: a population-based longitudinal study. Breast Cancer Res Treat. 2010;121:91–100.
18. Jenkins V, Shilling V, Deutsch G, et al. A 3-year prospective study of the effects of adjuvant treatments on cognition in women with early stage breast cancer. Br J Cancer. 2006;94: 828–34.
19. Ahles TA, Saykin AJ, McDonald BC, et al. Cognitive function in breast cancer patients prior to adjuvant treatment. Breast Cancer Res Treat. 2008;110:143–52.
20. Schilder CM, Seynaeve CM, Linn SC, et al. Cognitive functioning of postmenopausal breast cancer patients before adjuvant systemic therapy, and its association with medical and psychological factors. Crit Rev Oncol Hematol. 2010;76:133–41.
21. Cheung YT, Shwe M, Chui WK, et al. Effects of chemotherapy and psychosocial distress on perceived cognitive disturbances in Asian breast cancer patients. Ann Pharmacother. 2012;46:1645–55.
22. Reid-Arndt SA, Cox CR. Stress, coping and cognitive deficits in women after surgery for breast cancer. J Clin Psychol Med Settings. 2012;19:127–37.
23. Hermelink K, Untch M, Lux MP, et al. Cognitive function during neoadjuvant chemotherapy for breast cancer: results of a prospective, multicenter, longitudinal study. Cancer. 2007;109:1905–13.
24. Zheng Y, Luo J, Bao P, et al. Long-term cognitive function change among breast cancer survivors. Breast Cancer Res Treat. 2014;146:599–609.
25. Yamada TH, Denburg NL, Beglinger LJ, et al. Neuropsychological outcomes of older breast cancer survivors: cognitive features ten or more years after chemotherapy. J Neuropsychiatry Clin Neurosci. 2010;22:48–54.
26. Koppelmans V, de Ruiter MB, van der Lijn F, et al. Global and focal brain volume in long-term breast cancer survivors exposed to adjuvant chemotherapy. Breast Cancer Res Treat. 2012;132:1099–106.
27. Amidi A, Christensen S, Mehlsen M, et al. Long-term subjective cognitive functioning following adjuvant systemic treatment: 7–9 years follow-up of a nationwide cohort of women treated for primary breast cancer. Br J Cancer. 2015;113:794–801.
28. Broadbent DE, Cooper PF, FitzGerald P, et al. The Cognitive Failures Questionnaire (CFQ) and its correlates. Br J Clin Psychol. 1982;21:1–16.
29. Hutchinson AD, Hosking JR, Kichenadasse G, et al. Objective and subjective cognitive impairment following chemotherapy for cancer: a systematic review. Cancer Treat Rev. 2012;38:926–34.
30. Boykoff N, Moieni M, Subramanian SK. Confronting chemobrain: an in-depth look at survivors' report of impact on work, social networks and health care response. J Cancer Surviv. 2009;3:223–32.
31. Von Ah D, Habermann B, Carpenter JS, et al. Impact of perceived cognitive impairment in breast cancer survivors. Eur J Oncol Nursing. 2013;17:236–41.
32. Player L, Mackenzie L, Willis K, et al. Women's experiences of cognitive changes or 'chemobrain' following treatment for breast cancer: a role for occupational therapy? Aust Occup Ther J. 2014;61:230–40.
33. Ferguson RJ, McDonald BC, Saykin AJ, et al. Brain structure and function differences in monozygotic twins: possible effects of breast cancer chemotherapy. J Clin Oncol. 2007; 25:3866–70.

34. McDonald BC, Conroy SK, Ahles TA. Gray matter reduction associated with systemic chemotherapy for breast cancer: a prospective MRI study. Breast Cancer Res Treat. 2010;123: 819–28.
35. McDonald BC, Conroy SK, Smith DJ, et al. Frontal gray matter reduction after breast cancer chemotherapy and association with executive symptoms: a replication and extension study. Brain Behav Immun. 2013;30:S117–25.
36. Cheung YT, Ng T, Shwe M, et al. Association of pro-inflammatory cytokines and chemotherapy-associated cognitive impairment in breast cancer patients: a multi-centered, prospective, cohort study. Ann Oncol. 2015. doi:10.1093/annonc/mdv206.
37. Simó M, Rifà-Ros X, Rodriguez-Fornells A, et al. Chemobrain: a systematic review of structural and functional neuroimaging studies. Neuroscience Biobehav Rev. 2013;37:1311–21.
38. Koppelmans V, Groot MD, de Ruiter MB, et al. Global and focal white matter integrity in breast cancer survivors 20 years after adjuvant chemotherapy. Hum Brain Mapp. 2014;35:889–99.
39. Deprez S, Billiet T, Sunaert S, et al. Diffusion tensor MRI of chemotherapy-induced cognitive impairment in non-CNS cancer patients: a review. Brain Imaging Behav. 2013;7:409–35.
40. Deprez S, Amant F, Smeets A, et al. Longitudinal assessment of chemotherapy-induced structural changes in cerebral white matter and its correlation with impaired cognitive functioning. J Clin Oncol. 2012;30:274–81.
41. Kesler S, Janelsins M, Koovakkattu D, et al. Reduced hippocampal volume and verbal memory performance associated with interleukin-6 and tumor necrosis factor-alpha levels in chemotherapy-treated breast cancer survivors. Brain Behav Immun. 2013;30:S109–16.
42. Lopez Zunini RA, Scherling C, Wallis N, et al. Differences in verbal memory retrieval in breast cancer chemotherapy patients compared to healthy controls: a prospective fMRI study. Brain Imaging Behav. 2013;7:460–77.
43. Menning S, de Ruiter MB, Veltman DJ, et al. Multimodal MRI and cognitive function in patients with breast cancer prior to adjuvant treatment-the role of fatigue. Neuroimage Clin. 2015;7:547–54.
44. Janelsins MC, Mustian KM, Palesh OG, et al. Differential expression of cytokines in BCS receiving different chemotherapies: implications for cognitive impairment research. Support Care Cancer. 2012;20:831–9.
45. Ganz PA, Bower JE, Kwan L, et al. Does tumor necrosis factor-alpha (TNF-α) play a role in post-chemotherapy cerebral dysfunction? Brain Behav Immun. 2013;30:S99–108.
46. Tsavaris N, Kosmas C, Vadiaka M, et al. Immune changes in patients with advanced breast cancer undergoing chemotherapy with taxanes. Br J Cancer. 2002;87:21–7.
47. Pomykala KL, Ganz PA, Bower JE, et al. The association between pro-inflammatory cytokines, regional cerebral metabolism, and cognitive complaints following adjuvant chemotherapy for breast cancer. Brain Imaging Behav. 2013;7:511–23.
48. Mills PJ, Ancoli-Israel S, Parker B, et al. Predictors of inflammation in response to anthracycline-based chemotherapy for breast cancer. Brain Behav Immun. 2008;22:98–104.
49. Squire L. Memory and the hippocampus: a synthesis from findings with rats, monkeys, and humans. Psychol Rev. 1992;99:195–231.
50. Alves S, McEwen B. Estrogen and brain function: implications for aging and dementia. New York: Springer; 1999.
51. Roselli CE, Klosterman SA, Fasasi TA. Sex differences in androgen responsiveness in the rat brain: regional differences in the induction of aromatase activity. Neuroendocrinology. 1996;64:139–45.
52. Breuer B, Anderson R. The relationship of tamoxifen with dementia, depression and dependence in activities of daily living in elderly nursing home residents. Women Health. 2000;31:71–85.
53. Ernst T, Chang L, Cooray D, et al. The effects of tamoxifen andestrogen on brain metabolism in elderly women. J Natl Cancer Inst. 2002;94:592–7.
54. Bender CM, Sereika SM, Brufsky AM, et al. Memory impairments with adjuvant anastrozole versus tamoxifen in women with early-stage breast cancer. Menopause. 2007;14:995–8.

55. Boele FW, Schilder CMT, De Roode ML, et al. Cognitive functioning during long-term tamoxifen treatment in postmenopausal women with breast cancer. Menopause. 2015;22:17–25.
56. Jenkins V, Shilling V, Fallowfield L, et al. Does hormone therapy for the treatment of breast cancer have a detrimental effect on memory and cognition? A pilot study. Psycho Oncol. 2004;13:61–6.
57. Fisher B, Costantino JP, Wickerham DL, et al. Tamoxifen for prevention of breast cancer: report of the National Surgical Adjuvant Breast and Bowel Project P-1 Study. J Natl Cancer Inst. 1998;90:1371–88.
58. Schilder CM, Eggens PC, Seynaeve C, et al. Neuropsychological functioning in postmenopausal breast cancer patients treated with tamoxifen or exemestane after AC-chemotherapy: cross-sectional findings from the neuropsychological TEAM-side study. Acta Oncol. 2009;48:76–85.
59. Phillips K, Aldridge J, Ribi K, et al. Cognitive function in postmenopausal breast cancer patients one year after completing adjuvant endocrine therapy with letrozole and/or tamoxifen in the BIG 1–98 trial. Breast Cancer Res Treatment. 2011;126:221–6.
60. Jenkins VA, Ambroisine LM, Atkins L, et al. Effects of anastrozole on cognitive performance in postmenopausal women: a randomised, double-blind chemoprevention trial (IBIS II). Lancet Oncol. 2008;9:953–61.
61. Chan RJ, McCarthy AL, Devenish J, et al. Systematic review of pharmacologic and non-pharmacologic interventions to manage cognitive alterations after chemotherapy for breast cancer. Eur J Cancer. 2015;51:437–50.
62. Davis J, Ahlberg FM, Berk M, et al. Emerging pharmacotherapy for cancer patients with cognitive dysfunction. BMC Neurol. 2013;13:153.
63. Dolbeault S, Cayrou S, Brédart A. The effectiveness of a psycho-educational group after early-stage breast cancer treatment: results of a randomized French study. Psych Oncol. 2009;18:647–56.
64. Ferguson RJ, McDonald BC, Rocque MA, et al. Development of CBT for chemotherapy-related cognitive change: Results of a waitlist control trial. Psycho Oncol. 2012;21:176–86.
65. Von Ah D, Carpenter JS, Saykin A, et al. Advanced cognitive training for breast cancer survivors: a randomized controlled trial. Breast Cancer Res Treat. 2012;135:799–809.
66. Kesler SR, Hadi Hosseini SM, Heckler C, et al. Cognitive training for improving executive function in chemotherapy-treated breast cancer survivors. Clin Breast Cancer. 2013;13:299–306.
67. Ercoli LM, Petersen L, Hunter AM, et al. Cognitive rehabilitation group intervention for breast cancer survivors: results of a randomized clinical trial. Psycho Oncol. 2015;24:1360–7.
68. Damholdt MF, Mehlsen M, O'Toole MS, et al. Web-based cognitive training for breast cancer survivors with cognitive complaints – a randomized controlled trial. Psych Oncol. 2016. doi:10.1002/pon.4058.
69. Alvarez J, Meyer FL, Granoff DL, et al. The effect of EEG biofeedback on reducing postcancer cognitive impairment. Integr Cancer Ther. 2013;12:475–87.
70. Johns SA, Von Ah D, Brown LF. Randomized controlled pilot trial of mindfulness-based stress reduction for breast and colorectal cancer survivors: effects on cancer-related cognitive impairment. J Cancer Surviv. 2016;10:437–48. doi:10.1007/s11764-015-0494-3.
71. Derry HM, Jaremka LM, Bennet JM, et al. Yoga and self-reported cognitive problems in breast cancer survivors: a randomized controlled trial. Psycho Oncol. 2015;24:958–66.
72. Wefel JS, Vardy J, Ahles T, et al. International Cognition and Cancer Task Force recommendations to harmonise studies of cognitive function in patients with cancer. Lancet Oncol. 2011;12:703–8.

# Chapter 19
# Psychological Issues in Breast Cancer Survivorship

**Richard Towers**

**Abstract** This Chapter will explore the common psychological and emotional impact of a breast cancer diagnosis and its bearing on survivorship. An understanding of the psychological processes from the point of diagnosis aims to shed light on the needs of breast cancer survivors. Challenges, psychological issues and coping mechanisms will be explored and communication skills considered.

**Keywords** Psychological • Support • Listening • Self-management • Person-centered communication • Depression • Body-image • Uncertainty

## Introduction

There is no standard psychological or emotional response to a cancer diagnosis but many patients experience the emotional consequences to be the hardest to deal with [1]. Adjustment to survivorship can be influenced by: response to diagnosis; the treatment experience; individual coping style and prior experience with illness, cancer and loss. People mostly adapt well in the long term, but the transition at end of treatment remains challenging [2].

Cancer diagnosis is a shocking experience disrupting the lives of the strongest individuals and causing sadness, disbelief and sometimes depression, anxiety and family breakdown. Having cancer means exposure to an alien hospital environment where investigations and treatments are delivered in invasive and challenging circumstances. Many undergo surgery, chemotherapy, radiotherapy and an increasingly diverse range of interventions. Patients tend to engage with treatment with the primary aim of survival and have the expectation that normal life will resume

R. Towers, DNurs, MSc, BSc (Hons), RN
Deputy team leader Psychological Support service/Lecturer Practitioner Marsden School, Royal Marsden NHS Foundation Trust,, London, UK
e-mail: richard.towers@rmh.nhs.uk

 
A. Ring, M. Parton (eds.), *Breast Cancer Survivorship*,
DOI 10.1007/978-3-319-41858-2_19

following treatment. Survivorship however is a challenge and health professionals can help by meaningful engagement with psychological, social and emotional issues.

## Reactions to Breast Cancer Diagnosis and Coping

Many people with a diagnosis of breast cancer consider themselves to be healthy, with few or no symptoms. Diagnosis generates thoughts of mortality and with treatment lasting over a year for some, long term coping is demanding for all.

Following diagnosis people often experience numbness, disbelief, fear and vulnerability which affect normal thinking and functioning. Some experience high distress, profound uncertainty, sleeplessness and fear and it is in this unsettled period that challenging treatment choices are made. A significant loss of control is experienced when confronted with cancer [3] and in some cases support is required to enable people to engage with aspects of their normal lives. Retaining control supports adaptation and health professional communication can aid empowered reactions. A low sense of control can result in negative thoughts and feelings, resulting in a reduced ability to cope and greater distress [4].

A degree of denial or 'psychological buffering' can help people cope with the magnitude of a cancer diagnosis and its consequences. This buffering should be considered to be a normal and functional mechanism, enabling people to manage an otherwise unbearable situation. Most denial helps people manage challenging emotions and thoughts but can be confusing for health professionals who see unusual reactions or ambivalence in situations where a different reaction is expected. There can be concerning levels of denial, for example someone denying they have cancer at all. This happens because they are not able to confront and manage the situation effectively. Broad support and gentle exploration of fears are required to support adaptation in cases where there is concerning denial. The same treatment and options should be available and careful documentation is important to support a holistic and multi-professional approach. Professional psychological support should be offered sensitively. Denial can come and go, for example in a conversation about prognosis and it is always important to differentiate denial from a lack of understanding.

Patients frequently reflect upon the diagnosis and treatment period as an unreal and bewildering experience. This emotional detachment or numbness results from a profound psychological disturbance and is influenced by the impact of powerful drug treatment and side effects. People can adopt a singular focus on getting through their treatment, helping them to endure the physical side effects, but potentially storing up challenging thoughts and feelings. Once treatment ends people often begin to process their experiences and try to make sense of their future. Some dependence upon contact with hospital staff and the busy schedule of treatments, investigations and appointments may have developed.

Several people start to make lifestyle changes during treatment, possibly involving diet. These changes can be viewed as part of coping and such actions may contribute positively to a sense of control. Sometimes people seek to make ambitious changes and attempt to change too much, losing a sense of emotional balance and stability. Exploration and gentle guidance can help people judge what is achievable and helpful. More in-depth psychological support may help people realize the origin of the desire to control future risk and plans to change might be reformulated as a result.

Beliefs about the causes of cancer can be helpful in driving attitude and behavior change towards more healthy living but can sometimes be troublesome. Patients often believe that psychosocial factors influence cancer outcomes [5] and there is some evidence of their influence upon survival [6]. It can however be damaging to encourage people to adopt certain attitudes, as there is no proven psychological state to adopt.

## Uncertainty

A significant challenge in cancer is the sense of uncertainty that develops. Uncertainty inhibits coping, it causes distress and can reduce quality of life [7]. The end of cancer treatment reveals a future marked by pervasive thoughts about recurrence [8] and mortality. Constant active acknowledgement of life's uncertainty is not normal and such unsettling thoughts can persist long after cancer treatment has ended [9]. Patients can be left with the feeling that they are living with imminent risk and their concepts of life and hope are disrupted [10]. Acclimatizing to the awareness of uncertainty or returning to a healthy ignorance of its implications takes time and is dependent on individual circumstance. If uncertainty is generating troublesome anxiety or low mood then counseling may help people adjust. Uncertainty can sometimes be viewed positively, its vagueness helpful in avoiding fears (if the future is uncertain, fears are unconfirmed). After cancer treatment, people have the opportunity to make significant and positive changes to the way they have lived their lives, establishing a 'new normal' and resolving much of their personal uncertainty.

Clarity of knowledge influences the nature of uncertainty and its association with distress [9]. The trust that patients have with health professionals is likely to influence their ability to come to terms with the inherent ambiguity in survivorship. Patients can be frustrated by professionals' who fail to acknowledge uncertainty, but they also actively seek reassurance which can make striking the right balance of information challenging. Giving generic untailored and technical information is of limited value [11] as is sharing too much or too little. Professionals can put the person in charge of what information they acquire and regularly clarify what they want to know, giving information clearly and honestly to avoid confusion. The type, amount and delivery of information are crucial to helping patients adjust.

Indecision and confusion can emerge around specific issues, for example younger women face loss or uncertainty about fertility and this can be as challenging and traumatic as the diagnosis of cancer itself. Pregnancy increases cancer risks for some, and pregnancy rates clearly drop following cancer treatment in young women [12].

Professionals therefore need to keep an open mind and explore what uncertainties there are for individuals in order to be able to support their needs effectively.

## Family Considerations

The structure of families and their ability to adjust to illness varies considerably. Roles generally need to change to accommodate cancer treatment and misunderstandings and disagreements can emerge. All family members are affected and will have fears for the future [13]. At treatments end, many families assume that old roles will be restored which might conflict with the cancer patients' new view of their life priorities and their on-going experience of physical and psychological consequences. Professionals often assume that patients talk to their family members about feelings, fears and concerns and families might equally assume that professionals are addressing these issues. Patients can sometimes therefore feel quite isolated and struggle to find someone to hear their concerns (See section "Supportive Communication").

Distress in relationships can be experienced during diagnosis, treatment and the survivorship period and this often remains hidden from professionals [14]. A lower quality of life and anxiety are precipitated by poor family adaptation to a diagnosis [15] and social and emotional support is crucial in supporting patient adjustment [16, 17].

## Mood Disorders

More significant and potentially lasting psychological difficulties like anxiety, depression and adjustment disorders arise in a significant proportion of cancer patients [18, 19]. These difficulties have a profound impact upon quality of life and are under-recognized, with major depression occurring in around 9 % of the breast cancer population [20].

Depression is a clinical condition where people display some of the following symptoms: low mood; lack of motivation; anxiety; sleep disturbance; early morning waking; loss of interest, appetite and libido; a sense of hopelessness and negativity [21]. People may become withdrawn, sad and lose interest in their appearance. Many of the symptoms of low mood are caused by treatment and its side effects. Patients and family members may expect low mood, but this doesn't mean that support isn't required and further assessment is essential to establish whether therapeutic or medical interventions are needed. Patients who have experienced a significant symptom burden and functional impairment during treatment or who continue to suffer longer term impacts are vulnerable to low mood [21].

Feelings of anxiety are understandable e.g. leading up to review appointments or awaiting scan results. Anxiety links to a sense of control and uncertainty and therefore can respond to empowerment and self-help techniques like relaxation exercises.

A sense of control generally improves with medical reassurances, time and the re-emergence of a sense of self. One challenge many patients face is interpreting physical sensations, many of which are new following surgery and other medical interventions. Patients will inevitably be over-vigilant to physical sensations and fears are frequently triggered by symptomatic experiences. Health professionals need to show their understanding and pay proper attention to concerns, whilst giving realistic reassurance. Exploring fears can help – see section "Supportive Communication".

It is important to develop a trusting relationship and be non-judgmental about experiences of low mood and anxiety. It can help to normalize the feelings expressed, but care must be taken to avoiding trivializing patient experiences. Risk factors for mood problems include having a history of mood disturbance, being younger at diagnosis, having poor social support and in patients who experience poor symptom control. Low level depression depression is still challenging and many people will benefit from counseling to help them through difficult periods.

## Body Image

A range of body changes can occur with cancer treatment, most obviously those associated with hair loss from chemotherapy and longer term changes caused by surgery. The resulting changed body image requires adjustment. Cosmetic surgery can significantly improve outcomes but self-image and identity remain subjective and relatively minor changes or scarring can have a significant and negative impact on some people. Due to the sexual association of the breast and its place as a societal identifier of a woman's sexuality [22] feelings of attractiveness and feminine identity can be affected. Depression and anxiety might affect body image but such influences are bi-directional, with mood affected by self-perceptions. Prior self-image and social/relationship factors will influence adjustment to body image change. In younger women with breast cancer, body image concerns are directly linked to the type and extent of surgery, e.g. lumpectomy, with or without reconstruction generates fewer problems than mastectomy [23]. There can be an assumption that reconstructive surgery is more suitable for younger women but there are potentially equivalent benefits in well-being and self-image in an older population [24].

The effect of hair loss can be supported by the use of headscarves, wigs and makeup but health care professionals should not think this fixes or resolves the discomfort and the sense of difference that occurs. Many women struggle with the identification with the characteristic 'bald' cancer patient. Talking through such feelings can be of benefit. Some actions and support are suggested to support confidence and self-esteem [25].

Lymphoedema is a particular challenge due to its permanence, potential functional restriction and need to manage as a long-term consequence. The wearing of supportive stockings and visible limb swelling can make this a very conspicuous and difficult problem to adjust to problem. Getting specialist advice on management is likely to benefit a sense of control, improve management and result in a better quality of life.

## Should People Have Counseling?

Many patients talk of presenting themselves as 'well' to health professionals, even when they are struggling with symptoms and mood at home. Speigal [26] suggest that psychotherapeutic interventions have a role in promoting quality of life and length of survival in breast cancer, especially when depression and significant stress are present. Evidence however is mixed and the specific type of intervention remains unclear.

A significant percentage of breast cancer patients do opt to have some counseling to help them cope with treatment, process strong emotions and address personal challenges. Patients should always be informed of the support services available to them, but frequently manage with social support and caring health professionals with good communication skills (see section "Supportive Communication").

Counseling can support adjustment to identity, body image, coping with losses and address specific mood problems like anxiety and depression [27]. It can help people to identify their feelings and thoughts and support the development of a new sense of self in survivorship. Successful psychosocial interventions have an impact upon quality of life and can reduce costs from hospital follow up, community services and GP visits, especially in those patients with significant mood disturbance [28].

## Supportive Communication Skills for Health Professionals

Getting our communication right has the potential to support self-management, reduce inequalities in access to care and promote recovery to an optimal quality of life [29]. Bad communication can lead to negative patient experience, poor satisfaction and result in costly interventions and overuse of health services in the longer term [30].

Finding the time to explore and support patients' psychological and social needs can be challenging in hospital environments where there is an overriding focus upon physical issues and treatment advances. Survival is everyone's priority but the dominance of biomedical agendas can compromise the transfer of good psychological care into health professional practice [31]. Improving survival rates leads to increased chronic physical and psychological sequelae and greater collaboration and support are therefore required [11]. Health professionals have a tendency to favor information exchange as the primary focus of communication, but patients prefer trusting relationships and an appropriate emotional tone [32].

Breast patients have had a life changing experience and have lived through a range of emotions that need expression. Part of recovery involves the articulation of these experiences and feelings and having them listened to, acknowledged and understood. Health professionals spend far too much time focusing on the physical and all too frequently fail to address this agenda. If we ask people what they need and we listen and act in accordance with their wishes, we will not go too far wrong. Person centered communication approaches, where individuals are placed in a context of their own meaning and values [33] should be what health professionals aim for.

A plan for providing support (examples in italics)

1. Protect time. Even very short amounts of time can be beneficial, but it is important to declare a specific psychological/emotional focus. '*I would like now to spend 5 min to concentrate on how you have been feeling*.'
2. Pick up on cues (listening out for what people are really saying i.e. the meaning behind the words, paying attention to non-verbal and verbal cues).
   '*I noticed you seem a little down today*'
3. Explore with a mixture of open and closed questions, responding to the psychological or emotional agenda. '*What is concerning you the most?*'
4. Listening. The most underrated skill is being quiet! Even when we are silent we must remain present and attentive. Stop interrupting and periodically summarize or paraphrase your understanding of what is being said (aim to talk for less than 50 % of the time).
5. Be prepared to sit with distress. Don't try to stop people if they are upset but do acknowledge it: '*I can see its challenging and upsetting to talk about this*'
6. Avoid jumping in to solve problems. Listen first and then explore the patients solutions.
7. Close your conversation sensitively and effectively. Indicate you need to end the conversation e.g. '*I am going to need to end our meeting shortly*'. Summarize your conversation, especially if there has been distress '*It's been difficult and upsetting for you since...*'
8. Let people know where they can go for support. Can they talk to you again? When? If not you, who can they speak to? Signpost to information, pastoral, complementary, and counseling services (this means informing people what is available, not passing the buck).

If mood is obviously low or there are high levels of anxiety without an immediate cause, establish the duration and severity of symptoms. It can be useful to ask if they or others are concerned about their mood. Consider the symptoms of anxiety and low mood and impact of treatment and follow point 8 above. Expressions of hopelessness or concerning statements should be explored to exclude risk and if in doubt seek advice from a mental health professional.

People may respond well to self-selected, self-help resources and activities (see NHS choices link) like yoga, meditation and mindfulness, often run at cancer centers. There is growing evidence of the benefit of activity and the safety of exercise for cancer survivors. It is suggested to improve cancer outcomes and benefit those suffering from low mood [34, 35].

## Cognitive Behavioral Interventions

Health professionals can make use of cognitive behavioral interventions (CBT) but should seek training before changing their practice. In principle CBT aims to develop people's awareness of their thinking, emotions and behavior and the links between them. Unconscious repetitive thoughts can cause unpleasant mood states and block positive change. Patients can be helped to see how certain thoughts or behaviors maintain problems or thwart progress towards change. The approach involves breaking down and structuring problems into smaller parts. Using an example of someone with anxiety at the time of their cancer follow-up appointment, the approach would gather suitable descriptions of the situation and the difficult or unwanted actions and feelings experienced. A structured process of exploring the relationship between the situation and the difficulties aims to reveal some negative or fearful thoughts e.g. '*the cancer will return*' or '*I will get bad news*'. Working gently through these thoughts, the patient is encouraged to 'test out' their accuracy, revealing how one-sided or negative they may be. More balanced, realistic thoughts are sought that lead to less anxiety and more stable and tolerant mood states e.g. '*there is a good chance I will be reassured*', '*I have no reason to expect the worst*'. The changes and words have to be from the patient, it is not about giving advice and changing people's thoughts for them. Adopting this approach takes practice and training. There are self-help CBT resources available (see below).

## Supporting Self-Management

There is a suggested relationship between self-efficacy (a sense of control) and coping with diagnosis and survivorship [2]. If health professionals can support self-management it is likely to improve long term symptoms, clinical outcomes and alter the way that health services are accessed [36].

Health professionals are experts at helping and are eager to support people in their time of need. The tools we use to help are ones we feel familiar with, commonly those involving fixing problems through investigations, treatments, information, advice and plans. Most health professionals get reward from helping others and such interventions are mostly welcomed by patients. The skills to motivate others to self manage however conflict with the traditional helping dynamic. By seeking to fix peoples problems for them, we promote and maintain a degree of dependence.

Person centered communication skills and a strong emphasis upon collaboration and empowering people to be more involved in decisions and care are the bedrock of supporting self-management. Facilitating people to resolve and support their own challenges with our assistance is the shift in practice required. Communication training around being person centered and motivating others to self manage will help to develop suitable skills.

The sort of skills you would use would be: inviting the patient to set the agenda: '*What do you want to get out of our meeting today*? Encouraging people to tell you about their current situation, hearing reasons for and against making changes and showing your understanding. Avoid advice giving. Displaying accurate empathy is an important and underrated skill in supporting self-care. Changing communication to support self-management, also takes practice and training.

## Information and Support Resources

Patients should be encouraged to develop a relationship with their GP and to include discussions about their mood if possible. Some GP practices have counseling services and all currently have access to community Cognitive Behavioral Therapy services (IAPT) suitable to support depression and anxiety.

Many hospitals offer information and support/counseling services, sometimes these are cancer specific. Some geographical areas have dedicated breast cancer services providing a range of holistic interventions. Explore what is around you locally so that you can inform patients of available services. Avoid referral without primary assessment and consideration with the patient first – consider a holistic needs assessment. Clinical nurse specialists are key workers and can do much to support psychological and emotional issues.

Sources of support

| Organization | Website/contact | Services offered |
|---|---|---|
| Breast Cancer Care | https://www.breastcancercare.org.uk/ Freephone 0808 800 6000 | Information, support and can signpost to local support |
| Cancer Research UK | http://www.cancerresearchuk.org/about-cancer/type/breast-cancer/ | Information about disease and treatment. Chat forums |
| Look good, feel better | http://www.lookgoodfeelbetter.co.uk/ | Services for well-being, appearance and confidence building |
| Lymphoedema Support | http://www.lymphoedema.org/ | Information self-help promotion. Support network |
| Macmillan Cancer Support | Macmillan Cancer Support http://www.macmillan.org.uk/ Freephone 0808 808 00 00 | Advice, information support |
| The Haven | http://thehaven.org.uk/ | A range of holistic services |
| NHS choices: | http://www.nhs.uk/NHSEngland/NSF/Pages/Cancer.aspx http://www.nhs.uk/conditions/counselling/pages/talking-therapies.aspx Includes links to other sources of support and self-help e.g. 'Big White Wall' 'MoodGym', 'Living life to the full' 'Samaritans' Sources of counseling | Helpful advice on: cancer related issues; coping and psychological health issues |

## References

1. Macmillan. Worried sick: the emotional impact of cancer. 2006. http://www.macmillan.org.uk/Documents/GetInvolved/Campaigns/Campaigns/Impact_of_cancer_english.pdf. Accessed 20 June 15.
2. Jones JM, Cheng T, Jackman M, Rodin G, Walton T, Catton P. Self-efficacy, perceived preparedness, and psychological distress in women completing primary treatment for breast cancer. J Psychosoc Oncol. 2010;28(3):269–90.
3. Holland JC, Alici Y. Management of distress in cancer patients. J Support Oncol. 2010;8:1.
4. Henselmans I, Fleer J, de Vries J, Baas PC, Sanderman R, Ranchor AV. The adaptive effect of personal control when facing breast cancer: cognitive and behavioural mediators. Psychol Health. 2010;25(9):1023–40.
5. Thorne SE, Armstrong EA, Oglov V, Hislop TG. Cancer care communication: the power to harm and the power to heal? Patient Educ Couns. 2008;71:34–40.
6. Satin JR, Linden W, Phillips MJ. Depression as a predictor of disease progression and mortality in cancer patients: a meta-analysis. Cancer. 2009;115:5349–61.
7. Larsen PD, editor. Lubkin's chronic illness: impact and intervention. 9th ed. Burlington: Jones & Bartlett; 2016.
8. Waldrop DP, O'Connor TL, Trabold N. Waiting for the other shoe to drop distress and coping during and after treatment for breast cancer. J Psychosoc Oncol. 2011;29(4):450–73.
9. Miller LE. Sources of uncertainty in cancer survivorship. J Cancer Surviv Res Pract. 2012;6(4):431–40.
10. Perz J, Ussher J, Gilbert E. Loss, uncertainty, or acceptance: subjective experience of changes to fertility after breast cancer. Eur J Cancer Care. 2014;23:514–22.
11. Coulter A, Ellins J. Patient-focused interventions. A review of the evidence. London: The Health Foundation and Picker Institute; 2006.
12. Duffy C, Allen S. Medical and psychosocial aspects of fertility after cancer. Cancer J. 2009;15:27–33.
13. Watson M, St James-Roberts I, Ashley S, Tilney C, Brougham B, Edwards L, Baldus C, Romer G. Factors associated with emotional and behavioural problems among school age children of breast cancer patients. Br J Cancer. 2006;94(1):43–50.
14. Sprung BR, Janotha BL, Steckel AJ. The lived experience of breast cancer patients and couple distress. J Am Acad Nurse Pract. 2011;23:11.
15. Edwards B, Clarke V. The psychological impact of a cancer diagnosis on families: the influence of family functioning and patients' illness characteristics on depression and anxiety. Psychooncology. 2004;13(8):562–76.
16. Borstelmann NA, Rosenberg SM, Ruddy KJ, Tamimi RM, Gelber S, Schapira L, Come S, Partridge AH. Partner support and anxiety in young women with breast cancer. Psychooncology. 2015;15:(published online March 2015).
17. Leung J, Pachana NA, McLaughlin D. Social support and health-related quality of life in women with breast cancer: a longitudinal study. Psychooncology. 2014;23(9):1014–20.
18. Massie MJ. Prevalence of depression in patients with cancer. J Natl Cancer Inst Monogr. 2004;32:57–71.
19. Mitchell AJ, Chan M, Bhatti H, Halton M, Grassi L, Johansen C, Meader N. Prevalence of depression, anxiety, and adjustment disorder in oncological, haematological, and palliative-care settings: a meta-analysis of 94 interview-based studies. Lancet Oncol. 2011;12(2):160–74.
20. Walker J, Hansen CH, Martin P, Symeonides S, Ramessur R, Murray G, Sharpe M. Prevalence, associations, and adequacy of treatment of major depression in patients with cancer: a cross-sectional analysis of routinely collected clinical data. Lancet Psychiatry. 2014;1(5):343–50.
21. NICE. CG 90 depression in adults. 2009. http://www.nice.org.uk/guidance/cg90/resources accessed 29-7-15. Accessed 29 July 2015.

22. Falvo DR. Medical and psychosocial aspects of chronic illness and disability. Burlington: Jones & Bartlett Learning; 2014.
23. Rosenberg SM, Tamimi RM, Gelber S, Ruddy KJ, Kereakoglow S, Borges VF, Come SE, Partridge AH, et al. Body image in recently diagnosed young women with early breast cancer. Psychooncology. 2013;22(8):1849–55.
24. Sisco M, Johnson DB, Wang C, Rasinski K, Rundell VL, Yao KA. The quality-of-life benefits of breast reconstruction do not diminish with age. J Surg Oncol. 2015;111(6):663–8.
25. Look Good feel Better Survey. 2012. http://www.lookgoodfeelbetter.co.uk/. Accessed 6 Aug 2015.
26. Spiegel D. Minding the body: psychotherapy and cancer survival. Br J Health Psychol. 2014;19(3):465–85.
27. Morgan C, Cooper M. Helpful and unhelpful aspects of counselling following breast cancer: a qualitative analysis of post-session Helpful Aspects of Therapy forms. Counselling Psychother Res. 2015;15(3):197–206.
28. Carlson LE, Bultz BD. Efficacy and medical cost offset of psychosocial interventions in cancer care: making the case for economic analyses. Psychooncology. 2004;13:837–49.
29. Department for Health. Improving outcomes: a strategy for cancer. 2011. http://www.dh.gov.uk/en/Publicationsandstatistics/Publications/PublicationsPolicyAndGuidance/DH. Accessed 27 Apr 2015.
30. Macmillan. Psychological and emotional support provided by Macmillan Professionals: an evidence review [Online]. 2011. http://www.macmillan.org.uk/Documents/AboutUs/Commissioners/PsychologicalandEmotionalSupportProvidedbyMacmillanProfessionalsEvidenceReviewJuly2011.pdf. Accessed 24 Apr 2015.
31. Hack TF, Carlson L, Butler L, Degner LF, Jakulj F, Pickles T, Ruether JD, Weir L. Facilitating the implementation of empirically valid interventions in psychosocial oncology and supportive care. Support Care Cancer. 2011;19:1097–105.
32. Bensing J, Rimondini M, Visser A. What patients want. Patient Educ Couns. 2013;90(3):287–90.
33. Drach-Zahavy A. Patient-centred care and nurses health: the role of nurses caring orientation. J Adv Nurs. 2009;65:1463–74.
34. Rock CL, Doyle C, Demark-Wahnefried W, Meyerhardt J, Courneya KS, Schwartz AL, Bandera EV, Gansler T, et al. Nutrition and physical activity guidelines for cancer survivors. Cancer J Clin. 2012;62(4):242–74.
35. Stanton R, Reaburn P, Happell B. Is cardiovascular or resistance exercise better to treat patients with depression? A narrative review. Issues Ment Health Nurs. 2013;34(7):531–8.
36. Health Foundation. Ideas into action: person-centred care in practice. 2014. http://www.health.org.uk/publication/ideas-action-person-centred-care-practice. Accessed 1 Sept 2015.

# Chapter 20
# Fatigue in Breast Cancer Survivors

**Belinda Kingston and Marta Capelan**

**Abstract** Fatigue is a common symptom amongst cancer survivors which can have a significant impact on quality of life even in those who have completed treatment many years previously. It appears that a combination of genetic predisposition, environmental exposure, tumor and treatment factors combine to put women at increased risk of fatigue, but the precise mechanisms are not well understood. The fatigue experienced by cancer survivors is best regarded as a multidimensional symptom involving the subjective experience of tiredness, weakness and lack of energy. However there is a lack of consensus as to the optimal means by which to measure fatigue, and partly as a consequence of this, interventions to ameliorate this distressing symptom are not well established. This chapter examines what is known of the prevalence and natural history of fatigue amongst breast cancer survivors, with guidance as to the differential diagnosis and potential management strategies.

**Keywords** Breast cancer • Fatigue • Cancer-related fatigue • Cytokines

## Introduction

Fatigue is a common symptom amongst cancer survivors which can have a significant impact on quality of life even in those who have completed treatment many years previously [1, 2]. Despite this, relatively little is understood about the underlying pathophysiology and risk factors. Cancer-related fatigue is best regarded as a distressing, persistent, subjective sense of physical, emotional, and/or cognitive tiredness or exhaustion related to cancer and/or cancer treatment that is not proportional to recent activity and interferes with usual functioning [3]. However there is a lack of consensus as to the optimal means by which to measure fatigue, and partly as a consequence of this, interventions to ameliorate this distressing symptom are

B. Kingston, MBChB, BSc • M. Capelan, MD (✉)
The Breast Unit, The Royal Marsden NHS Foundation Trust, Surrey, UK
e-mail: Belinda.kingston@rmh.nhs.uk; capelanrodriguez@gmail.com, marta.capelan@rmh.nhs.uk

 
A. Ring, M. Parton (eds.), *Breast Cancer Survivorship*,
DOI 10.1007/978-3-319-41858-2_20

not well established. This chapter examines what is known of the prevalence and natural history of fatigue amongst breast cancer survivors, with guidance as to the differential diagnosis and potential management strategies.

## Epidemiology

Fatigue is one of the most common symptoms experienced during chemotherapy and radiotherapy, and as a direct effect of treatment one would anticipate that fatigue will be experienced by patients during and immediately after treatment [4]. However fatigue in breast cancer survivors appears to persist well beyond this initial treatment phase. Fatigue has been reported by up to 30–50% of breast cancer survivors in the first 5 years from completion of treatment [5–7], and whilst fatigue may be a common complaint in the general population these rates are significantly higher than in age matched controls [1, 8]. Bower et al assessed the persistence of fatigue up to 10 years from diagnosis [9]. Fatigue was assessed using the RAND-36 Item Health Survey questionnaire, which asks participant how much time in the proceeding 4 weeks they had felt 'full of pep', 'had a lot of energy', 'worn out' and 'felt tired'. The women were assessed at two time points, within 5 years and within 10 years of completing treatment. The investigators found that within 763 disease-free breast cancer survivors, there was only 1% difference in the prevalence of fatigue at the 1–5 year follow up compared to the 5–10 year follow up (35% versus 34% respectively). It is clear from this and other long term follow up studies [6], that fatigue can be a persistent symptom in approximately a third of individuals who have been diagnosed with breast cancer more than 5 years previously [5, 9].

## Causes and Associations

### *Risk Factors for Fatigue in Breast Cancer Survivors*

In order to fully inform patients and to plan interventions it is important to be able to identify those patients at risk of persistent fatigue. Bower et al. [10] investigated fatigue in nearly 2,000 breast cancer survivors in the first 5 years from diagnosis. The investigators used the RAND 36-Item Health Survey to establish levels of fatigue in 1,957 breast cancer survivors. Younger age, lower income, pain, depression, single relationship status, and presence of comorbidities were associated with increased fatigue levels. In contrast, ethnicity, educational attainment and employment status which were not significantly associated with being more fatigued [10]. Furthermore, women treated with chemo- and radiotherapy or chemotherapy alone were more likely to be fatigued than those treated with radiotherapy or surgery alone. Tamoxifen and other endocrine therapies are often believed to contribute to fatigue in clinical practice, but there was no association between tamoxifen use and fatigue identified in this study [10].

The risk factors for later (post 5 years) fatigue could potentially be different to those for fatigue earlier following diagnosis and in a subsequent study the only risk factor associated with persistent fatigue at 5–10 years post diagnosis was having a lower income (P=0.05). Women with persistent fatigue were also more likely to experience depressive symptoms, body pain, hypertension, and were more likely to have been treated with chemo-radiotherapy rather that radiotherapy alone [9]. This association of cancer-related fatigue with depression and treatment with chemotherapy is a frequent finding in other studies [11]. This highlights a high risk category of women in whom increased vigilance and earlier intervention aimed at fatigue management might be particularly useful.

## *Depression, Anxiety, Catastrophizing Personality*

A number of studies have identified the close relationship between depression, anxiety, coping strategies and cancer-related fatigue [12]. Specifically in breast cancer survivors the presence of an anxiety, low mood or adjustment disorder and depression has been found to correlate with fatigue severity in breast cancer survivors [1, 9]. There is also some evidence that pre-morbid personality may play a role in increasing the risk of fatigue. Individuals who use 'catastrophizing' as a coping strategy (having lower self-confidence and a tendency to adopt a negative outcome expectation) tended to experience more severe fatigue in one age-matched control study [1]. Furthermore, presence of this personality type has been shown to predict cancer-related fatigue at 42 months post treatment [13] and fatigue severity [14].

## *The Role of Cytokines*

Research investigating the possible underlying cause of cancer-related fatigue has identified an association between an increase in pro-inflammatory cytokines and fatigue. This pro-inflammatory state has been demonstrated in some tumor types to precede surgery, chemo- or radiotherapy (in other words to reflect the effects of the cancer *per se*), but in early breast cancer has also been observed to only occur following treatment [15, 16].

In the post-treatment setting, multiple studies in large numbers of disease-free breast cancer survivors have identified an association between higher levels of circulating cytokines such as IL-6, IL-1β and acute phase proteins, such as CRP, and fatigue [7, 17–21]. It is also clear that some women with fatigue have increased expression of genes associated with pro-inflammatory response, and this may provide a means by which to identify women at increased risk of fatigue [17, 18]. A further underlying driver to the increase in inflammation found in breast cancer survivors may be reactivation of latent viruses [22] such as CMV [23]. It may also be that genetic predisposition also puts some women at greater risk of cancer-related fatigue [24, 25]. Overall, these studies suggest that a combination of genetic predisposition, environmental exposure, tumor and treatment factors combine to put women at increased risk of fatigue.

### *Hypothalamic-Pituitary-Adrenal (HPA) Axis*

The HPA Axis controls production of the stress hormone cortisol. It is thought that production of this hormone modulates the body's inflammatory system [26]. Normally the body has two peaks of cortisol concentration within a 24 h period. In breast cancer survivors, however, the concentration of cortisol falls slower after the second peak [27]. Furthermore, the slower the decline, the more likely the patient is to be fatigued [27]. Alterations in the HPA axis may therefore be an alternative or complementary mechanism underlying the inflammatory component of fatigue. A clearer understanding of the mechanisms underlying fatigue will be vital in planning effective interventions.

## Diagnostic Evaluation

Clinical studies have been limited by the use of multiple different assessment methods to define cancer-related fatigue, making comparisons between studies difficult [28]. The subjective nature of the symptom and wide differential necessitates a comprehensive approach to assessment. The American Society of Clinical Oncology has published guidelines recommending that all patients are screened for cancer-related fatigue from the point of diagnosis onwards, including in the post-treatment setting [3]. A first step in any assessment is a thorough history of the fatigue. The ASCO guidelines [3] recommend the history should evaluate the severity, correlates, time course and impact of the symptom upon the patient's functional ability. One recommended screening method is asking all patients to score their fatigue levels on a scale of 1–10 (10 being high fatigue levels). Any score from 4 to 6 indicates moderate fatigue and a score of 7–10 qualifies as severe fatigue, with the group suggesting that all scores indicating moderate to severe fatigue require further assessment [3]. A number of more complex validated scales for measuring fatigue are also available, including: the Brief Fatigue Inventory (BFI), European Organisation for Research and Treatment of Cancer Quality-of-Life Questionnaire Core 30 (EORTC QLQ C30), Functional Assessment of Cancer Therapy-Fatigue (FACT-F), Multifunctional functional intervention (MFI), SF Medical Outcome Study 36-Item (SF-36) Short Health Survey. and Profile of Mood States-Fatigue (POMS-F) [29]. None of these scales has become established as a gold-standard, and their use is largely limited to clinical studies.

In conjunction with assessment of the symptom of fatigue itself, the history should also focus on identifying and excluding other causes of fatigue, including the possibility of disease relapse (Table 20.1). An important additional diagnosis to

**Table 20.1** Underlying causes of fatigue in breast cancer survivors

| |
|---|
| Past medical history |
| Anemia<br>Chronic disease<br>Hypothyroidism, diabetes, or other endocrine causes<br>Inflammatory conditions<br>Hypertension, heart disease and cardiac disorders<br>Electrolyte disturbances and renal failure<br>Mood disorders, especially depression<br>Cancer recurrence |
| Drug history |
| Any drugs known to cause fatigue such as aromatase inhibitors, beta blockers, antihypertensives, statins, benzodiazepines, antihistamines, SSRIs. |
| Social history |
| Alcohol and drug use<br>Social stressors such as work and relationships<br>Sleeping patterns<br>Functional ability and exercise tolerance |

consider is that of a coexisting depressive disorder may contribute to cancer-related fatigue. Thus, a screening for depression is recommended as part of the differential diagnoses [30].

Following history and examination, basic laboratory tests should be undertaken. This should include hemoglobin (with comparison to pre-treatment levels), renal and liver function, thyroid function, and electrolytes [3]. Any further investigations should be undertaken as directed by the history and examination.

## Interventions for Managing Cancer-Related Fatigue in Breast Cancer Survivors

Several interventions have shown significant efficacy in managing cancer-related fatigue, but none of them is considered as a gold standard intervention. Thus, it would seem appropriate to discuss with patients a multimodal approach which includes different interventions based on patients' preferences and physical conditions. This approach can be monitored and adjusted for efficacy and patients´ preferences over time.

The interventions for managing fatigue in breast cancer survivors are classified in five main groups:

1. Exercise or physical activity
2. Acupuncture
3. Cognitive behavioral therapy
4. Mind-body interventions
5. Pharmacological interventions

## Physical Activity

As for the general population breast cancer survivors are recommended to take a combination of moderate aerobic exercise (150 min per week) with two or three sessions of resistance training per week (see Chap. 8). There is evidence that physical activity, in addition to potential effects on recurrence, also reduces fatigue in breast cancer survivors. Several meta-analyses including randomized controlled clinical trials (RCTs) have shown that regular physical activity- particularly aerobic exercise- reduces fatigue in cancer survivors [31–35] (Table 20.2). One potential explanation for these observations is that long-term exercise reduces mononuclear cell production of proinflamatory cytokines such as IL-6, TNF-α and IL-1β, which are known to be associated with cancer-related fatigue [36].

Whilst it is apparent that exercise may reduce cancer-related fatigue (at least in those able and sufficiently motivated to enter clinical studies) there is limited consensus regarding the type of exercise (aerobic and/or resistance exercise) frequency, intensity and duration of exercise sessions. In addition, several studies have shown that patients with higher adherence to exercise achieve better outcomes in terms in managing cancer-related fatigue and that counseling and motivational interviews increase long-term physical activity in cancer survivors [37, 38]. Thus, motivation programs are likely to be crucial to ensure adherence to exercise, especially for those survivors who are fatigued and therefore less likely to be active.

## Acupuncture

Acupuncture is a key component of traditional Chinese Medicine, which involves inserting needles through the skin at specific points of the body to balance the flow of energy (chi). The role of acupuncture in managing treatment-related side effects such as nausea or vomiting, xerostomia, arthralgia and hot flushes in cancer patients is well-known [39, 40]; however there is still limited data about the role of acupuncture in treating cancer-related fatigue. The effectiveness of acupuncture in managing cancer-related fatigue is thought to be linked to its role in decreasing pro-inflammatory cytokines and increase of T-lymphocytes production. Several randomized trials have evaluated the effectiveness of acupuncture in managing fatigue in breast cancer survivors (Table 20.3). These studies demonstrate that breast cancer survivors with moderate or persistent fatigue, treated with acupuncture experience a significant reduction in fatigue, including physical and mental fatigue, (as well as anxiety, depression and well-being) during the intervention and several weeks after completing it when compared with usual care (Table 20.3).

## Cognitive-Behavioral Interventions

Cognitive behavioral therapy is a common type of talk therapy (psychotherapy) in which the mental counselor works closely with the patient helping them to be aware of their negative or inaccurate thoughts and also to change these thoughts (cognitive patterns) to

**Table 20.2** Meta-analysis and randomized-clinical trials evaluating the role of exercise in breast cancer survivors

| Type of study | Author, journal and year | N | Population characteristics | Randomized arms | Scale | Intervention | Outcome |
|---|---|---|---|---|---|---|---|
| Meta-analysis | Meneses-Echavez et al. *BMC Cancer* (2015) [33] | 9 RCTs (1156) | Breast cancer and survivors | n=556 Exercise<br>n=460 Waiting list control | FACT-B<br>POMS<br>EORT -QLQ C30 | Aerobic and resistance training | **Exercise vs. control**<br>Aerobic exercise (p=0.001) and resistance training (p=0.02) associated lower fatigue |
| Randomized-Clinical | Hagstrom et al. *Eur J Cancer* (2015) [34] | 39 | Breast cancer survivors (stage I-III)<br>Mainstream treatment completed within 11–13 months | n=20 strength training<br>(n=19 waiting list control | FACIT | 16-week resistance exercise training<br>3 times per week | **Exercise vs. control**<br>Resistance training associated with lower levels fatigue<br>(p =0.006) |
| | Cantero- Villanueva et al. *Arch Phys Med Rehab* (2013) [35] | 68 | Breast cancer survivors | n=32 water aquatic<br>n=32 control group | Piper Fatigue scale<br>POMS | 8-week aquatic exercise session<br>(3 times per week) | **Exercise vs. control**<br>Immediately after the exercise:<br>Fatigue (d=.087), endurance (d=0.92) and strength (d=1.0) improved in exercise group. Fatigue score effects maintained at 6 months |

*EORTC QLQ C-30* European Organization for Research and Treatment of Cancer Quality of Life Questionnaire, *FACIT* Functional Assessment of Chronic Illness Therapy –Fatigue, *FACT-B* Functional Assessment of breast cancer therapy, *POMS* Profile of Mood

**Table 20.3** Randomized-clinical trials evaluating the role of acupuncture in breast cancer survivors

| Author, journal and year | N | Population characteristics | Randomized arms | Scale | Intervention duration | Outcome |
|---|---|---|---|---|---|---|
| Mao *Cancer* (2014) [67] | 67 | Breast cancer survivors (stage I-III)<br>Mainstream treatment completed at least 3 months before enrolment | **n**=22 Electroacupunture (EA)<br>**n**=22 Sham acupuncture (SA)<br>**n**=23 Wait list control (WLC) | BFI | 8 week of EA followed by 4-week -follow-up vs.<br>8 weeks of SA<br>Wait list control | **EA vs. WLC p=0.095**<br>At week 8 (p=0.034);<br>**SA vs. WLC**<br>At week 8 (p=0.18) |
| Smith *Acupuncture Med* (2013) [67, 68] | 30 | Breast cancer survivors<br>After completing chemotherapy | True acupuncture (A)<br>Sham acupuncture (SA) | FACIT | 8 weeks of true acupuncture<br>8 weeks of sham acupuncture | **Acupuncture vs. sham acupuncture**<br>at 2 weeks (p=0.05) |
| Molassiotis *JCO* (2012) [69] | 302 | Breast cancer survivors (stage I-III)<br>1 month and up to 5 years after completing chemotherapy | 3:1<br>n = 227 Acupuncture<br>n = 75 Control arm | MFI | 6-week acupuncture vs. usual care | **Acupuncture vs. usual care** (p<0.001).<br>Physical fatigue score (p <0.001)<br>Mental fatigue score-(p <0.001) |

*BFI* Brief Fatigue Inventory, *EA* electroacupunture, *FACIT-F* Functional Assessment of Chronic Illness Therapy-Fatigue, *MFI* multidimensional fatigue inventor, *SA* Sham acupuncture modify their emotional state or behavior. Several meta-analysis and RCTs which evaluated cognitive behavioral therapy in managing fatigue in cancer survivors, and have demonstrated significant reductions in persistent fatigue [32, 41, 42].

## *Mind-Body Interventions*

### Mindfulness-Based Stress Reduction (MBSR)

Mindfulness-based stress reduction programs consist of 6 or 8 week-group mindfulness training practice which includes body (awareness) scan, gentle yoga, sitting meditation, group discussion and home practice. Several studies have shown that mindfulness-based stress reduction (MBSR) programs can improve mood and reduce fatigue in cancer survivors with persistent fatigue ($p < 0.001$) [43, 44]. Hoffman and Lengacher evaluated MBSR programs by conducting randomized studies in breast cancer survivors [45, 46] (Table 20.4). Both studies showed significant improvements in cancer-related fatigue; however the effect was moderate and did not persist over time. The reason for the moderate effect might be explained by the fact that breast cancer survivors included in these two studies had a cluster of symptoms, including fatigue but neither severe nor persistent fatigue. A further limitation of Hoffman´s study was the absence of recording of mindfulness practice by breast cancer survivors after completing the 8-week program. Regarding the effectiveness of MBSR program over time, Hoffman´s findings diverge with the results of an unrandomized study conducted by Appling and colleagues which demonstrated that the benefit of their program remained 6-months after completing the MBSR training [44, 45] (Table 20.4). In the short term it appears that MSBR may be an effective intervention to reduce cancer-related fatigue but it may be that continued practice of MBSR tools after completing MBSR training might be necessary to ensure longer term benefit.

### Yoga

Yoga is a mind-body technique which combines the practice of posture "asanas" along with breathing techniques "pranayama" and meditation. Several RCT studies have shown the positive effects of regular yoga practice on cancer patients and survivors [47–51]. These studies were primarily conducted in breast cancer populations and showed that the regular practice of yoga was associated with significant improvements in quality of life, stress, anxiety and depression, well-being- and also improvement in physical symptoms such as pain and fatigue [48, 51].

A meta-analysis conducted by Buffart el al. included 13 RCTs (12 conducted in patients with breast cancer) revealed a significant moderate reduction in CRF ($d = -0.51$) [47]. Furthermore, RCTs conducted by Kiecolt et al. [52] and Bower et al. [53] demonstrated that regular yoga practice not only reduced cancer-related fatigue but also inflammation-related gene expression and pro-inflammatory cytokines such as IL-6 and IL- 1β and NF-kβ ($p < 0.05$) (Table 20.4).

**Table 20.4** Randomized clinical trials evaluating the role of mind-body techniques in breast cancer survivors

| Intervention | Author and year | N | Population characteristics | Randomized arms | Assessment | Intervention | Outcome |
|---|---|---|---|---|---|---|---|
| Mindfulness based stress reduction (MBSR) | Hoffman *JCO* (2012) [45] | 229 | Breast cancer survivors (stage 0-III) | n = 103 MBSR<br>n = 111 control | FACT-B<br>FACT-ES<br>POMS<br>Assessment baseline, at week8 and at week 12 | 8-week-MBSR program | **Fatigue MBSR vs. control ($p<0.001$)**<br>**Baseline:**<br>MBSR 11.17 vs. control 11.75<br>**At week 8**:<br>MBSR 8.7 vs. control ($p<0.05$)<br>**At week 12**:<br>MBSR 9.27 vs. control 11.39 ($p>0.05$) |
| | Lengacher et al. *J Behav Med* (2012) [46] | 84 | Breast cancer survivors (stage 0-III)<br>Mainstream treatment completed within 18 months before enrolling onto the study<br>85 % have CRF | n = 41 MBSR<br>n = 43 control | MDASI<br>Assessment baseline and at week 6 | 6-week MBSR program | **MBSR vs. control ($p<0.01$)**<br>**Baseline:**<br>MBSR 3.6 vs. control 3.6<br>**At week 6:**<br>MBSR 2.0 vs. control 3.0 ($p<0.01$) |

| | | | | | | | |
|---|---|---|---|---|---|---|---|
| | Appling et al. *Oncolog Nurs* (2012) [44] | 68 | Breast cancer survivors (stage 0-III)<br>Mainstream treatment completed at least within 6 months before enrolling onto the study<br>CRF inclusion criteria | Single arm | SF-36 Health Survey<br>Assessment: baseline, at week 10 and 6 month | 10-week mind body medicine program | **$p < 0.001$**<br>**Baseline**: 6<br>**At week 10**: 4.2; ($p < 0.001$).<br>**At 6 months:** 3.2 ($p < 0.001$) |
| Yoga | Bower et al. *Cancer* (2012, 2014) [53] | 31 | Breast cancer survivors (stage 0-II)<br>Mainstream treatment completed at least 6 months before enrolling onto the study<br>Severe CRF was an inclusion criteria | 1:1<br>n=16: Iyengar yoga<br>n=15: Health education (control) | SF-36 vitality scale score<br>Blood and saliva samples<br>Assessment: baseline and at month 3 | 12-week of Iyengar yoga twice per week. Assessment baseline and at 3 months | **Yoga group vs. control group**<br>(a) **CRF at 3 month follow-up** declined significantly in the yoga group ($p = 0.032$)<br>(b) **Cytokines after 3 months**:<br>Activity of NF-kβ reduce ($p < 0.05$)<br>Activity of the anti-inflammatory glucorticoids receptor increase ($p < 0.05$) |

(continued)

**Table 20.4** (continued)

| Intervention | Author and year | N | Population characteristics | Randomized arms | Assessment | Intervention | Outcome |
|---|---|---|---|---|---|---|---|
| | Kiecolt-Glaser et al. *JCO* (2014) [52] | 200 | Breast cancer survivors (stage 0-III)<br>Mainstream treatment completed within 3 years (except for Tamoxifen and aromatase inhibitors) before enrolling onto the study<br>CRF was NOT an inclusion criteria | 1:1<br>n=100 Hatha yoga<br>n=100 wait-list | SF-36<br>MFSI-SF (fatigue)<br>Blood samples<br>Assessment: baseline and at 3 months | 12-week of Hatha yoga twice per week | **Fatigue: yoga vs. control group**<br>(a) Immediately after the treatment ($p > 0.5$)<br>(b) At 3 months follow-up ($p < 0.001$)<br>**Vitality: yoga vs. control group**<br>(a) Immediately after the treatment ($p = 0.01$).<br>(b) At 3 months follow-up ($p = 0.0045$)<br>**After 3 months cytokines reduction**:<br>TNF-α: ($p = 0.63$),<br>IL-6 and IL-β: ($p < 0.1$) |
| Massage | Listing et al. *Psychooncology* (2009) [56] | 115 | Breast cancer survivors stage I-II<br>Mainstream treatment completed at least 3 months before enrolling onto the study<br>CRF was not an inclusion criteria | n=58 (50 eligible) classical massage<br>n=57 (36 eligible) control | EORTC QLQ-BR23<br>GBB<br>Baseline, at the end of the intervention (week 5) and follow-up week 11 | Bi-weekly 30 min classical massage (back, head-neck area) for 5 weeks | **Massage vs. control**<br>At week 5 (end of the intervention): $p = 0.06$<br>At week 11 (follow-up): $p = 0.048$ |
| | Fernandez-Lao et al. *Eur J Care* (2009) [57] | 20 | Breast cancer survivors stage I-III<br>Moderate to high CRF | Cross-over with usual care | POMS | Bi-weekly myofascial release massage | After intervention fatigue reduced ($p < 0.036$) |

*CRF* Cancer-related fatigue, *EORTC QLQ-BR23* European Organization of Research and Treatment of Cancer quality of life questionnaire breast module, *FACT-B* Functional Assessment of Cancer Therapy Breast, *FACT-ES* Functional Assessment of Cancer Therapy-Endocrine symptoms, *GBB* Giessen Complaint Inventory, *MBSR* Mindfulness-Based Stress Reduction, *MDASI* M.D. Anderson Symptom Inventory, *MFSI-SF* Muldimensional Fatigue symptom Inventory Short form, *PMOS* Profile of Mood State questionnaire and fatigue, *SF-36* Medical Outcome Study 36-item short health survey

### Massage

Massage has been used to enhance well-being and health for many years. However, more recently massage has shown its efficacy in helping breast cancer patients to cope with treatment related-side effects such as pain and psychological distress during and after treatment [54, 55]. Pan et al. conducted a meta-analysis (18 RCTs, including 950 patients with breast cancer) which demonstrated that patients receiving regular massage had significant reductions in cancer-related fatigue [55]. These findings are consistent with two studies conducted in women with early breast cancer [56, 57] (Table 20.4).

## *Pharmacological Interventions*

Methylphenidate, guarana and ginseng are some of the pharmacological interventions which have been formally evaluated as therapies to help manage cancer-related fatigue.

### Methylphenidate

Some preliminary data suggests the use of psychostimulants such as methylphenidate may be useful in the treatment of cancer-related fatigue. Methylphenidate increases the levels of dopamine in the central nervous system, hence has the potential to improve fatigue levels. A Cochrane systematic review which included 31 studies (7,104 patients) with all types of cancer during and after mainstream treatment showed that methylphenidate improved fatigue vs. placebo ($p=0.005$) in patients receiving chemotherapy or with advanced disease [58]. However, there is much less data concerning the use of methylphenidate in cancer survivors to treat cancer-related fatigue. Lower et al conducted an RCT ($n=144$), mainly in breast and ovarian survivors, which showed that methylphenidate improved significantly fatigue ($p=0.02$) with minor adverse events [59] (Table 20.5). Larger RCTs will be required to confirm the effectiveness and long-term safety of methylphenidate before this therapy can be recommended in cancer survivors.

### Guarana

Guarana (Paullinia cupana) is a native plant from the Amazon forest which contains caffeine and has been used by the Amazonian Indians for than more than 3,000 years. Despite its medicinal use for centuries, there is very limited data regarding its use in managing cancer-related fatigue. In two small studies guarana apparently reduced fatigue in some breast cancer survivors on chemotherapy and radiotherapy [60, 61] (Table 20.5). At present, guarana should not be recommended to manage fatigue in breast cancer survivors until further larger RCTs confirm the results seen in these studies.

**Table 20.5** Trials evaluating pharmacological interventions in cancer patients (mainly cancer survivors)

| Author and year | N | Population characteristics | Randomized arms | Scale | Intervention | Outcome |
|---|---|---|---|---|---|---|
| Barton et al. *JNCI* (2013) [64] | 364 | Patients with different types of cancer (64 % breast cancer, 49 % still on main stream treatment)<br>Severe or persistent CRF | n = 183 American ginseng<br>n = 181 placebo | MFSI-SF<br>POMS<br>Baseline, at 4 weeks and 8 weeks | Wisconsin ginseng (American ginseng) 2,000 mg PO BD for 8 weeks<br>Placebo for 8 weeks | **Ginseng vs. placebo**<br>At 4 weeks ($p = 0.07$)<br>At 8 weeks ($p = 0.003$) |
| Lower et al. *J Pain Symptom Mange* (2009) [59] | 154 | Cancer survivors (mainly breast and ovarian)<br>Severe or persistent CRF present | n = 77 Dexmethlyphenidate<br>n = 77 placebo | FACIT-F | Dexmethlyphenidate (D-MPH) 5 mg BD up to 20 mg OD for 8 weeks<br>Placebo for 8 weeks | **Dexmethylphenidate vs. placebo** ($p = 0.02$) |
| De Oliveira et al. *J Alt Comp Med* (2011) [61] | 82 | Breast cancer patients on chemotherapy with progressive CRF after fist cycle of chemotherapy | n = 32 guarana<br>n = 43 placebo | FACIT-F<br>FACT-ES<br>BFI<br>Chalder | Guarana 50 mg PO BD for 21 days<br>Placebo for 21 days<br>Cross over after a 7-day washout period | **Guarana vs. placebo**<br>Using FACIT-F, FACT-ES and BFI: on day 21 and day 49 ($p < 0.01$)<br>**Guarana vs. placebo**<br>Using Chalder: on day 21 ($p < 0.01$), on day 49 ($p = 0.27$) |
| Da Costa et al. *J Alt Comp Med* (2009) [60] | 36 | Breast cancer patients undergoing adjuvant radiotherapy | Double –blind crossover trial | | Guarana 75 mg PO OD during radiotherapy<br>Placebo during radiotherapy | **Guarana vs. placebo**<br>$P < 0.05$ |

*BFI* Brief Fatigue Inventory, *CFS* Chalder fatigue scale, Chalder fatigue scale, *FACIT-F* Functional Assessment of Chronic Illness Therapy-Fatigue, *FACT-ES* Functional Assessment of Chronic Illness Therapy-Endocrine Systems, *MFSI-SF* Muldimensional Fatigue symptom Inventory Short form, *PMOS* Profile of Mood State questionnaire and fatigue

### Ginseng

Ginseng root seems to be the most effective pharmacological intervention to manage CRF. There are two major types of ginseng: Asian (Panax gingseng) and American/Wisconsin (Panax quinquefolius). Ginseng has been found to have anti-inflammatory and cortisol modulatory properties in in-vitro studies [62, 63], which may justify a potential role in managing cancer-related fatigue. Barton et al. evaluated the efficacy of root powder American ginseng in a multi-centre phase III RCT in fatigued cancer patients, 64 % of whom had breast cancer. This study showed that ginseng was associated with reductions in fatigue, but only after 8 weeks of starting the treatment [64] (Table 20.5). However it is important to recognize that there are preclinical data regarding ginseng estrogenic activity, which therefore has the potential to induce cell proliferation in hormone-sensitive breast cancer [65, 66]. Although this is not a universal finding we recommend that breast cancer survivors with previous hormone receptor positive breast cancer should avoid taking ginseng.

## Conclusion

Cancer-related fatigue is defined as a persistent physical, emotional, and/or cognitive tiredness related to cancer and/or cancer related treatments. It is commonly part of a cluster of symptoms including anxiety and depression. The prevalence of cancer-related fatigue is 30 %–50 % for breast cancer survivors in the first 5 years after completing initial treatment. It is a distressing symptom with a significant impact on daily activities and quality of life.

Over the last decade many attempts have been made to evaluate interventions to manage fatigue in cancer survivors. The studies which have been conducted have been challenging to design, and control, and are hampered by small sample sizes. Nonetheless meta-analyses and RCTs suggest that: exercise, acupuncture, mind-body techniques such as yoga, Tai-chi, MBSR and massage, as well as cognitive-behavioral therapy and some pharmacological interventions may have a role to play in managing cancer-related fatigue. (A suggested management plan is provided in Table 20.6).

In the future a better understanding of the immunological mechanisms underlying cancer-related fatigue will be invaluable in designing interventions and clinical trials. Studies with a larger sample size will be also required to generate reliable results, and provide reassurance as to the safety of some approaches. It is essential that these avenues are pursued in order to ameliorate this debilitating symptom and its impact on the daily life of breast cancer survivors.

**Table 20.6** Management plan for breast cancer survivors with fatigue

| |
|---|
| **1. Rule out order causes of fatigue** |
| Such as anemia, hypothyroidism or cardiac disease |
| **2. Sleep** |
| Sleep for just long enough to feel refreshed the following day but not excessive sleep<br>Taking short naps (30 min or less) rather than one long rest period<br>Waking up and going to bed at the same time every day to get a good sleep routine |
| **3. Regular exercise** |
| Regular exercise (aerobic and resistance exercise as well as yoga and Tai-chi) has demonstrated to be one of the most effective interventions in managing cancer related fatigue<br>Exercise needs to be tailored according to survivor´s physical conditions and preferences |
| **4. Acupuncture** |
| Acupuncture has also shown that it can be effective in managing fatigue<br>Acupuncture may be very helpful for extremely exhausted survivors who find exercise difficult, and may raise levels of energy enabling some survivors to start exercise following acupuncture sessions |
| **5. Healthy eating** |
| Drinking plenty of water and juices<br>Ensuring a healthy diet which includes proteins and at least five serving of fruits and vegetables every day |
| **6. Stress, anxiety and depression management** |
| Stress, anxiety and depression make fatigue worse<br>Mindfulness- based stress reduction; meditation and counseling such as cognitive behavioral therapy are invaluable tools to learn relaxation techniques, be more resilient and to cope better with stress, anxiety and fatigue |
| **7. Massage and music-therapy** |
| Massage and music-therapy may be helpful tools for some patients<br>Music-therapy can also produce uplifting emotions such as joy and hope |
| **8. American ginseng for hormone receptor negative breast cancer** |
| American Ginseng may improve fatigue<br>Ginseng has some estrogenic properties and should be avoided in breast cancer survivors with previous hormone receptor positive breast cancers |
| **9. Planning everyday according energy levels and type of activities** |
| Planning daily activities is essential in order not to get exhausted<br>Spreading activities across the day and not doing activities for long time is crucial |
| **10. Getting support** |
| Suffering alone makes fatigue even worse<br>Facilitating information regarding local support groups, counseling, and local complimentary centers might be helpful for some breast cancer survivors |

## References

1. Broeckel JA, Jacobsen PB, Horton J, Balducci L, Lyman GH. Characteristics and correlates of fatigue after adjuvant chemotherapy for breast cancer. J Clin Oncol Off J Am Soc Clin Oncol. 1998;16(5):1689–96.
2. Curt GA, Breitbart W, Cella D, Groopman JE, Horning SJ, Itri LM, et al. Impact of cancer-related fatigue on the lives of patients: new findings from the Fatigue Coalition. Oncologist. 2000;5(5):353–60.
3. Bower JE, Bak K, Berger A, Breitbart W, Escalante CP, Ganz PA, et al. Screening, assessment, and management of fatigue in adult survivors of cancer: an American Society of Clinical Oncology Clinical Practice guideline adaptation. J Clin Oncol. 2014;32(17):1840–50.

4. Smets EM, Garssen B, Schuster-Uitterhoeve AL, de Haes JC. Fatigue in cancer patients. Br J Cancer. 1993;68(2):220–4.
5. Lindley C, Vasa S, Sawyer WT, Winer EP. Quality of life and preferences for treatment following systemic adjuvant therapy for early-stage breast cancer. J Clin Oncol Off J Am Soc Clin Oncol. 1998;16(4):1380–7.
6. Cella D, Davis K, Breitbart W, Curt G. Fatigue Coalition. Cancer-related fatigue: prevalence of proposed diagnostic criteria in a United States sample of cancer survivors. J Clin Oncol Off J Am Soc Clin Oncol. 2001;19(14):3385–91.
7. Alexander S, Minton O, Andrews P, Stone P. A comparison of the characteristics of disease-free breast cancer survivors with or without cancer-related fatigue syndrome. Eur J Cancer. 2009;45(3):384–92.
8. Servaes P, Verhagen S, Bleijenberg G. Determinants of chronic fatigue in disease-free breast cancer patients: a cross-sectional study. Ann Oncol Off J Eur Soc Med Oncol ESMO. 2002;13(4):589–98.
9. Bower JE, Ganz PA, Desmond KA, Bernaards C, Rowland JH, Meyerowitz BE, et al. Fatigue in long-term breast carcinoma survivors: a longitudinal investigation. Cancer. 2006;106(4):751–8.
10. Bower JE, Ganz PA, Desmond KA, Rowland JH, Meyerowitz BE, Belin TR. Fatigue in breast cancer survivors: occurrence, correlates, and impact on quality of life. J Clin Oncol Off J Am Soc Clin Oncol. 2000;18(4):743–53.
11. Andrykowski MA, Schmidt JE, Salsman JM, Beacham AO, Jacobsen PB. Use of a case definition approach to identify cancer-related fatigue in women undergoing adjuvant therapy for breast cancer. J Clin Oncol Off J Am Soc Clin Oncol. 2005;23(27):6613–22.
12. Prue G, Rankin J, Allen J, Gracey J, Cramp F. Cancer-related fatigue: a critical appraisal. Eur J Cancer. 2006;42(7):846–63.
13. Andrykowski MA, Donovan KA, Laronga C, Jacobsen PB. Prevalence, predictors, and characteristics of off-treatment fatigue in breast cancer survivors. Cancer. 2010;116(24):5740–8.
14. Lukkahatai N, Saligan LN. Association of catastrophizing and fatigue: a systematic review. J Psychosom Res. 2013;74(2):100–9.
15. Bower JE. Cancer-related fatigue—mechanisms, risk factors, and treatments. Nat Rev Clin Oncol. 2014;11(10):597–609.
16. Pertl MM, Hevey D, Boyle NT, Hughes MM, Collier S, O'Dwyer A-M, et al. C-reactive protein predicts fatigue independently of depression in breast cancer patients prior to chemotherapy. Brain Behav Immun. 2013;34:108–19.
17. Bower JE, Ganz PA, Aziz N, Fahey JL. Fatigue and proinflammatory cytokine activity in breast cancer survivors. Psychosom Med. 2002;64(4):604–11.
18. Collado-Hidalgo A, Bower JE, Ganz PA, Cole SW, Irwin MR. Inflammatory biomarkers for persistent fatigue in breast cancer survivors. Clin Cancer Res Off J Am Assoc Cancer Res. 2006;12(9):2759–66.
19. Bower JE, Ganz PA, Irwin MR, Kwan L, Breen EC, Cole SW. Inflammation and behavioral symptoms after breast cancer treatment: do fatigue, depression, and sleep disturbance share a common underlying mechanism? J Clin Oncol. 2011;29(26):3517–22.
20. Bower JE, Ganz PA, Aziz N, Olmstead R, Irwin MR, Cole SW. Inflammatory responses to psychological stress in fatigued breast cancer survivors: relationship to glucocorticoids. Brain Behav Immun. 2007;21(3):251–8.
21. Orre IJ, Reinertsen KV, Aukrust P, Dahl AA, Fosså SD, Ueland T, et al. Higher levels of fatigue are associated with higher CRP levels in disease-free breast cancer survivors. J Psychosom Res. 2011;71(3):136–41.
22. Fagundes CP, Glaser R, Alfano CM, Bennett JM, Povoski SP, Lipari AM, et al. Fatigue and herpesvirus latency in women newly diagnosed with breast cancer. Brain Behav Immun. 2012;26(3):394–400.
23. Kuo C-P, Wu C-L, Ho H-T, Chen CG, Liu S-I, Lu Y-T. Detection of cytomegalovirus reactivation in cancer patients receiving chemotherapy. Clin Microbiol Infect. 2008;14(3):221–7.
24. Bower JE, Ganz PA, Irwin MR, Castellon S, Arevalo J, Cole SW. Cytokine genetic variations and fatigue among patients with breast cancer. J Clin Oncol. 2013;31(13):1656–61.

25. Collado-Hidalgo A, Bower JE, Ganz PA, Irwin MR, Cole SW. Cytokine gene polymorphisms and fatigue in breast cancer survivors: Early findings. Brain Behav Immun. 2008;22(8):1197–200.
26. Kronfol Z, Nair M, Zhang Q, Hill EE, Brown MB. Circadian immune measures in healthy volunteers: relationship to hypothalamic-pituitary-adrenal axis hormones and sympathetic neurotransmitters. Psychosom Med. 1997;59(1):42–50.
27. Bower JE, Ganz PA, Dickerson SS, Petersen L, Aziz N, Fahey JL. Diurnal cortisol rhythm and fatigue in breast cancer survivors. Psychoneuroendocrinology. 2005;30(1):92–100.
28. Smith E, Lai J-S, Cella D. Building a measure of fatigue: the functional assessment of chronic illness therapy fatigue scale. PM&R. 2010;2(5):359–63.
29. Minton O, Stone P. A systematic review of the scales used for the measurement of cancer-related fatigue (CRF). Ann Oncol Off J Eur Soc Med Oncol ESMO. 2009;20(1):17–25.
30. Cancer-related fatigue: epidemiology, pathogenesis, diagnosis, and treatment. Dtsch Aerzteblatt Online [Internet]. 2012 Mar 2 [cited 2016 Jan 14]. http://www.aerzteblatt.de/10.3238/arztebl.2012.0161.
31. Puetz TW, Herring MP. Differential effects of exercise on cancer-related fatigue during and following treatment: a meta-analysis. Am J Prev Med. 2012;43(2):e1–24.
32. Duijts SFA, Faber MM, Oldenburg HSA, van Beurden M, Aaronson NK. Effectiveness of behavioral techniques and physical exercise on psychosocial functioning and health-related quality of life in breast cancer patients and survivors—a meta-analysis. Psychooncology. 2011;20(2):115–26.
33. Meneses-Echávez JF, González-Jiménez E, Ramírez-Vélez R. Effects of supervised exercise on cancer-related fatigue in breast cancer survivors: a systematic review and meta-analysis. BMC Cancer. 2015;15:77.
34. Hagstrom AD, Marshall PWM, Lonsdale C, Cheema BS, Fiatarone Singh MA, Green S. Resistance training improves fatigue and quality of life in previously sedentary breast cancer survivors: a randomised controlled trial. Eur J Cancer Care (Engl). 2015. Nov 23 (Epub ahead of print)
35. Cantarero-Villanueva I, Fernández-Lao C, Cuesta-Vargas AI, Del Moral-Avila R, Fernández-de-Las-Peñas C, Arroyo-Morales M. The effectiveness of a deep water aquatic exercise program in cancer-related fatigue in breast cancer survivors: a randomized controlled trial. Arch Phys Med Rehabil. 2013;94(2):221–30.
36. Kasapis C, Thompson PD. The effects of physical activity on serum C-reactive protein and inflammatory markers. J Am Coll Cardiol. 2005;45(10):1563–9.
37. Bennett JA, Lyons KS, Winters-Stone K, Nail LM, Scherer J. Motivational interviewing to increase physical activity in long-term cancer survivors: a randomized controlled trial. Nurs Res. 2007;56(1):18–27.
38. Ligibel JA, Meyerhardt J, Pierce JP, Najita J, Shockro L, Campbell N, et al. Impact of a telephone-based physical activity intervention upon exercise behaviors and fitness in cancer survivors enrolled in a cooperative group setting. Breast Cancer Res Treat. 2012;132(1):205–13.
39. O'Regan D, Filshie J. Acupuncture and cancer. Auton Neurosci Basic Clin. 2010; 157(1–2):96–100.
40. Chao L-F, Zhang AL, Liu H-E, Cheng M-H, Lam H-B, Lo SK. The efficacy of acupoint stimulation for the management of therapy-related adverse events in patients with breast cancer: a systematic review. Breast Cancer Res Treat. 2009;118(2):255–67.
41. Gielissen MFM, Verhagen S, Witjes F, Bleijenberg G. Effects of cognitive behavior therapy in severely fatigued disease-free cancer patients compared with patients waiting for cognitive behavior therapy: a randomized controlled trial. J Clin Oncol. 2006;24(30):4882–7.
42. Heckler CE, Garland SN, Peoples AR, Perlis ML, Shayne M, Morrow GR, et al. Cognitive behavioral therapy for insomnia, but not armodafinil, improves fatigue in cancer survivors with insomnia: a randomized placebo-controlled trial. Support Care Cancer Off J Multinatl Assoc Support Care Cancer. 2016;24(5):2059–66.
43. Carlson LE, Garland SN. Impact of mindfulness-based stress reduction (MBSR) on sleep, mood, stress and fatigue symptoms in cancer outpatients. Int J Behav Med. 2005;12(4):278–85.

44. Appling SE, Scarvalone S, MacDonald R, McBeth M, Helzlsouer KJ. Fatigue in breast cancer survivors: the impact of a mind-body medicine intervention. Oncol Nurs Forum. 2012;39(3):278–86.
45. Hoffman CJ, Ersser SJ, Hopkinson JB, Nicholls PG, Harrington JE, Thomas PW. Effectiveness of mindfulness-based stress reduction in mood, breast- and endocrine-related quality of life, and well-being in stage 0 to III breast cancer: a randomized, controlled trial. J Clin Oncol Off J Am Soc Clin Oncol. 2012;30(12):1335–42.
46. Lengacher CA, Reich RR, Kip KE, Barta M, Ramesar S, Paterson CL, et al. Influence of Mindfulness-Based Stress Reduction (MBSR) on Telomerase activity in women with Breast Cancer (BC). Biol Res Nurs. 2014;16(4):438–47.
47. Buffart LM, van Uffelen JGZ, Riphagen II, Brug J, van Mechelen W, Brown WJ, et al. Physical and psychosocial benefits of yoga in cancer patients and survivors, a systematic review and meta-analysis of randomized controlled trials. BMC Cancer. 2012;12:559.
48. Culos-Reed SN, Mackenzie MJ, Sohl SJ, Jesse MT, Zahavich ANR, Danhauer SC. Yoga & cancer interventions: a review of the clinical significance of patient reported outcomes for cancer survivors. Evid-Based Complement Alternat Med ECAM. 2012;2012:642576.
49. Bower JE, Woolery A, Sternlieb B, Garet D. Yoga for cancer patients and survivors. Cancer Control J Moffitt Cancer Cent. 2005;12(3):165–71.
50. Culos-Reed SN, Carlson LE, Daroux LM, Hately-Aldous S. A pilot study of yoga for breast cancer survivors: physical and psychological benefits. Psychooncology. 2006;15(10):891–7.
51. Büssing A, Khalsa SBS, Michalsen A, Sherman KJ, Telles S. Yoga as a therapeutic intervention. Evid-Based Complement Alternat Med ECAM. 2012;2012:174291.
52. Kiecolt-Glaser JK, Bennett JM, Andridge R, Peng J, Shapiro CL, Malarkey WB, et al. Yoga's impact on inflammation, mood, and fatigue in breast cancer survivors: a randomized controlled trial. J Clin Oncol Off J Am Soc Clin Oncol. 2014;32(10):1040–9.
53. Bower JE, Greendale G, Crosswell AD, Garet D, Sternlieb B, Ganz PA, et al. Yoga reduces inflammatory signaling in fatigued breast cancer survivors: A randomized controlled trial. Psychoneuroendocrinology. 2014;43:20–9.
54. Krohn M, Listing M, Tjahjono G, Reisshauer A, Peters E, Klapp BF, et al. Depression, mood, stress, and Th1/Th2 immune balance in primary breast cancer patients undergoing classical massage therapy. Support Care Cancer. 2011;19(9):1303–11.
55. Pan YQ, Yang KH, Wang YL, Zhang LP, Liang HQ. Massage interventions and treatment-related side effects of breast cancer: a systematic review and meta-analysis. Int J Clin Oncol. 2014;19(5):829–41.
56. Listing M, Reisshauer A, Krohn M, Voigt B, Tjahono G, Becker J, et al. Massage therapy reduces physical discomfort and improves mood disturbances in women with breast cancer. Psychooncology. 2009;18(12):1290–9.
57. Fernández-Lao C, Cantarero-Villanueva I, Díaz-Rodríguez L, Cuesta-Vargas AI, Fernández-Delas-Peñas C, Arroyo-Morales M. Attitudes towards massage modify effects of manual therapy in breast cancer survivors: a randomised clinical trial with crossover design. Eur J Cancer Care (Engl). 2012;21(2):233–41.
58. Minton O, Richardson A, Sharpe M, Hotopf M, Stone P. Drug therapy for the management of cancer-related fatigue. In: The Cochrane Collaboration, editor. Cochrane Database Syst Rev. [Internet]. Chichester: Wiley; 2010 [cited 2016 Apr 26]. http://doi.wiley.com/10.1002/14651858.CD006704.pub3.
59. Lower EE, Fleishman S, Cooper A, Zeldis J, Faleck H, Yu Z, et al. Efficacy of dexmethylphenidate for the treatment of fatigue after cancer chemotherapy: a randomized clinical trial. J Pain Symptom Manage. 2009;38(5):650–62.
60. da Costa MV, Trufelli DC, Santos J, Campos MP, Nobuo M, da Costa MM, et al. Effectiveness of guaraná (Paullinia cupana) for postradiation fatigue and depression: results of a pilot double-blind randomized study. J Altern Complement Med N Y N. 2009;15(4):431–3.
61. de Oliveira Campos MP, Riechelmann R, Martins LC, Hassan BJ, Casa FBA, Del Giglio A. Guarana (Paullinia cupana) improves fatigue in breast cancer patients undergoing systemic chemotherapy. J Altern Complement Med N Y N. 2011;17(6):505–12.

62. Jin Y, Hofseth AB, Cui X, Windust AJ, Poudyal D, Chumanevich AA, et al. American ginseng suppresses colitis through p53-mediated apoptosis of inflammatory cells. Cancer Prev Res (Phila Pa). 2010;3(3):339–47.
63. Yang C-S, Ko S-R, Cho B-G, Shin D-M, Yuk J-M, Li S, et al. The ginsenoside metabolite compound K, a novel agonist of glucocorticoid receptor, induces tolerance to endotoxin-induced lethal shock. J Cell Mol Med. 2008;12(5A):1739–53.
64. Barton DL, Liu H, Dakhil SR, Linquist B, Sloan JA, Nichols CR, et al. Wisconsin ginseng (Panax quinquefolius) to improve cancer-related fatigue: a randomized, double-blind trial, N07C2. JNCI J Natl Cancer Inst. 2013;105(16):1230–8.
65. King ML. Extraction-dependent effects of American ginseng (Panax quinquefolium) on human breast cancer cell proliferation and estrogen receptor activation. Integr Cancer Ther. 2006;5(3):236–43.
66. Lee Y, Jin Y, Lim W, Ji S, Choi S, Jang S, et al. A ginsenoside-Rh1, a component of ginseng saponin, activates estrogen receptor in human breast carcinoma MCF-7 cells. J Steroid Biochem Mol Biol. 2003;84(4):463–8.
67. Mao JJ, Farrat JT, Bruner D, Zee J, Seluzicki C, De Michele A. Electroacupunture for fatigue, sleep and psychological distress in breast cancer patients with aromatase inhibitor related fatigue. Cancer. 2014;120:3744–51.
68. Smith C, Carmady B, Thornthon C, Perz J, Ussher JM. The effect of acupuncture on cancer related fatigue and well-being for women recovering from BC. Acupuncture Med. 2013; 31:9–5.
69. Malassiotis A, Bardy J, Finegan-John J, Mackereth P. Acupuncture for cancer-related fatigue in patients with breast cancer: a pragmatic randomised controlled trial. J. Clic Oncol 2012;30:4470–6.

# Index




A. Ring, M. Parton (eds.), *Breast Cancer Survivorship*,
DOI 10.1007/978-3-319-41858-2

The manufacturer's authorised representative in the EU is Springer Nature Customer Service Centre GmbH, Europaplatz 3, 69115 Heidelberg, Germany. If you have any concerns regarding our products, please contact ProductSafety@springernature.com

Printed and bound by CPI Group (UK) Ltd, Croydon, CR0 4YY
25/09/2026
02222841-0007